Handbook of Incidents and Essential Topics in Pediatric Anesthesiology

Edited by
David A. Young
Associate Professor of Anesthesiology
Baylor College of Medicine/Texas Children's Hospital, Houston, TX, USA

Olutoyin A. Olutoye
Associate Professor of Anesthesiology
Baylor College of Medicine/Texas Children's Hospital, Houston, TX, USA

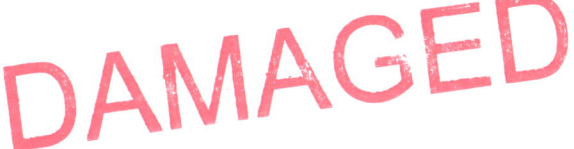

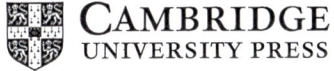

CAMBRIDGE
UNIVERSITY PRESS

University Printing House, Cambridge CB2 8BS, United Kingdom

Cambridge University Press is part of the University of Cambridge.

It furthers the University's mission by disseminating knowledge in the pursuit of education, learning and research at the highest international levels of excellence.

www.cambridge.org
Information on this title: www.cambridge.org/9781107687585

© Cambridge University Press 2015

This publication is in copyright. Subject to statutory exception and to the provisions of relevant collective licensing agreements, no reproduction of any part may take place without the written permission of Cambridge University Press.

First published 2015

Printed and bound in the United Kingdom by Clays, St Ives plc

A catalogue record for this publication is available from the British Library

Library of Congress Cataloguing in Publication data

ISBN 978-1-107-68758-5 Paperback

Cambridge University Press has no responsibility for the persistence or accuracy of URLs for external or third-party internet websites referred to in this publication, and does not guarantee that any content on such websites is, or will remain, accurate or appropriate.

....

Every effort has been made in preparing this book to provide accurate and up-to-date information which is in accord with accepted standards and practice at the time of publication. Although case histories are drawn from actual cases, every effort has been made to disguise the identities of the individuals involved. Nevertheless, the authors, editors and publishers can make no warranties that the information contained herein is totally free from error, not least because clinical standards are constantly changing through research and regulation. The authors, editors and publishers therefore disclaim all liability for direct or consequential damages resulting from the use of material contained in this book. Readers are strongly advised to pay careful attention to information provided by the manufacturer of any drugs or equipment that they plan to use.

Handbook of Critical Incidents and Essential Topics in Pediatric Anesthesiology

This book is dedicated to all anesthesiologists who provide perioperative care to pediatric patients.

Contents

List of contributors xv
Preface xix
Acknowledgments xx
Legal disclaimer xxi

Section 1 – Critical incidents

1 **Crisis management: general principles** 3
Mary A. Felberg

Part A – Airway/Pulmonary

2 **Airway fire** 5
Tae W. Kim

3 **Airway foreign body** 7
John E. Fiadjoe

4 **Bronchospasm** 9
Luigi Viola and Senthilkumar Sadhasivam

5 **Difficult airway** 11
Diane Gordon and Jacquelyn Morillo-Delerme

6 **Difficult ventilation** 14
John E. Fiadjoe

7 **Hemoptysis** 17
Lisa D. Heyden

8 **Hypercarbia** 19
Rajeev Subramanyam and Senthilkumar Sadhasivam

9 **Hypocarbia** 22
Rajeev Subramanyam and Senthilkumar Sadhasivam

10 **Hypoxemia** 24
Normidaris Jimenez and Jacquelyn Morillo-Delerme

11 **Increased peak airway pressures** 26
Normidaris Jimenez and Jacquelyn Morillo-Delerme

12 **Laryngospasm** 28
Kha M. Tran

13 **Pulmonary aspiration of gastric contents** 30
Mary A. Felberg

14 **Stridor** 33
John E. Fiadjoe

15 **Tension pneumothorax** 35
Amanda K. Brown and Rhonda A. Alexis

16 **Respiratory acidosis** 37
Amy Graham-Carlson

17 **Respiratory alkalosis** 39
Amy Graham-Carlson

18 **Upper airway obstruction** 41
Carlos Rodriguez

Part B – Cardiac

19 **Anaphylaxis** 43
Kha M. Tran

20 **Asystole** 45
Joanna Rosing and Jacquelyn Morillo-Delerme

21 **Bradycardia** 47
Amanda K. Brown and Rhonda A. Alexis

22 **Heart failure** 49
Stephen Robert Hays

23 **Hypertension** 52
Catherine P. Seipel

24 **Hypotension** 54
Catherine P. Seipel

25 **Inability to obtain vascular access** 57
Graciela Argote-Romero and Jacquelyn Morillo-Delerme

26 **Local anesthetic toxicity** 59
Smokey Clay and Senthilkumar Sadhasivam

27 **Myocardial ischemia** 62
Stephen Robert Hays

28 **Pericardial tamponade** 65
Lisa D. Heyden

29 **Prolonged QT interval** 67
Catherine P. Seipel

30 **Pulmonary hypertensive crisis** 69
Stephen Robert Hays

31 **Pulseless electrical activity** 72
Julia Chen

32 **Sinus tachycardia** 74
Amanda K. Brown and Rhonda A. Alexis

33 **Supraventricular tachycardia** 76
Catherine P. Seipel

34 **Tetralogy of Fallot spell** 78
Lisa D. Heyden

35 **Thrombotic pulmonary embolism** 80
Lisa D. Heyden

36 **Venous air embolism** 82
Amanda K. Brown and Rhonda A. Alexis

37 **Ventricular fibrillation** 84
Kha M. Tran

38 **Ventricular tachycardia** 86
Matthew Mitchell and Jacquelyn Morillo-Delerme

Part C – Metabolic

39 **Acute adrenal insufficiency** 89
Julia Chen

40 **Hypercalcemia** 91
Julia Chen

41 **Hyperglycemia** 94
Mary A. Felberg

42 **Hyperkalemia** 96
Luigi Viola and Senthilkumar Sadhasivam

43 **Hypernatremia** 98
Andrew J. Costandi and Senthilkumar Sadhasivam

44 **Hyperthermia** 100
Lisa D. Heyden

45 **Hypocalcemia** 102
Kha M. Tran

46 **Hypoglycemia** 104
Mary A. Felberg

47 **Hypokalemia** 106
Amanda K. Brown and Rhonda A. Alexis

48 **Hypomagnesemia** 108
Amanda K. Brown and Rhonda A. Alexis

49 **Hyponatremia** 110
Andrew J. Costandi and Senthilkumar Sadhasivam

50 **Hypothermia** 112
Paul A. Stricker

51 **Malignant hyperthermia** 114
Tae W. Kim

52 **Metabolic acidosis** 116
Paul A. Stricker

53 **Metabolic alkalosis** 118
Lisa D. Heyden

54 **Thyrotoxicosis** 120
Julia Chen

Part D – Neurologic

55 **Altered mental status** 123
Normidaris Jimenez and Jacquelyn Morillo-Delerme

56 **Blindness and perioperative vision loss** 125
Yang Liu

57 **Delayed emergence** 127
David A. Young

58 **Emergence agitation** 129
David Moore and Senthilkumar Sadhasivam

59 **Increased intracranial pressure** 131
Yang Liu

60 **Intraoperative awareness** 134
Carlos Rodriguez

61 **Peripheral nerve injury** 136
Vidya Chidambaran and Senthilkumar Sadhasivam

62 **Seizure** 139
Yang Liu

63 **Stroke** 141
Yang Liu

Part E – Equipment

64 **Anesthesia machine failure** 145
Carlos Rodriguez

65 **Line isolation monitor activation** 147
Stephen Robert Hays

66 **Power failure** 149
Stephen Robert Hays

Part F – Hematology

67 **Coagulopathy** 151
Paul A. Stricker

68 **Massive hemorrhage** 153
Paul A. Stricker

69 **Sickle cell crisis** 156
Tae W. Kim

70 **Transfusion reaction** 158
Tae W. Kim

Part G – Renal

71 **Oliguria** 161
Amy Graham-Carlson

72 **Polyuria** 163
Amy Graham-Carlson

Section 2 – Essential topics

Part A – Basic concepts in pediatric anesthesiology

73 **Development: general concepts** 167
Shakeel Siddiqui

74 **Anatomy: general concepts** 171
Shakeel Siddiqui

75 **Anatomy: airway** 173
Rachel A. Koll and Jacquelyn Morillo-Delerme

76 **Anatomy: central** 175
Nitin Wadhwa

77 **Anatomy: peripheral** 178
Nitin Wadhwa

78 **Pharmacology: general concepts** 181
Carlos Rodriguez

79 **Pharmacology: inhaled anesthetic agents** 183
Carlos Rodriguez

80 **Pharmacology: hypnotics and anxiolytics** 186
Kha M. Tran

81 **Pharmacology: opioids, antagonists, and non-opioids** 190
Luigi Viola and Senthilkumar Sadhasivam

82 **Pharmacology: neuromuscular blocking and reversal agents** 194
Julia Chen

83 **Pharmacology: cardiovascular agents** 198
Premal M. Trivedi and Pablo Motta

84 **Pharmacology: local anesthetics** 203
Smokey Clay and Jacquelyn Morillo-Delerme

85 **Pharmacology: other** 206
Shakeel Siddiqui

86 **Fluid management: general concepts** 210
Mary A. Felberg

87 **Fluid management: crystalloid/colloid** 214
Rebecca Laurich and Jacquelyn Morillo-Delerme

88 **Fluid management: blood products** 217
Premal M. Trivedi and Pablo Motta

89 **Regional anesthesia: general concepts** 221
Nitin Wadhwa

90 **Regional anesthesia techniques: central** 224
Amanda K. Brown and Rhonda A. Alexis

91 **Regional anesthesia techniques: peripheral** 227
Diane Gordon and Jacquelyn Morillo-Delerme

92 **Airway management: general concepts** 231
Graciela Argote-Romero and Jacquelyn Morillo-Delerme

93 **Airway management techniques: direct** 234
Paul A. Stricker

94 **Airway management techniques: indirect** 236
Paul A. Stricker

95 **Malignant hyperthermia: general concepts** 240
Tae W. Kim

96 **Resuscitation: general concepts** 243
Matthew D. Sjoblom and Jacquelyn Morillo-Delerme

97 **Monitoring: general concepts** 247
Olutoyin A. Olutoye

98 **Monitoring: neurophysiologic monitors** 250
Veronica O. Busso, Senthilkumar Sadhasivam and Mohamed Mahmoud

99 **Preoperative care: general concepts** 254
Mary A. Felberg

100 **Preoperative care: separation anxiety/upper respiratory infections** 258
Nancy S. Hagerman and Senthilkumar Sadhasivam

101 **Postoperative care: general concepts** 262
Carlos Rodriguez

102 **Postoperative care: emergence agitation/PONV** 264
David Moore and Senthilkumar Sadhasivam

103 **Pediatric critical care medicine: general concepts** 267
Amanda K. Brown and Rhonda A. Alexis

104 **Pediatric critical care medicine: ECMO** 270
Kha M. Tran

105 **Medical genetics: general concepts** 274
Vidya Chidambaran and Senthilkumar Sadhasivam

106 **Medical genetics: Down syndrome** 277
Julia Chen

107 **Medical genetics: other conditions** 280
Shakeel Siddiqui

Part B – System-based topics in pediatric anesthesiology

108 **Respiratory system: anatomy and physiology** 285
Vanessa A. Olbrecht and Senthilkumar Sadhasivam

109 **Respiratory system: medical conditions** 287
Vanessa A. Olbrecht and Senthilkumar Sadhasivam

110 **Respiratory system: reactive airway disease/cystic fibrosis** 290
Vanessa A. Olbrecht and Senthilkumar Sadhasivam

111 **Cardiovascular system: anatomy and physiology** 293
Premal M. Trivedi and Pablo Motta

112 **Cardiovascular system: medical conditions** 297
Premal M. Trivedi and Pablo Motta

113 **Cardiovascular system: valvular disorders/rhythm disorders** 301
Premal M. Trivedi and Pablo Motta

114 **Cardiovascular system: pulmonary hypertension/heart failure** 308
Premal M. Trivedi and Pablo Motta

115 **Nervous system: anatomy and physiology** 312
Yang Liu

116 **Nervous system: medical conditions** 315
Yang Liu

117 **Nervous system: seizure disorder/cerebral palsy/autism** 319
Amanda K. Brown and Rhonda A. Alexis

118 **Renal system: anatomy and physiology** 322
Julia Chen

119 **Renal system: medical conditions** 324
Julia Chen

120 **Gastrointestinal system: anatomy and physiology** 327
Amanda K. Brown and Rhonda A. Alexis

121 **Gastrointestinal system: medical conditions** 329
Amanda K. Brown and Rhonda A. Alexis

122 **Hepatic system: anatomy and physiology** 333
Yang Liu

123 **Hepatic system: medical conditions** 336
Paul A. Stricker

124 **Endocrine system: anatomy and physiology** 338
Tae W. Kim

125 **Endocrine system: medical conditions** 342
Tae W. Kim

126 **Endocrine system: diabetes mellitus/diabetes insipidus/ SIADH** 346
Tae W. Kim

127 **Endocrine system: thyroid disorders/adrenal disorders** 351
Tae W. Kim

128 **Hematology system: anatomy and physiology** 355
Shakeel Siddiqui

129 **Hematology system: medical conditions** 358
Shakeel Siddiqui

130 **Hematology system: sickle cell disease/von Willebrand/ hemophilia** 362
Tae W. Kim

Part C – Clinical-based areas in pediatric anesthesiology

131 **Cardiac surgery: general considerations** 367
Erin A. Gottlieb

132 **Cardiac surgery: acyanotic lesions** 371
Premal M. Trivedi and Pablo Motta

133 **Cardiac surgery: cyanotic lesions** 375
Premal M. Trivedi and Pablo Motta

134 **Cardiac surgery: non-cardiac surgery** 379
Erin A. Gottlieb

135 **Cardiac surgery: pacemaker/ICD management** 383
Erin A. Gottlieb

136 **Cardiac surgery: cardiac bypass** 387
Premal M. Trivedi and Pablo Motta

137 **Cardiac surgery: cardiac transplantation** 391
Premal M. Trivedi and Pablo Motta

138 **Fetal surgery: general considerations** 396
Kha M. Tran

139 **Fetal surgery: EXIT procedure** 400
Kha M. Tran

140 **General surgery: general considerations** 403
Mary A. Felberg

141 **General surgery: laparoscopy/abdominal procedures** 405
Mary A. Felberg

142 **Neonatal surgery: general considerations** 408
Carlos Rodriguez

143 **Neonatal surgery: PDA ligation/CDH** 410
Carlos Rodriguez

144 **Neonatal surgery: necrotizing enterocolitis/abdominal wall defects** 412
Carlos Rodriguez

145 **Neurosurgery: general considerations** 414
Yang Liu

146 **Neurosurgery: hydrocephalus/VP shunts** 417
Julia Chen

147 **Neurosurgery: brain tumors/neural tube defects** 420
Yang Liu

148 **Ophthalmologic surgery: general considerations** 423
Mary A. Felberg

149 **Ophthalmologic surgery: retinopathy of prematurity/strabismus surgery** 426
Mary A. Felberg

150 **Orthopedic surgery: general considerations** 430
Andrew J. Costandi and Senthilkumar Sadhasivam

151 **Orthopedic surgery: scoliosis surgery** 433
Luigi Viola and Senthilkumar Sadhasivam

152 **Otolaryngology: general considerations** 437
John E. Fiadjoe

153 **Otolaryngology: adenotonsillectomy/otologic procedures** 439
John E. Fiadjoe and Senthilkumar Sadhasivam

154 **Otolaryngology: airway surgery/airway foreign body** 442
John E. Fiadjoe

155 **Pain medicine: general considerations** 446
Andrew J. Costandi and Senthilkumar Sadhasivam

156 **Pain medicine: acute pain management** 449
Vidya Chidambaran and Senthilkumar Sadhasivam

157 **Pain medicine: chronic pain management** 453
Alexandra Szabova and Kenneth Goldschneider

158 **Plastic surgery: general considerations** 457
Rajeev Subramanyam and Senthilkumar Sadhasivam

159 **Plastic surgery: craniofacial reconstruction** 460
Rajeev Subramanyam and Senthilkumar Sadhasivam

160 **Plastic surgery: cleft lip and palate surgery** 463
Smokey Clay and Jacquelyn Morillo-Delerme

161 **Providing anesthesia in remote locations: general considerations** 466
David Moore and Senthilkumar Sadhasivam

162 **Thoracic surgery: general considerations/lung isolation techniques** 469
Kha M. Tran

163 **Thoracic surgery: mediastinal masses** 474
Andrew J. Costandi and Senthilkumar Sadhasivam

164 **Thoracic surgery: video thoracoscopic procedures/pectus excavatum** 478
Jagroop Mavi and Senthilkumar Sadhasivam

165 **Transplant surgery: general considerations** 481
Paul A. Stricker

166 **Transplant surgery: hepatic** 483
Yang Liu

167 **Transplant surgery: renal** 487
Paul A. Stricker

168 **Trauma surgery: general considerations** 490
Carlos Rodriguez

169 **Trauma surgery: burn surgery** 492
Carlos Rodriguez

170 **Urologic surgery: general considerations** 496
Kha M. Tran

Index 499

Contributors

Rhonda A. Alexis, MD
Assistant Professor, Department of Anesthesiology and Critical Care Medicine, Perelman School of Medicine at the University of Pennsylvania, The Children's Hospital of Philadelphia, Philadelphia, Pennsylvania

Graciela Argote-Romero, MD
Assistant Professor, Department of Anesthesiology, The Ohio State University, Nationwide Children's Hospital, Columbus, Ohio

Amanda K. Brown, MD
Assistant Professor, Department of Anesthesiology, Mercer University School of Medicine, Macon, Georgia

Veronica O. Busso, MD
Assistant Professor, Department of Anesthesiology and Pediatrics, University of Cincinnati College of Medicine, Cincinnati Children's Hospital and Medical Center, Cincinnati, Ohio

Julie Chen, MD
Assistant Professor, Department of Anesthesiology, Division of Pediatric Anesthesiology, Baylor College of Medicine, Texas Children's Hospital, Houston, Texas

Vidya Chidambaran, MB, BS, MD
Associate Professor, Department of Anesthesiology and Pediatrics, University of Cincinnati College of Medicine, Cincinnati Children's Hospital Medical Center, Cincinnati, Ohio

Smokey J. Clay, MD
Assistant Professor, Department of Anesthesiology and Pediatrics, University of Cincinnati College of Medicine, Cincinnati Children's Hospital Medical Center, Cincinnati, Ohio

Andrew J. Costandi, MD
Assistant Professor, Department of Anesthesiology and Pediatrics, University of Cincinnati College of Medicine, Cincinnati Children's Hospital Medical Center, Cincinnati, Ohio

Mary A. Felberg, MD, FAAP
Assistant Professor, Department of Anesthesiology, Division of Pediatric Anesthesiology, Baylor College of Medicine, Texas Children's Hospital, Houston, Texas

John Fiadjoe, MD
Assistant Professor, Department of Anesthesiology and Critical Care Medicine, Perelman School of Medicine at the University of Pennsylvania, The Children's Hospital of Philadelphia, Philadelphia, Pennsylvania

Kenneth R. Goldschneider, MD, FAAP
Professor, Department of Anesthesiology and Pediatrics, University of Cincinnati College of Medicine, Cincinnati Children's Hospital Medical Center, Cincinnati, Ohio

Diane Gordon, MD
Assistant Professor, Department of Anesthesiology and Pediatrics, University of Cincinnati College of Medicine, Cincinnati Children's Hospital Medical Center, Cincinnati, Ohio

Erin A. Gottlieb, MD
Assistant Professor, Department of Anesthesiology, Division of Pediatric Cardiovascular Anesthesiology, Baylor

College of Medicine, Texas Children's
Hospital, Houston, Texas

Amy Graham-Carlson, MD
Assistant Professor, Department of
Anesthesiology, The University of Texas
Health Science Center at Houston,
Children's Memorial Hermann Hospital,
Houston, Texas

Nancy S. Hagerman, MD
Department of Anesthesiology and
Pediatrics, University of Cincinnati College
of Medicine, Cincinnati Children's Hospital
Medical Center, Cincinnati, Ohio

Stephen Robert Hays, MS, MD, FAAP
Associate Professor, Department of
Anesthesiology and Pediatrics, Vanderbilt
University School of Medicine, Monroe
Carell Jr. Children's Hospital at Vanderbilt,
Nashville, Tennessee

Lisa D. Heyden, MD
Assistant Professor, Department of
Anesthesiology, Division of Pediatric
Anesthesiology, Baylor College of
Medicine, Texas Children's Hospital,
Houston, Texas

Normidaris Jimenez, MD
Department of Anesthesiology, Nemours
Health System, Wolfson Children's
Hospital, Jacksonville, Florida

Tae W. Kim, MD
Professor, Department of Anesthesiology,
University of Minnesota School of
Medicine, University of Minnesota
Children's Hospital, Minneapolis,
Minnesota

Rachel A. Koll, MD
Assistant Professor, Department of
Anesthesiology and Pediatrics, University
of Cincinnati College of Medicine,
Cincinnati Children's Hospital Medical
Center, Cincinnati, Ohio

Rebecca Laurich, MD
Assistant Professor, Department of
Anesthesiology, Texas A&M Health
Science Center College of Medicine,
McLane Children's Hospital,
Temple, Texas

Yang Liu, MD
Assistant Professor, Department of
Anesthesiology, Division of Pediatric
Anesthesiology, Baylor College of
Medicine, Texas Children's Hospital,
Houston, Texas

Mohamed Mahmoud, MD
Associate Professor, Department of
Anesthesiology and Pediatrics, University
of Cincinnati College of Medicine,
Cincinnati Children's Hospital Medical
Center, Cincinnati, Ohio

Jagroop Mavi, MD
Assistant Professor, Department of
Anesthesiology and Pediatrics, University
of Cincinnati College of Medicine,
Cincinnati Children's Hospital Medical
Center, Cincinnati, Ohio,

Matthew Mitchell, DO
Assistant Professor, Department of
Anesthesiology, The Ohio State University,
Nationwide Children's Hospital,
Columbus, Ohio

David L. Moore, MD
Associate Professor, Department of
Anesthesiology and Pediatrics, University
of Cincinnati College of Medicine,
Cincinnati Children's Hospital Medical
Center, Cincinnati, Ohio

Jacquelyn W. Morillo-Delerme, MD
Associate Professor, Department of
Anesthesiology and Pediatrics, University
of Cincinnati College of Medicine,
Cincinnati Children's Hospital Medical
Center, Cincinnati, Ohio

List of contributors

Pablo Motta, MD
Assistant Professor, Department of Anesthesiology, Division of Pediatric Cardiovascular Anesthesiology, Baylor College of Medicine, Texas Children's Hospital, Houston, Texas

Vanessa A. Olbrecht, MD
Assistant Professor, Department of Anesthesiology and Pediatrics, University of Cincinnati College of Medicine, Cincinnati Children's Hospital Medical Center, Cincinnati, Ohio

Olutoyin A. Olutoye, MD, MSc, FAAP
Associate Professor, Department of Anesthesiology, Division of Pediatric Anesthesiology, Baylor College of Medicine, Texas Children's Hospital, Houston, Texas

Carlos L. Rodriguez, MD
Assistant Professor, Department of Anesthesiology, Division of Pediatric Anesthesiology, Baylor College of Medicine, Texas Children's Hospital, Houston, Texas

Joanna L. Rosing, MD
Assistant Professor, Department of Anesthesiology and Pediatrics, University of Cincinnati College of Medicine, Cincinnati Children's Hospital Medical Center, Cincinnati, Ohio

Senthilkumar Sadhasivam, MD, MPH
Professor, Department of Anesthesiology and Pediatrics, University of Cincinnati College of Medicine, Cincinnati Children's Hospital Medical Center, Cincinnati, Ohio

Catherine P. Seipel, MD
Assistant Professor, Department of Anesthesiology, Division of Pediatric Anesthesiology, Baylor College of Medicine, Texas Children's Hospital, Houston, Texas

Shakeel A. Siddiqui, MD, FAAP
Assistant Professor, Department of Anesthesiology, Division of Pediatric Anesthesiology, Baylor College of Medicine, Texas Children's Hospital, Houston, Texas

Matthew D. Sjoblom, MD
Assistant Professor, Department of Anesthesiology and Pediatrics, University of Cincinnati College of Medicine, Cincinnati Children's Hospital Medical Center, Cincinnati, Ohio

Paul Stricker, MD
Assistant Professor, Department of Anesthesiology and Critical Care Medicine, Perelman School of Medicine at the University of Pennsylvania, The Children's Hospital of Philadelphia, Philadelphia, Pennsylvania

Rajeev Subramanyam MBBS, DNB, MNAMS, MD, MS
Assistant Professor, Department of Anesthesiology and Pediatrics, University of Cincinnati College of Medicine, Cincinnati Children's Hospital Medical Center, Cincinnati, Ohio

Alexandra Szabova, MD
Assistant Professor, Department of Anesthesiology and Pediatrics, University of Cincinnati College of Medicine, Cincinnati Children's Hospital Medical Center, Cincinnati, Ohio

Kha M. Tran, MD
Assistant Professor, Department of Anesthesiology and Critical Care Medicine, Perelman School of Medicine at the University of Pennsylvania, The Children's Hospital of Philadelphia, Philadelphia, Pennsylvania

Premal M. Trivedi, MD
Assistant Professor, Department of Anesthesiology, Division of Pediatric

Cardiovascular Anesthesiology, Baylor College of Medicine, Texas Children's Hospital, Houston, Texas

Luigi Viola, MD
Assistant Professor, Department of Anesthesiology, Division of Pediatric Anesthesiology, Baylor College of Medicine, Texas Children's Hospital, Houston, Texas

Nitin Wadhwa, MD
Assistant Professor, Department of Anesthesiology, The University of Texas Health Science Center at Houston, Children's Memorial Hermann Hospital, Houston, Texas

David A. Young MD, MEd, MBA, FAAP
Associate Professor, Department of Anesthesiology, Division of Pediatric Anesthesiology, Baylor College of Medicine, Texas Children's Hospital, Houston, Texas

Preface

There has been an exponential increase in the amount of knowledge expected of physicians. This increase in required knowledge has especially occurred in subspecialty areas such as pediatric anesthesiology. Novice learners find it very challenging to correctly identify the essential topics to master. Advanced learners find it equally challenging to rapidly acquire vital facts. Furthermore, many learners feel that the ideal format for review is not the same as for initial exposure to a topic.

A significant portion of providing anesthesia care in pediatric anesthesiology is focused around risk identification, early detection, and immediate management of critical incidents. None of the previously available books in pediatric anesthesiology provide a mixture of essential topics and can also act as a bedside reference to manage a critical incident. This was the main driving force for the creation of the *Handbook of Critical Incidents and Essential Topics in Pediatric Anesthesiology*.

Handbook of Critical Incidents and Essential Topics in Pediatric Anesthesiology is the first book written by practicing full-time pediatric anesthesiologists that will provide the reader with a bedside reference for the management of critical incidents and an effective approach for mastering the key topics within pediatric anesthesiology. The purpose of this book was to develop a two-step approach for providing a focused reference to the essential topics and the most commonly encountered critical incidents within pediatric anesthesiology.

The first main section of *Handbook of Critical Incidents and Essential Topics in Pediatric Anesthesiology* consists of the Critical Incidents section related to the anesthetic management of pediatric patients. The Critical Incidents are listed in alphabetical order to allow rapid identification by the reader. Seventy of the most common critical incidents in pediatric anesthesiology are presented in a standardized format consisting of presentation, differential diagnosis, risk factors, management and prevention, which should aid the reader in the quick and accurate management of patients while also improving the safety for future patients. The second main section of the book contains Essential Topics in a focused and very efficient review format. The 100 most common issues in pediatric anesthesiology are presented in a condensed format, identifying key facts for the novice reader and also providing a quick reference review for the experienced clinician.

We truly hope that you will be able to incorporate this book into your practice to more effectively care for your patients while also promoting life-long learning.

David A. Young
Olutoyin A. Olutoye

Acknowledgments

We gratefully acknowledge the continued encouragement from our families, participation of the authors, and support from Cambridge University Press which all together made this book become a reality.

David A. Young
Olutoyin A. Olutoye

Legal disclaimer

Medicine is an ever-changing field. New research and clinical experiences may result in changes to treatment and drug therapy. All readers are advised to check the most current product information provided by the drug manufacturer of each drug to be administered to verify the recommended indications, dose, duration of administration, and contraindications. It is the responsibility of the treating physician, relying on experience, judgment, and knowledge of the specific patient, to determine the best treatment for each individual patient. Neither the publisher, editors, nor contributors assume any liability for any injury and/or damage to persons or property arising from this publication.

Section 1
Critical incidents

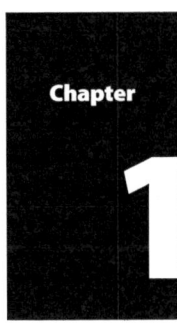

Chapter 1

Crisis management
General principles

Mary A. Felberg

1. Presentation
   a) Critical incident definition: An event which puts the patient in imminent danger and cannot be resolved without active intervention
   b) Two broad categories of critical incidents
      i) Sudden, brief and intense event (e.g., uncontrolled surgical hemorrhage, allergic reaction)
      ii) The culmination of a series of problems evolving into imminent danger (e.g., faulty anesthesia machine → incomplete machine check-out → alarms turned off → distraction during airway management → unrecognized esophageal intubation).
   c) Anesthesiologists assume the responsibility of detecting and correcting problems that occur in the perioperative period and thus help avoid critical incidents or minimize the extent of harm
   d) Crisis management involves early detection of a problem and instituting measures to minimize or eliminate harm
   e) Crisis management is based on the effective use of all available resources and effective team communication
   f) Resources, in addition to your abilities, include operating room personnel, equipment, cognitive aids, external resources, and plans of care
   g) Prevention is the most effective strategy for crisis management. Adequate preoperative patient assessment, room set-up, and communication with the surgeon and operating room staff increases identification of potential problems and also allows for the formulation of contingency plans prior to induction of anesthesia.
2. Risk factors
   Failure to recognize a problem before it evolves into a critical incident may be due to:
   a) Loss of vigilance (e.g., turning alarm monitors off, multitasking beyond clinical care, loud auditory stimulus, external distractions)
   b) Increased production pressure (e.g., incomplete machine check or preoperative evaluation)
   c) Failure of action
   d) Error of fixation: the persistent failure to revise a diagnosis or plan despite available evidence to the contrary

---

Handbook of Critical Incidents and Essential Topics in Pediatric Anesthesiology, ed. David A. Young and Olutoyin A. Olutoye. Published by Cambridge University Press. © Cambridge University Press 2015.

e) Fatigue
  f) Hazardous attitudes
     i) Antiauthority – resists rules/policies; feels the rules don't apply
     ii) Impulsivity – urge to act now, before appropriately evaluating the situation
     iii) Invulnerability – "It can't happen to me" thinking
     iv) Macho – need to prove you can handle the situation alone
     v) Resignation – feel hopeless in the situation.
3. Management
   a) Recognition of critical incident
   b) Mobilize all available resources
   c) Call for help early
   d) Assume a leadership role
   e) Initiate treatment using repeating loops of Observation, Decision, Action and Re-evaluation for response to treatment
   f) Leader should assign clear roles and tasks; leader should only do specific tasks if no other expertise is available
   g) Distribute the workload as evenly as possible among available resources (based on known skill sets of team members)
   h) Maintain awareness of the big picture (situational awareness)
   i) Maintain clear communication with all team members (closed loop communication)
   j) Listen to input from other team members
   k) Focus on what is right for the patient, not who is right
   l) Use all available information (e.g., electronic medical record)
   m) Utilize cognitive aids as appropriate (e.g., pediatric advanced life support algorithm)
   n) Avoid errors of fixation
   o) Avoid hazardous attitudes
   p) Utilize team debriefing after the critical incident to highlight strengths and areas for improvement.
4. Prevention
   a) Identification of individual risk for every anesthetic based on the patient's comorbidities, the planned procedure, and available resources
   b) Surgical time-outs or briefings are opportunities to verbalize contingency plans for probable events
   c) Develop effective communication skills with all members of the perioperative team
   d) Identify cognitive resources in advance of at-risk procedures (e.g., location of malignant hyperthermia treatment algorithm).

Further reading

Bracco D, Videlier E, Ramadori F. Anesthesia crisis resource management. *Anesthesiol Rounds.* 2009; 8(4):1–6.

Gaba DM, Fish KJ, Howard SK. *Crisis Management in Anesthesiology.* New York: Churchill Livingstone, 1994; 1–47.

Gregory GA, Andropoulos DB. *Gregory's Pediatric Anesthesia*, 5th edition. Hoboken: Wiley-Blackwell, 2012; 1221–5.

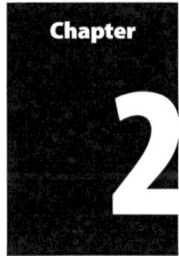

Part A: Airway/Pulmonary

Chapter 2: Airway fire

Tae W. Kim

1. Presentation
   Airway fires occur more frequently in patients undergoing airway surgical procedures. Adverse outcomes include inhalation injuries, spread of fire to nearby flammable materials, secondary infection, disfigurement and death.
2. Risk factors
   a) Presence of three components is required to generate fire: oxidizer, ignition source, and fuel
   b) Oxidizer: oxygen concentration above room air or any concentration of nitrous oxide
   c) Ignition source: use of electrocautery or any device emitting intense heat (e.g., laser, light source)
   d) Fuel
      i) Solids: tracheal tubes, sponges, drapes
      ii) Liquids: alcohol-containing prep solutions
      iii) Gases: methane (GI tract).
3. Differential diagnosis
   a) Surgical fire occurring but not within the airway
   b) Near miss that does not actually result in airway fire (e.g., spark).
4. Pathophysiology
   a) The interaction of all three elements – oxidizer, ignition source, and fuel – leads to combustion
   b) Intense heat and burning of tissue may lead to airway swelling and obstruction, scarring, severe disfigurement.
5. Management
   a) Treatment of an airway fire
      i) Immediately remove tracheal tube
      ii) Stop flow of all airway gases
      iii) Remove all flammable materials from airway
      iv) Pour saline into mouth and airway to extinguish fire
      v) Remove all burning and flammable materials from patient

Handbook of Critical Incidents and Essential Topics in Pediatric Anesthesiology, ed. David A. Young and Olutoyin A. Olutoye. Published by Cambridge University Press. © Cambridge University Press 2015.

- vi) Use fire extinguisher (carbon dioxide variety) in operating room and on patient if fire not extinguished with saline
- vii) If fire persists and does not involve patient: evacuate patient, close doors, turn off gas supply to room.

b) After fire is extinguished

- i) Re-establish ventilation
- ii) Avoid oxidizer-enriched atmosphere if clinically acceptable
- iii) Examine tracheal tube for damage and airway for any residual fragments
- iv) Assess airway for inhalation injury.

6. Prevention
   a) Determine the risk of fire prior to starting procedure
   b) Discuss strategy with team for prevention and management of fire prior to starting procedure
   c) Verify essential equipment immediately available prior to initiating case (e.g., sterile water, fire extinguisher)
   d) Place surgical drapes in a configuration to minimize the accumulation of oxidizers
   e) Moisten sponges and gauze when placed in proximity to any ignition source
   f) Minimize or avoid an oxidizer-enriched atmosphere when any ignition source is being utilized
   g) Communication is essential during the planned use of at-risk devices (e.g., 100% oxygen, laser)
   h) Reduce potential for oxygen-enriched environments, allow flammable skin-preparation solution to dry, use laser-resistant tracheal tubes and cuffed tracheal tubes
   i) Education
      i) Acquire knowledge of institutional fire safety protocols
      ii) Participate in institutional fire safety education including operating room fire drills that include the entire operating room team
      iii) Identify high-risk patients and procedures.

Further reading

Apfelbaum JL, Caplan RA, Barker SJ et al. Practice advisory for the prevention and management of operating room fires: an updated report by the American Society of Anesthesiologists Task Force 2013 on Operating Room Fires. *Anesthesiology.* 2013; 118(2):271–90.

Davis PJ et al. *Smith's Anesthesia for Infants and Children*, 8th edition. Philadelphia: Elsevier Mosby, 2011; 802.

Part A   Airway/Pulmonary

Chapter 3

Airway foreign body

John E. Fiadjoe

1. Presentation
   a) Stridor
   b) Wheezing
   c) Cough
   d) Witnessed choking episode (most sensitive finding)
   e) Acute respiratory distress
   f) Atelectasis
   g) Bronchiectasis
   h) Pneumonia, empyema
   i) Pneumothorax.

2. Risk factors
   a) Age less than 3 years
   b) Lack of molars before age 4
   c) Developmental delay
   d) Child neglect/abuse.

3. Differential diagnosis
   a) Asthma
   b) Chronic cough
   c) Pneumonia
   d) Bronchitis
   e) Atelectasis.

4. Pathophysiology
   a) Tracheal aspiration is associated with a mortality as high as 45%
   b) Most common item aspirated is food (peanuts, popcorn, grapes, hotdogs comprise > 60% of all choking episodes)
   c) Coins, toys, needles, pins, balloons, balls, and batteries are also common
   d) Batteries lead to corrosive damage and should be removed emergently
   e) Right main bronchus is a common location for the item to become lodged due to the larger diameter of the right bronchus and shallower angle from trachea.

Handbook of Critical Incidents and Essential Topics in Pediatric Anesthesiology, ed. David A. Young and Olutoyin A. Olutoye. Published by Cambridge University Press. © Cambridge University Press 2015.

5. Management
   a) Radiologic findings: most objects are radiopaque except food items
   b) Lateral decubitus radiographs confirm presence of obstruction as obstructed lung will not deflate in the dependent position
   c) Inspiratory and expiratory films may identify air trapping, hyperinflation, obstructive emphysema, atelectasis, and mediastinal shift
   d) Communication between care providers is essential, teamwork is mandatory, and the endoscopist should be familiar with equipment prior to induction of anesthesia
   e) Anticholinergic administration should be considered to minimize secretions and can easily be achieved if preoperative intravenous access is present
   f) General inhalation anesthesia with supplemental intravenous anesthesia while maintaining spontaneous ventilation is the preferred technique by most providers
   g) Topical aerosolization of the airway with local anesthetic by surgeon attenuates airway reflexes prior to foreign body extraction
   h) Rigid bronchoscopy is performed with administration of anesthetic gases through the side port
   i) Intraoperative intravenous steroid administration is commonly administered to decrease airway mucosal swelling
   j) Laryngeal/airway edema may occur after surgery, requiring racemic epinephrine.
6. Prevention
   a) Close supervision of children at risk
   b) Labeling of toys that may present a choking hazard.

Further reading

Ashcraft KW. *Pediatric Surgery*, 4th edition. Philadelphia: Elsevier, 2005; 137–40.

Coté CJ, Lerman J, Anderson BJ. *Coté and Lerman's A Practice of Anesthesia for Infants and Children*, 5th edition. Philadelphia, PA: Elsevier, 2013; 653–67.

Gregory GA, Andropoulos DB. *Gregory's Pediatric Anesthesia*, 5th edition. Hoboken: Wiley-Blackwell, 2012; 792–5.

Part A Airway/Pulmonary

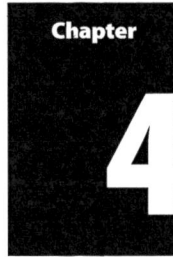

Chapter 4: Bronchospasm

Luigi Viola and Senthilkumar Sadhasivam

1. Presentation
    a) Intraoperative bronchospasm may present as hypoxemia, hypercarbia, and expiratory wheezing
    b) If using pressure-controlled ventilation, expired tidal volumes will decrease; with volume-controlled ventilation, peak inspiratory pressures will increase
    c) The display of the capnograph tracing changes from the appearance of a square wave to an upsloping pattern.
2. Risk factors
    a) Recent history of upper or lower respiratory tract infection
    b) History of reactive airway disease including asthma
    c) Passive or active exposure to parental smoking
    d) Anesthesia-related: endobronchial intubation, endotracheal intubation, airway instrumentation with inadequate levels of general anesthesia, carina irritation by the endotracheal tube, volatile agents (e.g., desflurane, isoflurane), medications (e.g., morphine, neostigmine)
    e) Airway foreign body, aspiration of gastric contents, mucous plug.
3. Differential diagnosis
    Wheezing is not always secondary to bronchospasm.
    a) Preoperative wheezing may be due to many causes including:
        i) Bronchiolitis, aspiration, asthma, bronchiectasis, chronic lung disease, vascular malformations, airway foreign bodies.
    b) Intraoperative wheezing:
        i) Bronchial stimulation due to a relatively inadequate level of general anesthesia
        ii) Bronchial reactivity from medications (e.g., desflurane) or gastric contents (i.e., aspiration after rapid sequence induction)
        iii) Mechanical airway obstruction (kinking or plugging of tracheal tube, inhaled airway foreign body, obstructive airway mass, pneumothorax, pulmonary edema).
4. Pathophysiology
    Bronchospasm results from the smooth muscle contraction and obstruction of intrathoracic small airways or main bronchi; this leads to forced expiration and generates turbulent airflow appreciated clinically as wheezing.

Handbook of Critical Incidents and Essential Topics in Pediatric Anesthesiology, ed. David A. Young and Olutoyin A. Olutoye. Published by Cambridge University Press. © Cambridge University Press 2015.

5. Intraoperative management
   a) Rapid identification of the cause:
      i) Inspect circuit, auscultate both lungs, exclude main stem bronchus intubation
      ii) Increase oxygen concentration to 100%
      iii) Suction tracheal tube, exclude tracheal tube obstruction
      iv) Deepen anesthesia (i.e., with a nonirritating volatile agent such as sevoflurane, or intravenous medications such as propofol and ketamine)
      iv) Review administered drugs particularly for histamine release and allergic reaction potential; discontinue all suspected medications.
   b) Administer a beta-2 agonist with a spacer device through the breathing circuit (e.g., albuterol 4–8 puffs)
   c) Consider administration of anticholinergic agents with a spacer device through the breathing circuit (e.g., ipratropium: 1–2 puffs)
   d) Administer an intravenous corticosteroid such as methylprednisolone (1 mg/kg) or hydrocortisone (2 mg/kg)
   e) Consider administration of lidocaine (1 mg/kg) to reduce airway reactivity
   f) Modify ventilation settings to avoid gas trapping (i.e., increase the expiratory time) and barotrauma (i.e., decrease tidal volume along with increasing respiratory rate)
   g) For severe or refractory bronchospasm:
      i) Administer epinephrine (1 µg/kg)
      ii) Magnesium sulfate (25–50 mg/kg over 10 minutes)
      iii) Consider high-dose volatile agents for status asthmaticus (i.e., 2–3 MAC).
   h) Consider obtaining an arterial blood gas and chest x-ray.
6. Prevention
   a) Avoid elective procedures within 2–6 weeks of a significant respiratory infection
   b) Consider preoperative administration (48–72 hours before anesthesia) of corticosteroids in poorly controlled asthmatic patients
   c) Strongly consider premedication with beta-2 agonists (e.g., albuterol) in high-risk patients
   d) Ensure adequate levels of general anesthesia, especially during airway management.
   e) Avoid histamine-releasing drugs (e.g., morphine)
   f) Consider anesthetic techniques that avoid tracheal intubation if appropriate
   g) Consider using a deep extubation technique if acceptable (i.e., not with a full stomach or suspected difficult airway)
   h) Consider empiric administration of intra-tracheal lidocaine (1–2 mg/kg).

Further reading

Bissonnette B. *Pediatric Anesthesia*. Shelton, CT: People's Medical Publishing House, 2011; 57(912).

Davis PJ, Cladis FP, Motoyama EK. *Smith's Anesthesia for Infants and Children*, 8th edition. Philadelphia: Mosby, 2011; 1114–20.

Woods BD, Sladen RN. Perioperative considerations for the patient with asthma and bronchospasm. *Br J Anaesth*. 2009;103(Suppl 1): i57–65.

Part A Airway/Pulmonary

Chapter 5 Difficult airway

Diane Gordon and Jacquelyn Morillo-Delerme

1. Presentation
   a) Difficult ventilation via face mask or supraglottic airway (SGA)
   b) Difficult placement of SGA after multiple attempts
   c) Difficult laryngscopy with inability to visualize the vocal cords
   d) Difficult endotracheal intubation including failure to insert the endotracheal tube
   e) Craniofacial abnormalities
   f) Patient may not present with any features suggestive of a difficult airway
   g) Mask ventilation may be adequate despite difficult intubation.

2. Risk factors
   a) Cervical instability
      i) Down syndrome
      ii) Achondroplasia
      iii) Trauma.
   b) Cervical inflexibility
      i) Treacher-Collins syndrome
      ii) Klippel–Feil syndrome
      iii) Arthrogryposis
      iv) Cornelia de Lange syndrome
      v) Turner syndrome
      vi) Trauma–cervical collar in place.
   c) Micrognathia/Retrognathia
      i) Pierre Robin syndrome
      ii) Nager syndrome
      iii) Goldenhar syndrome
      iv) Smith-Lemli-Opitz syndrome
      v) Rheumatoid arthritis.
   d) Macroglossia
      i) Beckwith-Wiedemann syndrome
      ii) Pompe disease.
   e) Soft tissue rigidity

Handbook of Critical Incidents and Essential Topics in Pediatric Anesthesiology, ed. David A. Young and Olutoyin A. Olutoye. Published by Cambridge University Press. © Cambridge University Press 2015.

- i) Mucopolysaccharidoses (Hurler syndrome, Hunter syndrome)
- ii) Head/neck radiation or burns
- iii) Scleroderma.
  - f) Soft tissue fragility
    - i) Epidermolysis bullosa
    - ii) Stevens–Johnson syndrome.
  - g) Airway masses
    - i) Laryngeal papillomatosis
    - ii) Airway foreign bodies
    - iii) Head and neck tumors that displace airway anatomy
    - iv) Retropharyngeal abscess.
  - h) Limited mouth opening
    - i) Trismus
    - ii) Mandible fracture
    - iii) Temporomandibular joint dysfunction.
3. Pathophysiology
   - a) Inability to align oral, pharyngeal and tracheal openings, prevents visualization of the glottis and successful insertion of an endotracheal tube
   - b) Obstruction of ventilation can occur due to relaxation of oropharyngeal soft tissues.
4. Management
   - a) Many difficult airways in pediatrics are known or suspected prior to induction
   - b) Communication and preoperative team planning is essential
   - c) Early recognition of difficulty and calling for help early is essential
   - d) Strongly consider an anesthetic technique that maintains spontaneous ventilation
     - i) Desaturation occurs much faster even in adequately preoxygenated pediatric patients compared to adults.
   - e) An SGA may be effective in a rescue situation to reestablish ventilation and may also serve as a conduit for endotracheal intubation
   - f) Consider early use of fiberoptic bronchoscopy or video laryngoscopes
   - g) Utilize the ASA difficult airway algorithm
   - h) Invasive airway techniques (cricothyrotomy, tracheostomy, and transtracheal jet ventilation) are less likely to be successful in the pediatric population unless performed by an experienced provider (i.e., pediatric ear, nose and throat surgeon).
5. Prevention
   - a) Adequate preoperative history, airway evaluation, and intraoperative preparation
   - b) Major airway disasters may be reduced by
     - i) Adequate preoxygenation
     - ii) Anticipation of a difficult airway and having a variety of airway adjuncts immediately available
     - iii) Immediate availability of experienced help prior to induction of anesthesia
     - iv) Maintenance of spontaneous ventilation.

Further reading

Apfelbaum JL, Hagberg CA, Caplan RA. Practice guidelines for management of the difficult airway: an updated report by the American Society of Anesthesiologists task Force on Management of the Difficult Airway. *Anesthesiology.* 2013; 118(2):251–70.

Coté CJ, Lerman J, Anderson BJ. *Coté and Lerman's A Practice of Anesthesia for Infants and Children*, 5th edition. Philadelphia, PA: Elsevier, 2013; 258–76.

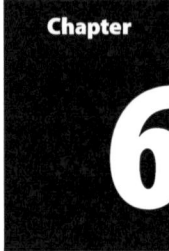

Part A Airway/Pulmonary

Chapter 6

Difficult ventilation

John E. Fiadjoe

1. Presentation
   a) Inability to generate adequate chest rise
   b) Increased peak airway pressures
   c) Hypoxemia and hypercarbia.

2. Risk factors
   a) Obesity
   b) Craniofacial dysmorphisms
   c) History of obstructive sleep apnea
   d) Previous radiation therapy to head and neck
   e) Limited jaw mouth opening or protrusion
   f) History of difficult tracheal intubation
   g) Trauma
   h) Reactive airway disease.

3. Differential diagnosis
   a) Bronchospasm
   b) Laryngospasm
   c) Endotracheal tube obstruction, dislodgement
   d) Esophageal intubation
   e) Equipment failure.

4. Pathophysiology
   a) Hypoxemia, barotrauma, and hypercarbia may result dependent on the etiology.

5. Management
   a) Difficult facemask ventilation
      i) Insert shoulder roll if < 2 years of age, place child in neutral position if older than 2 years
      ii) Increase fraction of inspired oxygen to 100%
      iii) Apply jaw thrust or chin lift
      iv) Insert oral or nasopharyngeal airway
      v) Employ two hand mask ventilation

Handbook of Critical Incidents and Essential Topics in Pediatric Anesthesiology, ed. David A. Young and Olutoyin A. Olutoye. Published by Cambridge University Press. © Cambridge University Press 2015.

vi) Rule out laryngospasm, bronchospasm (evaluate for inspiratory stridor, auscultation for expiratory wheezing)
vii) If above measures are ineffective, call for help
viii) Decompress stomach if distended
ix) If ventilation remains difficult despite above measures, insert a supraglottic airway device
x) Attempt tracheal intubation
xi) If tracheal intubation fails, move to an invasive airway (cricothyroidotomy or tracheostomy).

b) Laryngospasm
   i) Apply continuous positive airway pressure with 100% oxygen
   ii) Deepen anesthesia with intravenous agents (e.g., propofol 1–2 mg/kg IV)
   iii) If above not effective or if severe hypoxemia/bradycardia is present – consider succinylcholine 0.1–0.5 mg/kg IV or 2–5 mg/kg IM or rocuronium if IV access is present.

c) Difficult ventilation using a supraglottic airway device
   i) Confirm proper placement; remove and reinsert device
   ii) Rule out bronchospasm and laryngospasm
   iii) Remove supraglottic airway device and attempt tracheal intubation.

d) Difficult ventilation with endotracheal tube
   i) Rule out esophageal intubation: verify bilateral breath sounds
   ii) Rule out mucus plug- suction endotracheal tube
   iii) Rule out bronchospasm- auscultate lungs and consider deepening volatile anesthetic; consider beta agonist if wheezing present
   iv) Rule out equipment failure.

e) Persistent inability to ventilate
   i) Invasive airway techniques:
      (1) Cricothyroidotomy
         - Cricothyroid membrane more difficult to identify in small children
         - Overlap of cricoid and thyroid cartilages makes landmarks difficult to identify.
      (2) Needle cricothyrotomy
         - Place patient supine with neck extended, sterile preparation of area, drape neck, infiltrate local anesthesia if necessary
         - Have high pressure oxygen source ready (25–35 psi for children)
         - Attach 3 mL luer lock syringe to 14–18g angiocatheter
         - Insert needle with syringe attached at a 30–45° angle and aspirate; air bubbles indicate tracheal entry, slide catheter into trachea and attach high pressure oxygen source.
      (3) Surgical cricothyroidotomy
         - Incision is made in cricothyroid membrane and tracheostomy tube is inserted
         - Contraindicated in children less than 5 years of age because of small size of membrane.

(4) Complications of cricothyroidotomy
- Bleeding, catheter misplacement, catheter kinking
- Subcutaneous emphysema, barotrauma
- Pneumothorax, pneumomediastinum
- Laryngeal injury, esophageal injury.

6. Prevention
   a) Develop a routine for carrying out a complete airway history and examination
   b) In patients with abnormal facial anatomy: maintain spontaneous ventilation while securing airway.

Further reading

Gregory GA. *Gregory's Pediatric Anesthesia*, 5th edition. Hoboken: Wiley-Blackwell, 2012; 317.

Maces SE, Khan N. Needle cricothyrotomy. *Emerg Med Clin N Am.* 2008; 26(4):1085–1101.

Part A Airway/Pulmonary

Chapter 7

Hemoptysis

Lisa D. Heyden

1. Presentation
   Expectoration of blood from the respiratory tract
2. Risk factors
   a) Respiratory infections, foreign body aspiration, and bronchiectasis are the most common etiologies
   b) Vasculitic syndromes
   c) Congenital heart defects, (e.g., end-stage Eisenmenger syndrome – pulmonary hypertension secondary to prolonged excessive pulmonary blood flow)
   d) Lung malformations (e.g., bronchiectasis)
   e) Pulmonary vascular disorders
   f) Neoplasm
   g) Trauma (e.g., suctioning)
   h) Idiopathic
   i) Coagulopathy
   j) Other (e.g., cystic fibrosis, toxins, retained foreign body).
3. Differential diagnosis
   a) Nasopharyngeal bleeding
   b) Upper gastrointestinal bleeding (bright red color, alkaline pH, and/or thoracic pain can distinguish hemoptysis from blood originating from the gastrointestinal tract.
4. Pathophysiology
   a) The lung receives blood supply from the pulmonary arterial circulation (high volume, low pressure system) and the bronchial circulation (much smaller volume of oxygenated blood but at higher, systemic pressures)
   b) Bleeding can arise from either system but can be substantial when arising from the bronchial circulation.
5. Management
   a) For massive hemoptysis, securing the airway is mandatory; either selective intubation to the unaffected lung, the use of a combined bronchial blocker/tracheal tube, or a double lumen tube

---

Handbook of Critical Incidents and Essential Topics in Pediatric Anesthesiology, ed. David A. Young and Olutoyin A. Olutoye. Published by Cambridge University Press. © Cambridge University Press 2015.

b) Obtain laboratory testing including complete blood cell count, type/crossmatch, and coagulation studies
c) Coagulopathy should be corrected if present
d) Minimize coughing. Rigid or flexible bronchoscopy may be used to locate the source and control active bleeding.
e) Hemostasis may be achieved via:
   i) Application of cold saline or topical epinephrine, a mixture of fibrinogen and thrombin, or laser therapy
   ii) Angiography and bronchial artery embolization should be considered for persistent bleeding
   iii) Lung resection is the final resort for persistent severe bleeding refractory to therapy
   iv) Extracorporeal membrane oxygenation (ECMO) may be considered as a bridge to surgery.

6. Prevention

   Prevention depends on the cause of bleeding. Some options include:
   a) Cough suppressants (not in young children)
   b) Cessation of smoking
   c) Antibiotic therapy for bronchiectasis or infection
   d) Adjustment of coagulation medications.

Further reading

Davis PJ. *Smith's Anesthesia for Infants and Children*, 8th edition. Philadelphia: Mosby, Inc., 2011; 1128.

Morgan GE, Mikhail MS, Murray MJ. *Clinical Anesthesiology*, 4th edition. New York: Lange Medical Books, 2006; 868.

Part A: Airway/Pulmonary

Chapter 8: Hypercarbia

Rajeev Subramanyam and Senthilkumar Sadhasivam

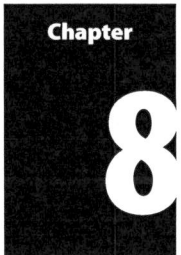

1. Presentation
   a) Hypercarbia is defined as an arterial carbon dioxide tension ($PaCO_2$) greater than 45 mmHg
   b) Permissive hypercarbia ($PaCO_2$ 45–55 mmHg) is a strategy used to minimize lung trauma (e.g., congenital diaphragmatic hernia)
   c) Symptoms depend on the rate of increase, degree of metabolic compensation, and the absolute $PaCO_2$ level
   d) Acute increases are associated with increases in cerebral blood flow and intracranial pressure
   e) Elevations of more than 80 mmHg may cause central nervous system depression
   f) Hypercarbia increases sympathetic output and may cause tachycardia, hypertension, as well as cardiac arrhythmias
   g) Hypercarbia is typically associated with a compensatory tachypnea in spontaneously breathing patients. Preterm infants with history of apnea do not typically increase their respiratory rate in response to hypercarbia; these patients may develop apnea
   h) Hypercarbia prolongs transitional fetal circulation and is a risk for intraventricular hemorrhage.
2. Risk factors
   See Differential diagnosis.
3. Differential diagnosis
   All the conditions listed are associated with either decreased CO_2 elimination or increased CO_2 production.
   a) Metabolic
      i) Shivering
      ii) Malignant hyperthermia
      iii) Neuroleptic malignant syndrome
      iv) Thyroid storm
      v) Severe sepsis
      vi) Hyperthermia.

b) Circulatory
   i) Tourniquet release
   ii) CO_2 insufflation (laparoscopy)
   iii) Treatment of metabolic acidosis (administration of sodium bicarbonate).
c) Respiratory
   i) Hypoventilation
   ii) Inadequate mechanical ventilation settings
   iii) Chronic obstructive pulmonary disease
   iv) Restrictive lung disease
   v) Pulmonary embolism.
d) Drug overdose
e) Overfeeding of carbohydrates/ total parenteral nutrition
f) Technical
   i) Exhausted CO_2 absorbant
   ii) Tracheal tube obstruction
   iii) Mechanical ventilator failure.

4. Pathophysiology
   a) $PaCO_2$ relates to the adequacy of alveolar ventilation and metabolic production of carbon dioxide
   b) Any condition which results in the reduction of alveolar ventilation or an increase in the production of carbon dioxide can result in the development of hypercarbia.

5. Management
   a) Initially evaluate the airway, breathing, vital signs, pupils, and neurologic status
   b) Quickly determine severity and onset of hypercarbia; severe/sudden onset may require cardiac resuscitation (e.g., thyroid storm, malignant hyperthermia)
   c) Consider assisted bag mask ventilation or endotracheal intubation and mechanical ventilation if not already present
   d) Suction tracheal tube if obstruction is suspected
   e) Determine if increased inspired CO_2 is present; this would suggest a mechanical etiology
   f) Attempt to increase minute ventilation of mechanical ventilator
   g) Determine the arterial to end-tidal CO_2 gradient; it is normally 5–10 with the arterial CO_2 being the larger value
   h) Treatment is aimed at the underlying cause (e.g., dantrolene for malignant hyperthermia)
   i) Consider emergent imaging (i.e., CT scan) if a neurologic insult is suspected.

6. Prevention
   a) Maintain vigilance for appropriate titration of mechanical ventilator settings
   b) Consider arterial blood gas testing for high-risk patients
   c) Set appropriate alarm limits for capnograph monitor
   d) Consider evaluation for conditions associated with hypercarbia (see Differential diagnosis).

Further reading

Davis PJ. *Smith's Anesthesia for Infants and Children*, 8th edition. Philadelphia: Elsevier, 2013; 523.

Hines RL, Marschall KE. *Stoelting's Anesthesia and Co-Existing Disease*, 6th edition. Philadelphia: Elsevier, 2013.

Kodali BS. Capnography outside the operating rooms. *Anesthesiology* 2013; 118(1):192–201.

Part A Airway/Pulmonary

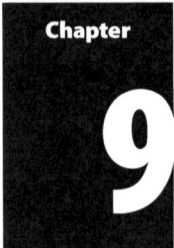

Chapter 9: Hypocarbia

Rajeev Subramanyam and Senthilkumar Sadhasivam

1. Presentation
   a) Hypocarbia is defined as an arterial carbon dioxide tension ($PaCO_2$) of ≤ 25 mmHg
   b) Hypocarbia is usually well tolerated when it is not acute. However, hypocarbia may be harmful to the brain and is a risk factor for intraventricular hemorrhage and cerebral ischemia. It may also predispose to cardiac dysrhythmias and apnea in spontaneously breathing patients
   c) Most conditions associated with hypocarbia occur due to a compensatory hyperventilation.
2. Risk factors
   See Differential diagnosis.
3. Differential diagnosis
   a) Metabolic acidosis
      i) Lactic acidosis
      ii) Diabetic acidosis
      iii) Renal acidosis.
   b) Respiratory
      i) Hyperventilation
      ii) Hypoxemia
      iii) Pneumonia
      iv) Interstitial lung disease
      v) Pulmonary edema
      vi) Pulmonary embolism
      vii) Asthma
      viii) Pneumothorax.
   c) Cardiac
      i) Decreased cardiac output
      ii) Heart failure
      iii) Cardiac arrest
      iv) Anaphylaxis
      v) Embolism.

Handbook of Critical Incidents and Essential Topics in Pediatric Anesthesiology, ed. David A. Young and Olutoyin A. Olutoye. Published by Cambridge University Press. © Cambridge University Press 2015.

d) Neurologic disorders
      i) Seizures
   e) Pain
   f) Fever/sepsis
   g) Hypothermia
   h) Anxiety.
4. Pathophysiology

   An increase in carbon dioxide elimination or a decrease in the production results in hypocarbia.
5. Management
   a) Initially evaluate the airway, breathing, vital signs, pupils, and neurologic status
   b) Quickly determine severity and onset of hypocarbia; severe/sudden onset may require cardiac resuscitation (e.g., cardiac arrest)
   c) Determine the arterial to end-tidal CO_2 gradient (a-ET) PCO_2; it is normally 5–10 with the arterial CO_2 being the larger value
   d) Adjust the ventilator settings to reduce the respiratory rate and/or tidal volume
   e) Hypocarbia-induced alkalosis can be used to reduce pulmonary vascular resistance
   f) Attempt to treat the underlying etiology.
6. Prevention
   a) Maintain vigilance for titration of mechanical ventilator settings
   b) Consider arterial blood gas testing for high-risk patients
   c) Set appropriate alarm limits for capnograph monitor
   d) Consider evaluation for conditions associated with hypocarbia (see Differential diagnosis).

Further reading

Davis PJ. *Smith's Anesthesia for Infants and Children*, 8th edition. Philadelphia: Elsevier, 2013; 709.

Kodali BS. Capnography outside the operating rooms. *Anesthesiology* 2013; 118(1):192–201.

Laffey JG, Kavanagh BP. Hypocapnia. *N Engl J Med*. 2002; 347(1):43–53.

Part A Airway/Pulmonary

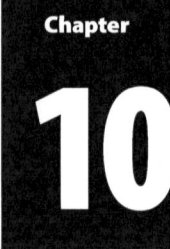

Hypoxemia

Normidaris Jimenez and Jacquelyn Morillo-Delerme

1. Presentation
    a) Most common cause of bradycardia in infants and children
    b) Fairly common occurrence in the perioperative period
    c) The incidence of intraoperative hypoxemia increases with younger ages, with the highest incidence in neonates
    d) Hypoxemia occurs easily in children because of physiologic differences in children compared to adults:
        i) Increased metabolic requirements
        ii) Decreased functional residual capacity.
2. Risk factors
    a) Inadequate ventilation
    b) Airway obstruction
    c) General anesthesia: infants and younger children are prone to airway closure and atelectasis. Atelectasis is a well-known cause of hypoxemia due to changes in the mechanics of the pediatric chest wall
    d) Intracardiac shunts
    e) Ventilation/perfusion (V/Q) mismatch.
3. Differential diagnosis
    a) Decreased cardiac output
    b) Decreased fraction of inspired oxygen
    c) Decreased minute ventilation
    d) Pulmonary conditions: pulmonary edema, pneumothorax, asthma, pulmonary hypertension
    e) Pulmonary aspiration.
4. Pathophysiology
    a) Acute hypoxemia may result in bradycardia
    b) Chronic hypoxemia results in polycythemia, increased blood viscosity, sludging and increased risk for thrombotic events, increased blood volume, altered oxygen uptake and delivery.

Handbook of Critical Incidents and Essential Topics in Pediatric Anesthesiology, ed. David A. Young and Olutoyin A. Olutoye. Published by Cambridge University Press. © Cambridge University Press 2015.

5. Management
   a) Identify the cause (most important step)
   b) Administer oxygen
      i) Hypoxemia secondary to shunts typically do not respond to increased inspired oxygen concentrations (FiO_2) in contrast to hypoxemia related to V/Q mismatch.
   c) Alleviate any existing airway obstruction (i.e., laryngospasm)
   d) Auscultate lungs and verify that appropriate ventilation is present
   e) Administer beta agonists if wheezing is present
   f) Consider obtaining an arterial blood gas and chest X-ray in refractory cases.
6. Prevention
   a) Identify predisposing conditions and treat promptly
   b) Maintain adequate oxygenation and ventilation in patients under sedation or general anesthesia
   c) Administer supplemental oxygen after extubation and during patient transportation to the recovery room
   d) Administer supplemental oxygen during the recovery period while the patient is asleep or for as long as clinically indicated.

Further reading

Coté CJ, Lerman J, Anderson BJ. *Coté and Lerman's A Practice of Anesthesia for Infants and Children*, 5th edition. Philadelphia, PA: Elsevier, 2013; 458.

de Graaff JC. Incidence of intraoperative hypoxemia in children in relation to age. *Anesth Analg.* 2013; 117(1):169–75.

Gregory GA. *Gregory's Pediatric Anesthesia*, 5th edition. Hoboken: Wiley-Blackwell, 2012; 303–27.

Part A Airway/Pulmonary

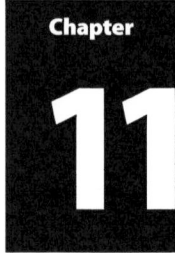

Increased peak airway pressures

Normidaris Jimenez and Jacquelyn Morillo-Delerme

1. Presentation
   a) High airway pressure alarm activated on mechanicalventilator
   b) Peaking of end-tidal carbon dioxide tracing on capnograph
   c) Hypoxemia
   d) Difficult ventilation
   e) Detection of decreased lung compliance during manual ventilation
   f) Bronchospasm
   g) Change in hemodynamics – hypotension, decreased cardiac output.

2. Risk factors
   a) Preexisting poor lung compliance, reactive airway disease
   b) Obesity
   c) History of drug allergies
   d) Head/neck/chest surgery:
      i) Thoracotomy and open lung surgery
      ii) Central venous catheter placement
      iii) Radical neck dissection.
   e) Neonates and infants with smaller diameter endotracheal tubes
   f) Trauma
   g) Pulmonary disorders (pneumonia, cystic fibrosis).

3. Differential diagnosis
   a) Inadequate (light) anesthesia
   b) Endobronchial intubation
   c) Obstruction or kinking of tracheal tube or anesthesia machine circuit
   d) Incorrect ventilator parameters (excessive tidal volumes)
   e) High-pressure delivery due to faulty pressure regulator on anesthesia machine
   f) Increased airway resistance due to anaphylaxis, aspiration, bronchospasm, or airway foreign body
   g) Decreased chest wall compliance (prone/trendelenburg position, obesity, abdominal/thoracic insufflation, ascites)

Handbook of Critical Incidents and Essential Topics in Pediatric Anesthesiology, ed. David A. Young and Olutoyin A. Olutoye. Published by Cambridge University Press. © Cambridge University Press 2015.

    h) Decreased lung compliance: pneumo/hemothorax, atelectasis, pulmonary edema, pleural effusion
    i) Compression of airway during surgery (e.g., open thoracotomy)
    j) Pneumothorax.
4. Pathophysiology
Increased peak airway pressure may lead to hypercarbia, hypoxemia, and barotrauma.
5. Management
    a) Auscultate lung fields, confirm bilateral breath sounds
    b) Quickly assess vital signs – blood pressure, heart rate, oxygen saturation and check for abnormalities
    c) Convert to 100% oxygen and manual ventilation
    d) Check circuit for kinks and endotracheal tube for obstruction, blood, sputum or secretions; suction the endotracheal tube (ETT) to verify patency
    e) Consider verifying appropriate tracheal tube position
    f) Check machine to confirm that ventilator settings are appropriate
    g) Inform surgeon and look at the surgical field for a possible explanation (e.g., pneumoperitoneum, retractors in the field, recent central line placement).
    h) Consider administration of neuromuscular blocking agents
    i) Consider increasing the depth of anesthesia
    j) Consider administration of bronchodilators if wheezing is present.
6. Prevention
    a) Confirm correct tracheal tube placement prior to securing it and immediately after any significant intraoperative change (position change, insufflation)
    b) Verify that a proper machine check takes place at the start of the day, between cases, and after changing circuits
    c) Monitor surgical field often during surgery; particularly during thoracotomy procedures in neonates and smaller children, consider suctioning the tracheal tube to prevent obstruction
    d) Support smaller diameter ETTs prior to application of surgical drapes to avoid kinking, compression or dislodgement by surgeon
    e) Have high suspicion in high-risk procedures or high-risk patients
    f) Activate ventilator high-pressure alarms and set limits close to current values.

Further reading

Davis PJ. *Smith's Anesthesia for Infants and Children*, 8th edition. Philadelphia: Mosby Inc., 2011; 1157.

Gregory GA. *Gregory's Pediatric Anesthesia*, 5th edition. Hoboken: Wiley-Blackwell, 2012; 963.

Part A Airway/Pulmonary

Chapter 12 Laryngospasm

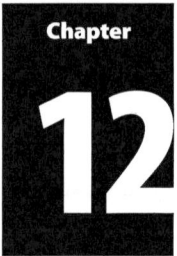

Kha M. Tran

1. Presentation
   a) Inability to effectively ventilate due to partial or complete glottic closure
   b) Ineffective inspiratory effort resulting in high-pitched inspiratory stridor, sternal retractions, paradoxical breathing pattern, reduced tidal volumes, apnea
   c) Incidence at least 1–5% in children < 9 years old.
2. Risk factors
   a) Presence of active (copious secretions or nasal congestion) or resolving respiratory infection
   b) Reactive airway disease
   c) Endotracheal intubation (greater risk when compared with supraglottic airway devices)
   d) Younger age
   e) Passive smoke exposure
   f) History of prior anesthetic complications
   g) Surgery in head or neck region
   h) Airway stimulation while receiving an inadequate depth of anesthesia.
3. Differential diagnosis
   a) Upper airway obstruction
   b) Severe bronchospasm
   c) Apnea
   d) Airway foreign body.
4. Pathophysiology
   a) Reflex closure of the vocal cords prevents air flow
   b) Prolonged laryngospasm may result in:
      i) Hypoxemia, bradycardia, post-obstructive negative pressure pulmonary edema, pulmonary aspiration due to regurgitation of gastric contents, cardiac arrest.
   c) Negative pressure pulmonary edema may occur following laryngospasm in children with muscular body habitus such as adolescents.

5. Management
   a) Ensure effective mask seal, apply 100% oxygen and continuous positive airway pressure (CPAP)
   b) Attempt to assist patient's spontaneous breaths
   c) May need to be very aggressive with CPAP; this may result in gastric insufflation
   d) In mild cases of partial laryngospasm (i.e., SPO_2 >90%), supportive measures and oropharyngeal suctioning only may be required
   e) In more severe cases and in the absence of intravenous access:
      i) Deepen volatile anesthetic (though likely to be ineffective due to airway obstruction)
      ii) Promptly secure intravenous (IV) access
      iii) Consider intramuscular succinylcholine (4–5 mg/kg)
      iv) Consider co-administration of atropine (0.02 mg/kg IM) if succinylcholine will be administered.
   f) In more severe cases and if intravenous access is present:
      i) Deepen anesthesia either with volatile and/or IV medications (propofol, rocuronium, succinylcholine)
      ii) Consider co-administration of atropine (0.02 mg/kg IV/IM) if succinylcholine will be administered (0.1–0.2 mg/kg IV).
   g) Consider emergent endotracheal intubation
   h) Consider gastric decompression
   i) Endotracheal intubation of short duration may be required in patients who are suspected to have developed negative pressure pulmonary edema.
6. Prevention
   a) Consider postponing elective procedures in the presence of active respiratory infections
   b) Maintain adequate depth of anesthesia for patients recovering from an upper respiratory tract infection or at increased risk for laryngospasm
   c) Institute prompt application of CPAP if coughing occurs during induction or emergence from anesthesia
   d) Ensure adequate depth of anesthesia prior to airway instrumentation
   e) Consider suctioning naso- and oropharynx under deep anesthesia if nasal congestion is present
   f) Consider deep extubation techniques for at-risk patients.

Further reading

Coté CJ, Lerman J, Anderson BJ. *Coté and Lerman's A Practice of Anesthesia for Infants and Children*, 5th edition. Philadelphia, PA: Elsevier, 2013; 243.

Davis PJ. *Smith's Anesthesia for Infants and Children*, 8th edition. Philadelphia: Elsevier, 2011; 38–9.

Gregory GA. *Gregory's Pediatric Anesthesia*, 5th edition. Hoboken: Wiley-Blackwell, 2012; 317.

Part A: Airway/Pulmonary

Chapter 13: Pulmonary aspiration of gastric contents

Mary A. Felberg

1. Presentation
   a) Active vomiting or passive regurgitation of gastric contents into the airway
   b) Incidence during elective surgery: 1:1,000 to 1:10,000
   c) Incidence increases during emergent surgery: 1:400 to 1:1,000
   d) Mortality from aspiration: 0 to 1:50,000
   e) May occur any time during the perioperative period, 80% occur during induction
   f) Confirmed by visualization or suctioning of gastric material from airway
   g) New onset respiratory distress
      i) Hypoxemia, hypercarbia, tachypnea
      ii) Increased ventilatory pressures/decreased compliance
      iii) Wheezing, rhonchi, and rales.
   h) The extent of presentation varies ranging from clinically asymptomatic to acute respiratory distress syndrome.

2. Risk factors
   a) Full stomach (e.g., recent food ingestion, trauma)
   b) Emergent surgery
   c) Impaired protective reflexes (e.g., altered mental status)
   d) Delayed gastric emptying (e.g., pyloric stenosis, bowel obstruction)
   e) Gastrointestinal dysmotility (e.g., gastroesophageal reflux)
   f) Abdominal distension (e.g., ascites)
   g) Difficult airway/multiple attempts to secure airway/prolonged mask ventilation.

3. Differential diagnosis
   a) Bronchospasm
   b) Pneumonia
   c) Airway foreign body
   d) Tracheal tube obstruction
   e) Pneumothorax.

Handbook of Critical Incidents and Essential Topics in Pediatric Anesthesiology, ed. David A. Young and Olutoyin A. Olutoye. Published by Cambridge University Press. © Cambridge University Press 2015.

4. Pathophysiology
   a) Aspiration or regurgitation of gastric contents into the airway may result in development of chemical pneumonitis
      i) Most studies based on animal data
      ii) Gastric contents with pH < 2.5 readily penetrates the mucosal surface causing inflammation, edema, and sloughing of airway mucosa
      iii) Volume of aspirate > 0.8 mL/kg is reportedly required to produce significant disease.
5. Management
   a) If patient vomits without tracheal tube:
      i) Place patient in lateral decubitus position
      ii) Suction oral pharynx
      iii) Secure airway with tracheal tube or consider trial with supplemental oxygen.
   b) If patient vomits with tracheal tube present:
      i) Suction tracheal tube
      ii) Consider fiberoptic bronchoscopy to evaluate airway
      iii) Consider rigid bronchoscopy for removal of particulate material
      iv) Consider normal saline lavage if particulate matter present
      v) Administer beta-2 agonists (e.g., albuterol) for bronchospasm
      vi) Administer positive end-expiratory pressure (PEEP) to increase alveolar recruitment
      vii) Anticipate potential for increased mechanical ventilatory support.
   c) Consider cancellation of non-emergent procedures
   d) Place oral gastric tube to evacuate stomach contents
   e) Consider obtaining arterial blood gas
   f) Extubate patient awake only if patient has acceptable vital signs, spontaneous ventilatory effort, oxygenation, and ventilation
   g) Consider obtaining chest X-ray although signs of aspiration may be delayed
   h) Clinically apparent symptoms are usually evident within several hours after event
   i) Empiric corticosteroid administration is not indicated
   j) Empiric antibiotic administration is not indicated.
6. Prevention
   a) Preoperative identification of at-risk patients
   b) Consider premedications (e.g., sodium citrate, metoclopramide)
   c) Consider gastric tube suctioning *before* induction of anesthesia
   d) Utilize anesthetic techniques that avoid gastric distension, especially during mask ventilation
   e) Consider use of rapid sequence induction techniques
   f) Use of cricoid pressure to reduce aspiration is controversial
   g) Utilize cuffed tracheal tubes for at-risk patients
   h) Consider gastric suctioning after induction and prior to emergence
   i) Strongly consider utilizing awake extubation techniques for at-risk patients.

Further reading

Coté CJ, Lerman J, Anderson BJ. *Coté and Lerman's A Practice of Anesthesia for Infants and Children*, 5th edition. Philadelphia, PA: Elsevier, 2013; 31–32, 569–70.

Gregory GA, Andropoulos DB. *Gregory's Pediatric Anesthesia*, 5th edition. Hoboken: Wiley-Blackwell, 2012; 211–23.

Kliegman RM. *Nelson Textbook of Pediatrics*, 19th edition. Philadelphia: Elsevier, Saunders, 2011; 517–531.

Raggavebdran M. Aspiration induced lung injury. *Crit Care Med.* 2011; 39(4):818–26.

Part A Airway/Pulmonary

Chapter 14

Stridor

John E. Fiadjoe

1. Presentation
    a) High-pitched respiratory noise caused by turbulent airflow commonly heard on inspiration
    b) May be present with inspiration and expiration.
2. Risk factors
    a) Infants and children with narrow airways
    b) Upper respiratory tract infections
    c) Foreign body aspiration
    d) Airway masses
    e) Congenital airway anomalies.
3. Differential diagnosis
    a) Laryngomalacia (most common cause of stridor in neonates)
    b) Croup (common cause of acute stridor in children 6 months to 2 years)
    c) Foreign body aspiration (children 1–2 years and patients with developmental delay)
    d) Retropharyngeal abscess (high fever, swallowing difficulty also present)
    e) Tracheomalacia
    f) Peritonsillar abscess
    g) Anaphylaxis
    h) Epiglottitis
    i) Vocal cord paresis (biphasic stridor)
    j) Subglottic stenosis
    k) Laryngeal web, tumors, cysts, papillomas
    l) Choanal atresia
    m) Laryngospasm
    n) Vascular rings
    o) Subglottic hemangioma.
4. Pathophysiology
    a) Inspiratory stridor indicates extrathoracic obstruction
    b) Expiratory stridor indicates intrathoracic obstruction

Handbook of Critical Incidents and Essential Topics in Pediatric Anesthesiology, ed. David A. Young and Olutoyin A. Olutoye. Published by Cambridge University Press. © Cambridge University Press 2015.

c) Biphasic stridor suggests glottic or subglottic obstruction
   d) As gas moves linearly through a narrowed airway, lateral pressure decreases, causing the airway to collapse and obstruct airflow thereby creating stridor.
5. Management
   a) Careful observation if patient is otherwise not in respiratory distress
   b) Consider use of humidified air/oxygen in mild cases
   c) Consider racemic epinephrine
   d) Consider imaging studies such as chest X-ray, flexible laryngoscopy, CT scan
   e) Evaluation in the operating room with rigid bronchoscopy may be required in cases with unclear etiologies
   f) Antibiotics for infectious causes
   g) Steroids to reduce inflammation.

Further reading

Coté CJ, Lerman J, Anderson BJ. *Coté and Lerman's A Practice of Anesthesia for Infants and Children*, 5th edition. Philadelphia, PA: Elsevier, 2013; 246–7.

Gregory GA, Andropoulos DB. *Gregory's Pediatric Anesthesia*, 5th edition. Hoboken: Wiley-Blackwell, 2012; 777–98.

Part A Airway/Pulmonary

Chapter 15
Tension pneumothorax
Amanda K. Brown and Rhonda A. Alexis

1. Presentation
   Presentation varies with extent of lung collapse, rate of collapse and presence of underlying medical conditions:
   a) Dyspnea
   b) Tachypnea
   c) Hypoxemia
   d) Pleuritic chest pain
   e) Cyanosis
   f) Decreased breath sounds on affected side
   g) Hyperresonance to percussion on affected side
   h) Tracheal deviation to the contralateral side
   i) Distended neck veins (jugular venous distension)
   j) Hypotension
   k) Pulseless electrical activity
   l) Trauma-induced pneumothorax; suspect in presence of chest wall contusion.

2. Risk factors
   a) Tall, thin body habitus (spontaneous pneumothorax)
   b) Apical lung blebs
   c) Trauma
   d) Mechanical ventilation using elevated peak airway pressures
   e) Pulmonary infections
   f) Overzealous cardiopulmonary resuscitation
   g) Surgical procedures in the chest region (central line placement).

3. Differential diagnosis
   a) Other causes of cardiac arrest (e.g., hypovolemic shock)
   b) Endobronchial intubation
   c) Tension gastrothorax secondary to diaphragmatic tear
   d) Pulmonary conditions (e.g., pneumonia, asthma, airway foreign body).

Handbook of Critical Incidents and Essential Topics in Pediatric Anesthesiology, ed. David A. Young and Olutoyin A. Olutoye. Published by Cambridge University Press. © Cambridge University Press 2015.

4. Pathophysiology
   a) Air enters the pleural space but cannot exit, resulting in progressive build-up of air and a one-way valve effect
   b) Increasing pressure in pleural space further obstructs venous return to the heart and also results in deviation of the mediastinum towards the opposite hemithorax
   c) Circulatory instability and cardiac arrest may occur due to lack of preload.
5. Management
   a) Patients without hemodynamic compromise: obtain chest X-ray for confirmation and to rule out endobronchial intubation
   b) Patients with cardiovascular instability: emergent decompression with needle thoracostomy (2nd intercostal space, above the rib, at the mid-clavicular line). Discontinue nitrous oxide if present. Cardiopulmonary resuscitation may also be required. Definitive treatment is chest tube placement.
6. Prevention
   a) Maintain increased vigilance for signs of a pneumothorax for at-risk patients
   b) Avoid excessive peak airway pressures in patients on mechanical ventilation.

Further reading

Butterworth JF. *Morgan and Mikhail's Clinical Anesthesiology*, 5th edition. New York: McGraw-Hill Company, Inc., 2013; 544.

Davis PJ. *Smith's Anesthesia for Infants and Children*, 8th edition. Philadelphia: Mosby, Inc., 2011; 981.

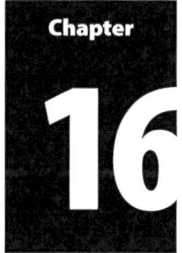

Part A Airway/Pulmonary

Chapter 16 Respiratory acidosis

Amy Graham-Carlson

1. Presentation
   a) Hypercarbia: PaCO$_2$ > 45 mmHg and acidemia pH (< 7.35)
   b) Signs and symptoms include dyspnea, confusion, somnolence, seizures, tachycardia, hypertension.
2. Risk factors
   a) Decreased carbon dioxide elimination (hypoventilation)
      i) Airway obstruction (asthma, tracheal secretions)
      ii) Lung or chest wall restriction (congenital diaphragmatic hernia, kyphoscoliosis, obesity)
      iii) Decreased skeletal muscle strength (partial neuromuscular blockade, muscular dystrophy)
      iv) Interstitial or parenchymal lung disease (pneumonia, pulmonary edema) and increased dead space
      v) Central nervous system depression (obstructive sleep apnea, opioids, benzodiazepines, encephalitis)
      vi) Inadequate mechanical ventilator settings.
   b) Increased carbon dioxide production (CO$_2$)
      i) Absorption of CO$_2$ from pneumoperitoneum during laparoscopic surgery
      ii) Rebreathing of exhaled CO$_2$ (exhausted soda lime, incompetent inspiratory or expiratory valve)
      iii) Malignant hyperthermia
      iv) Hyperthyroidism
      v) Hyperalimentation/total parenteral nutrition with high carbohydrate content
      vi) Hypermetabolic state (burn injury, fever).
3. Differential diagnosis
   See Risk factors.
4. Pathophysiology
   a) Hypercarbia results in the compensatory mechanism of increased hydrogen ion secretion as well as bicarbonate reabsorption and production
   b) There are acute and long-term (chronic) responses to hypercarbia:

Handbook of Critical Incidents and Essential Topics in Pediatric Anesthesiology, ed. David A. Young and Olutoyin A. Olutoye. Published by Cambridge University Press. © Cambridge University Press 2015.

i) Acute phase response is characterized by buffering from hemoglobin and exchange of extracellular hydrogen ion for intracellular sodium and potassium which may produce hyperkalemia ($\Delta pHa = 0.008 \times \Delta PaCO_2$)
   ii) Chronic phase response by the kidneys is characterized by a 4 mmol/L increase in plasma bicarbonate for each 10 mmHg increase in $PaCO_2$ above 40 mmHg ($\Delta pHa = 0.003 \times \Delta PaCO_2$).
5. Management
   a) Reverse the imbalance between CO_2 production and alveolar ventilation; obtain arterial blood gas to determine $PaCO_2$
   b) Increase minute ventilation:
      i) Increase tidal volume and/or ventilating pressures as well as respiratory rate
   c) Reduce CO_2 production (e.g., dantrolene therapy for malignant hyperthermia, antithyroid medications for thyrotoxicosis, acetaminophen for fever)
   d) Improve alveolar ventilation with bronchodilator therapy, suctioning of tracheal tube, reversal of opioids or administration of respiratory stimulant (caffeine) where applicable
   e) Consider prolonged mechanical ventilation for severe or refractory respiratory acidosis
   f) Relative intraoperative permissive hypercapnia should be considered for patients with preoperative chronic respiratory acidosis.
6. Prevention
   a) Meticulous attention to end tidal carbon dioxide ($EtCO_2$) monitoring in patients at increased risk for hypercarbia development
   b) Consider use of non-opioid analgesics and multimodal pain strategies in the opioid sensitive population.

Further reading

Barash P, Cullen B, Stoelting R. *Clinical Anesthesia*, 5th edition. Philadelphia: Lippincott Williams & Wilkins, 2006; 178–9.

Bissonnette B. *Pediatric Anesthesia: Basic Principles – State of the Art – Future*. Shelton, CT: People's Medical Publishing House, 2011; 150–1.

Stoelting R, Miller R. *Basics of Anesthesia*, 5th edition. Philadelphia: Churchill Livingstone, Elsevier Inc., 2007; 320–2.

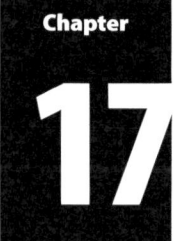

Part A Airway/Pulmonary

Chapter 17

Respiratory alkalosis

Amy Graham-Carlson

1. Presentation
   a) Hypocarbia: $PaCO_2 < 35$ mmHg and alkalosis pH (> 7.45)
   b) Apnea, dizziness, tinnitus although may be clinically asymptomatic
   c) Positive Trousseau sign, positive Chvostek sign resulting from hypocalcemia.
2. Risk factors
   a) Hyperventilation secondary to:
      i) Pain
      ii) Underlying anxiety disorder
      iii) Excessive mechanical ventilation.
   b) Overwhelming infection (increased basic metabolic rate)
   c) Metabolic acidosis (compensatory)
   d) Pulmonary disorders (interstitial or parenchymal disorders)
   e) Drug toxicities (salicylate, theophylline, sodium bicarbonate).
3. Differential diagnosis
   See Risk factors.
4. Pathophysiology
   a) Increased minute ventilation exceeds amount required to eliminate metabolic carbon dioxide (CO_2) production
   b) Metabolic compensation occurs by decreased reabsorption of bicarbonate ions from the renal tubules
   c) Hypokalemia and hypocalcemia may develop
   d) If minute ventilation doubles, it reduces partial pressure of arterial carbon dioxide ($PaCO_2$) and decreases cerebral blood flow by half.
5. Management
   a) Treat underlying cause (hyperventilation)
   b) For patients on mechanical ventilation:
      i) Decrease minute ventilation by decreasing rate of mechanical breaths
      ii) Decrease peak inspiratory pressure or tidal volume.

Handbook of Critical Incidents and Essential Topics in Pediatric Anesthesiology, ed. David A. Young and Olutoyin A. Olutoye. Published by Cambridge University Press. © Cambridge University Press 2015.

c) Obtain arterial blood gas (ABG) to determine $PaCO_2$ and compare to end-tidal carbon dioxide concentration ($EtCO_2$)
d) Condition may be self-limiting and therapy may not be required.

6. Prevention
   a) Adequate pain management with multimodal analgesia
   b) Recognition and prompt treatment of anxiety
   c) Meticulous attention to mechanical ventilation parameters and adherence to appropriate minute ventilation.

Further reading

Barash P, Cullen B, Stoelting R. *Clinical Anesthesia*. 5th edition. Philadelphia: Lippincott Williams & Wilkins, 2006; 178–9.

Bissonnette B. *Pediatric Anesthesia: Basic Principles – State of the Art – Future.* Shelton, CT: People's Medical Publishing House, 2011; 152.

Stoelting R, Miller R. *Basics of Anesthesia*, 5th edition. Philadelphia: Churchill Livingstone, Elsevier Inc., 2007; 320–2.

Part A Airway/Pulmonary

Chapter 18

Upper airway obstruction

Carlos Rodriguez

1. Presentation
   a) The presence of an increase in the upper airway resistance, which leads to the obstruction of airflow through the airway
   b) Inspiratory stridor is a sign of extrathoracic obstruction
   c) Signs include: high-pitched airway noise, silence (complete airway obstruction), hypoxemia, tachypnea, respiratory distress (nasal flaring), paradoxical breathing.

2. Risk factors
   a) Residual anesthetic agents (i.e., following deep extubation)
   b) Obesity
   c) Obstructive sleep apnea
   d) Down syndrome (due to macroglossia)
   e) Adenotonsillar hypertrophy
   f) Airway mass (e.g., laryngeal papilloma)
   g) Choanal atresia (neonate)
   h) Infections (e.g., epiglottitis).

3. Differential diagnosis
   a) Obstructive sleep apnea
   b) Laryngospasm
   c) Airway lesions
   d) Infectious etiology (epiglottitis, croup)
   e) Airway foreign body.

4. Pathophysiology
   Pathophysiology depends on the specific etiology of the obstruction.
   a) Reduction of airway tone during general anesthesia leads to collapse of the surrounding tissue and the development of airway obstruction
   b) Laryngospasm leads to partial or complete obstruction of airflow. Laryngospasm occurs when there is a stimulus (i.e., secretions) in the setting of an insufficient depth of anesthesia
   c) Epiglottitis is due to an infectious origin which results in progressive swelling of the epiglottis and upper airway

---

Handbook of Critical Incidents and Essential Topics in Pediatric Anesthesiology, ed. David A. Young and Olutoyin A. Olutoye. Published by Cambridge University Press. © Cambridge University Press 2015.

d) Croup is usually due to a viral infectious process that leads to edema within the upper airway.

5. Management
   a) Attempt to open/clear the airway by:
      i) Head extension
      ii) Jaw thrust
      iii) Insertion of an oral or nasal airway
      iv) Placing the patient in the lateral position
      v) Suctioning when indicated.
   b) Administer supplemental oxygen
   c) Consider administration of continuous positive airway pressure (CPAP)
   d) Consider positive pressure ventilation and tracheal intubation for refractory cases
   e) Consider removal of suspected foreign body or airway lesion
   f) Consider therapy to decrease edema when applicable (e.g., racemic epinephrine).

6. Prevention
   a) There are certain viral processes that can be prevented by the administration of vaccines such as for epiglottitis. This condition is rarely seen clinically but can present in patients who have not received the *H. influenzae* vaccination (most common pathogen to cause epiglottitis)
   b) Verify that adequate depths of general anesthesia are present during situations in which a tracheal tube is not present, such as during induction of general anesthesia. To reduce laryngospasm during extubation, one should assure that the patient is fully awake
   c) Patients will naturally obstruct in the presence of residual anesthetic agents due to loss of airway tonicity. Vigilance and prompt recognition of airway tone loss is critical to preventing prolonged airway obstruction as well as the development of severe hypoxemia.

Further reading

Coté, CJ, Lerman, J, Anderson, BJ. *Coté and Lerman's A Practice of Anesthesia for Infants and Children*, 5th edition. Philadelphia, PA: Elservier, 2013; 2298–312.

Gregory GA, Andropoulos DB. *Gregory's Pediatric Anesthesia*, 5th edition. Hoboken: Wiley-Blackwell, 2012; 281.

Miller RD. *Miller's Anesthesia*, 7th edition. Philadelphia: Churchill Livingstone, 2010; 3542–5.

Part B Cardiac

Chapter 19

Anaphylaxis

Kha M. Tran

1. Presentation
   a) Urticaria
   b) Erythema
   c) Bronchospasm
   d) Hypotension
   e) Tachycardia
   f) Cardiac arrest.
2. Risk factors
   a) History of anaphylaxis
   b) History of atopy
   c) Patients with multiple prior exposures to latex products
   d) Neuromuscular blocking agents, antibiotics, and latex products are common culprits.
3. Differential diagnosis
   a) Isolated urticaria
   b) Isolated bronchospasm
   c) Histamine release from medications (morphine, atracurium)
   d) Alternative causes of hypotension: cardiac, vasomotor, volume status
   e) Anaphylactoid reaction (clinically indistinguishable from anaphylaxis).
4. Pathophysiology
   a) IgE-mediated release of factors from mast cells following repeat antigen exposure
   b) Release of histamine, proteases, inflammatory and vasoactive mediators results in increased vascular permeability, decreased peripheral vascular resistance, flushing, urticaria, hypotension, and bronchoconstriction.
5. Management
   a) If possible identify offending antigen and discontinue administration
   b) Discontinue anesthetic agents if patient is unstable
   c) Administer 100% oxygen
   d) Secure airway if endotracheal tube not already in place
   e) Fluid resuscitation should occur using isotonic crystalloid

---

Handbook of Critical Incidents and Essential Topics in Pediatric Anesthesiology, ed. David A. Young and Olutoyin A. Olutoye. Published by Cambridge University Press. © Cambridge University Press 2015.

f) Epinephrine 1 µg/kg IV bolus for hypotension, 10 µg/kg or more for cardiovascular collapse; this may need to be repeated frequently
g) Consider epinephrine infusion (0.05–0.1 µg/kg/min) for persistent symptoms.
h) Histamine receptor blockers to block effect of histamine:
  i) H-1 receptor blocker: diphenhydramine 1 mg/kg IV
  ii) H-2 receptor blocker: ranitidine 0.5 mg/kg IV.
i) Steroid administration: hydrocortisone 1–5 mg/kg IV to diminish mediator formation and release
j) Administration of inhaled bronchodilators (albuterol) to treat bronchospasm
k) Obtain blood to check for serum tryptase levels (increased within 30 minutes to 2 hours following beginning of reaction)
l) Establish invasive monitoring
m) Strongly consider aborting all elective procedures
n) Arrange for patient transfer to intensive care unit for stabilization after initial resuscitation
o) Once the patient is stabilized in the postoperative period, strongly consider referral for performance of antigen-specific IgE testing.

6. Prevention
  a) Avoid administration of known allergens or medications allergies
  b) Heightened degree of vigilance after administration of medications known to be associated with anaphylaxis (antibiotics)
  c) Create latex-free operating rooms
  d) Consider consultation with an allergist to consider desensitization
  e) Recommend medical alert bracelets for identified patients.

Further reading

Cote CJ. *A Practice of Anesthesia for Infants and Children*, 4th edition. Philadelphia: Saunders, 2009; 38.

Davis PJ. *Smith's Anesthesia for Infants and Children*, 8th edition. Philadelphia: Elsevier, 2011; 1169.

Hepner DL, Castells MC. Anaphylaxis during the perioperative period. *Anesth Analg.* 2003; 97(5):1381–95.

Nel L, Eren E. Peri-operative anaphylaxis. *Br J Clin Pharmacol.* 2011; 71(5):647–58.

Part B Cardiac

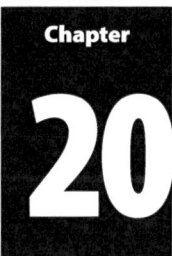

Chapter 20 Asystole

Joanna Rosing and Jacquelyn Morillo-Delerme

1. Presentation
   a) Full cardiac arrest with no electrical activity on electrocardiogram
   b) Symptoms may be nonspecific: apnea, unconsciousness, and unresponsiveness. Asystole is considered a terminal rhythm commonly presenting after refractory ventricular fibrillation or ventricular tachycardia.
2. Risk factors
   a) Infants less than one year of age are at increased risk in comparison to older children
   b) Preexisting electrolyte abnormalities (i.e., hyperkalemia, hypocalcemia)
   c) Metabolic conditions (i.e., hypoxemia, hypothermia)
   d) Recent administration of pharmacologic agents (i.e., inhaled anesthetic agents, succinylcholine, anticholinesterase inhibitors, intravascular local anesthetic injection)
   e) Drug toxicity
   f) Trauma.
3. Differential diagnosis
   a) Electrocardiogram lead misplacement
   b) Syncope following vagal reaction
   c) Junctional bradycardia.
4. Pathophysiology
   a) Asystole may result from failure of the cardiac conducting system to generate ventricular depolarization due to:
      i) Sino-atrial node dysfunction
      ii) Atrioventricular node dysfunction
      iii) Myocardial ischemia
      iv) Congenital heart block
      v) Tumor
      vi) Trauma
      vii) Cardiac reflexes (oculocardiac reflex).
   b) Factors external to the cardiac conducting system resulting in failure to generate electrical depolarization:
      i) Cardiovascular

Handbook of Critical Incidents and Essential Topics in Pediatric Anesthesiology, ed. David A. Young and Olutoyin A. Olutoye. Published by Cambridge University Press. © Cambridge University Press 2015.

(1) Cardiogenic shock
  (2) Cardiac tamponade
  (3) Thrombosis (coronary or pulmonary).

  ii) Progressive respiratory failure (most common cause of cardiopulmonary arrest in children):

  (1) Hypoxemia
  (2) Acidosis
  (3) Tension pneumothorax.

  iii) Metabolic

  (1) Tissue hypoxia
  (2) Electrolyte abnormalities.

  iv) Medication induced asystole is most commonly a result of cardiovascular depression

  (1) Volatile agents (previously halothane was the most common precipitating agent)
  (2) Succinylcholine
  (3) Neostigmine
  (4) Local anesthetic toxicity.

5. Management
   a) Declare intraoperative crisis, initiate Pediatric Advanced Life Support; immediately call for help and code cart
   b) Chest compressions (2 minute cycles followed by patient reassessment)
   c) Secure airway
   d) Administer 100% oxygen, fluid bolus, discontinue anesthetic agents
   e) Secure intravenous access
   f) Medications: epinephrine is the drug of choice in pediatric resuscitation (dose 10 µg/kg IV every 3 minutes).

6. Prevention
   a) Atropine is the drug of choice to treat bradycardia from excessive vagal stimulation and bradycardia induced by anesthetic drugs (dose 0.01–0.03 mg/kg IV/IM)
   b) Prompt management of predisposing electrolyte or metabolic abnormalities
   c) Early initiation of chest compressions for bradycardia (heart rate < 60) with palpable pulse is more likely to result in survival following hospital discharge compared to chest compressions for asystole.

Further reading

Bhananker S, Ramamoorthy C, Geiduschek JM. Anesthesia-related cardiac arrest in children: Update from the Pediatric Perioperative Cardiac Arrest Registry. *Anesth Analg.* 2007; 105(2):344–50.

Donoghue A, Berg RA, Hazinski F. Cardiopulmonary resuscitation for bradycardia with poor perfusion versus pulseless cardiac arrest. *Pediatrics.* 2009; 124(6):1541–8.

Gregory GA, Andropoulos DB. *Gregory's Pediatric Anesthesia*, 5th edition. Hoboken: Wiley-Blackwell, 2012; 255–65.

Kleinman ME, Chameides L, Schexnayder SM. Part 14: Pediatric advanced life support: 2010 American Heart Association Guidelines for Cardiopulmonary Resuscitation and Emergency Cardiovascular Care. *Circulation.* 2010; 122(18 Suppl 3):S876–908.

Part B **Cardiac**

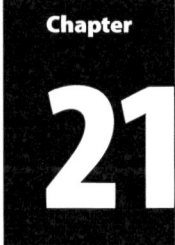

Bradycardia

Amanda K. Brown and Rhonda A. Alexis

1. Presentation
   a) Bradycardia is clinically significant only if signs of poor perfusion are present
   b) Heart rate lower than normal for the patient's age:
      i) Heart rate < 100 BPM (beats per minute) in infants
      ii) Heart rate < 80 BPM in children 1–5 years
      iii) Heart rate < 60 BPM in children > 5 years of age and adolescents.
   c) May be asymptomatic
   d) Symptoms vary with age when present:
      i) Infants/young children: poor feeding and lethargy
      ii) Children and adolescents: fatigue, exercise intolerance, dizziness or syncope.
2. Risk factors
   a) Prematurity
   b) Neurologic problems (e.g., intracranial tumors)
   c) Underlying heart disease or prior heart surgery.
3. Etiology
   a) Hypoxemia (most common cause)
   b) Cardiac: conduction defects (congenital, autoimmune diseases such as systemic lupus erythematous)
   c) Vagal stimulation, seen in the following settings:
      i) Nasopharyngeal/esophageal stimulation
      ii) Breath-holding spells
      iii) Gastroesophageal reflux in preterm infants
      iv) Increased intracranial pressure
      v) Traction on extraocular muscles during eye surgery (especially medial rectus muscle)
      vi) Medications which increase parasympathetic tone (neostigmine, succinylcholine).
   d) Negative chronotropes: β-blockers, calcium channel blockers, digoxin, amiodarone, clonidine, and verapamil
   e) Metabolic conditions: hyperkalemia, hypercalcemia, hypothermia, hypothyroidism.

Handbook of Critical Incidents and Essential Topics in Pediatric Anesthesiology, ed. David A. Young and Olutoyin A. Olutoye. Published by Cambridge University Press. © Cambridge University Press 2015.

4. Pathophysiology
   Varies with the etiology of the bradycardia but two main pathways exist:
   a) High vagal tone which slows the intrinsic pacing rate of the sino-atrial node
   b) Medications which act indirectly on the nervous system or directly on the sinus node.
5. Management
   Depends on clinical scenario:
   a) If related to hypoxemia: assess the airway, support airway management, oxygenation and ventilation
   b) Consider atropine if due to high vagal tone
   c) Initiate chest compressions if heart rate < 60 BPM with poor perfusion despite adequate ventilation and oxygenation
   d) Administer epinephrine at a dose of 0.01 mg/kg (1:10,000 concentration) for refractory cases
   e) Consider use of transcutaneous pacing
   f) Identify and treat other potentially reversible causes of bradycardia
   g) Perform thorough history and physical to determine etiology and administer definitive treatment while resuscitative efforts continue.
6. Prevention
   a) Maintain adequate oxygenation especially during induction and emergence from anesthesia
   b) Prevent high levels of volatile agents for long periods during induction (especially in children with Down syndrome)
   c) Recognize that most children with bradycardia are asymptomatic and this is normal
   d) Maintain continuous monitoring of heart rate with appropriate alarm settings and use of audible tone.

Further reading

Doniger SJ. *Pediatric Clinics of North America*. Philadelphia: Elsevier, 2006; 97–8.

Gregory GA, Andropoulos DB. *Gregory's Pediatric Anesthesia*, 5th edition. Hoboken: Wiley-Blackwell, 2012; 350.

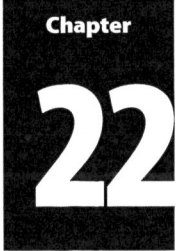

Part B Cardiac

Chapter 22 Heart failure

Stephen Robert Hays

1. Presentation
   Presentation may be nonspecific.
   a) Respiratory: tachypnea, dyspnea, grunting, retractions, crackles, wheezing, and respiratory failure
   b) Cardiac: tachycardia, dysrhythmias, new murmur, gallop, poor pulses/perfusion/hypotension, diaphoresis, exercise intolerance, fatigue
   c) Gastrointestinal: hepatosplenomegaly, poor feeding, failure to thrive
   d) Peripheral: jugular venous distension, edema.

2. Risk factors
   a) Asphyxia
   b) Sepsis
   c) Cardiomyopathy/myocardial ischemia
   d) Congenital heart disease (e.g., ventricular outflow obstruction)
   e) Valvular heart disease (e.g., severe aortic stenosis)
   f) Volume overload
   g) Severe shunting (e.g., arteriovenous shunt from vein of Galen or large patent ductus arteriosus)
   h) Severe anemia.

3. Differential diagnosis
   a) Systemic infection
   b) Pulmonary process
   c) Renal dysfunction
   d) Excessive or severe deficiency of intravascular volume.

4. Pathophysiology
   Pathophysiology is greatly dependent on the underlying mechanism.
   a) Inadequate or excessive systemic vascular resistance
   b) Inadequate or excessive pulmonary vascular resistance
   c) Misdirected blood flow, including valvar dysfunction
   d) Dysrhythmia
   e) Systolic dysfunction

Handbook of Critical Incidents and Essential Topics in Pediatric Anesthesiology, ed. David A. Young and Olutoyin A. Olutoye. Published by Cambridge University Press. © Cambridge University Press 2015.

f) Diastolic dysfunction
   g) Coronary artery compromise
      i) Congenital: anomalous coronary artery
      ii) Acquired: surgical compromise, Kawasaki disease, dissection, atherosclerosis.
5. Management
   Management is directed at the underlying etiology.
   a) Inadequate or excessive systemic vascular resistance
      i) Supplemental intravascular volume or diuresis as indicated
      ii) Systemic vasodilator or vasoconstrictor as indicated.
   b) Inadequate or excessive pulmonary vascular resistance
      i) Pulmonary vasodilator or vasoconstrictor as indicated, including nitric oxide
      ii) Manipulation of oxygenation, ventilation; may require mechanical ventilation.
   c) Misdirected blood flow
      i) Ductus-dependent lesion: prostaglandin infusion
      ii) Valvular dysfunction: manipulation of heart rate, vascular resistance, intravascular volume
      iii) Structural heart disease: percutaneous or surgical intervention.
   d) Dysrhythmia
      i) Bradycardia: vagolytic, adrenergic agent, pacing
      ii) Tachycardia: β-blocker, calcium channel blocker, anti-dysrhythmic
      iii) Abnormal conduction: anti-dysrhythmic, electrical cardioversion.
   e) Systolic dysfunction
      i) Supplemental intravascular volume or diuresis as indicated
      ii) Afterload reduction: β-blocker, calcium channel blocker, angiotensin converting enzyme inhibitor
      iii) Inotrope: adrenergic agent, phosphodiesterase inhibitor
      iv) Extracorporeal support: balloon pump, assist device, extracorporeal membrane oxygenation, cardiopulmonary bypass.
   f) Diastolic dysfunction
      i) Supplemental intravascular volume or diuresis as indicated
      ii) Management of comorbidities
      iii) Specific therapy lacking.
   g) Coronary artery compromise
      i) Pharmacologic: anti-dysrhythmic, nitrate, anticoagulant, thrombolytic agents
      ii) Percutaneous: angioplasty, stenting
      iii) Surgical: coronary reimplantation, coronary artery bypass.
6. Prevention
   a) Recognition of risk factors
   b) Continuation of preoperative therapies for patients at risk
   c) Avoidance of extremes in heart rate, blood pressure, vascular resistance, intravascular volume.

Further reading

Coté CJ, Lerman J, Anderson BJ. *Coté and Lerman's A Practice of Anesthesia for Infants and Children*, 5th edition. Philadelphia, PA: Elsevier, 2013; 300–1.

Gregory GA, Andropoulos DB ed. *Gregory's Pediatric Anesthesia*, 5th edition. Chichester, UK: Wiley-Blackwell, 2012; 601–2.

Mossad EB, Motta P, Rossano J, et al. Perioperative management of pediatric patients on mechanical cardiac support. *Paediatr Anaesth.* 2011;21(5):585–93.

Rosenthal DN, Hammer GB. Cardiomyopathy and heart failure in children: anesthetic implications. *Paediatr Anaesth.* 2011;21(5):577–84.

White MC. Approach to managing children with heart disease for noncardiac surgery. *Paediatr Anaesth.* 2011;21(5):522–9.

Part B Cardiac

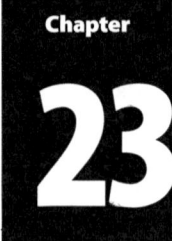

Hypertension

Catherine P. Seipel

1. Presentation
   a) Systolic or diastolic blood pressure (BP) > 99th %ile (based on height, age, and gender) + 5 mmHg (Table 23.1)
   b) Headache.
2. Risk factors
   Risk factors can be divided into four categories.
   a) Pharmacologic
      i) Medications (vasoactive, anticholinergic)
      ii) Light anesthesia or inadequate analgesia (i.e., pain)
      iii) Agitation or emergence delirium
      iv) Hypervolemia
      v) Medication administration error.
   b) Metabolic
      i) Hypoxemia
      ii) Hypercarbia
      iii) Hypermetabolic states (e.g., thyroid storm, pheochromocytoma).
   c) Anatomic
      i) Preexisting hypertension (i.e., renal disease)
      ii) Increased intracranial pressure (ICP)
      iii) Distended bladder
      iv) Coarctation of the aorta.
   d) Equipment related
      i) Incorrect BP cuff size (too small) or position (placed in dependent location).
3. Differential diagnosis
   See Risk factors.
4. Pathophysiology
   The pathophysiology of hypertension depends on the underlying etiology.
5. Management
   a) Ensure adequate oxygenation and ventilation

Handbook of Critical Incidents and Essential Topics in Pediatric Anesthesiology, ed. David A. Young and Olutoyin A. Olutoye. Published by Cambridge University Press. © Cambridge University Press 2015.

b) Review perioperative medications and fluid administration (ensure adequate anesthetic depth, administer medications if inadequate analgesia is suspected)
c) Confirm correct BP cuff size and position
d) Review preexisting conditions
e) Consider measures to lower ICP if increased ICP is suspected (raise head of bed, judicious increase in ventilation, and diuretics)
f) Encourage patient to void or place urine catheter
g) Compare upper and lower extremity blood pressures if previously undiagnosed coarctation of the aorta is suspected
h) If treatment of the underlying cause is ineffective, consider pharmacologic therapy including β-blockers, calcium channel blockers, hydralazine, and nitrates.

6. Prevention
   a) Close monitoring of patient's volume status and replacement of intravenous fluids
   b) Continue preoperative antihypertensive medications
   c) Consider placement of urine catheter for prolonged cases.

Table 23.1 Blood pressure ranges at the 99th %ile for boys aged 1 to 12 years. After age 12, hypertensive values begin to approximate those of adults.

Age (years)	Systolic pressure (mmHg)	Diastolic pressure (mmHg)
1	105–114	61–66
2	109–117	66–71
3	111–120	71–75
4	113–122	74–79
5	115–123	77–82
6	116–125	80–84
7	117–126	82–86
8	119–127	83–88
9	120–129	84–89
10	122–130	85–90
11	124–132	86–90
12	126–135	86–90

Further reading

The Fourth Report on the Diagnosis, Evaluation, and Treatment of High Blood Pressure in Children and Adolescents (online). Available at www.nhlbi.nih.gov/health/prof/heart/hbp/hbp_ped.htm (accessed September 21, 2013). Bethesda: NIH Publication No. 05-5267; 2005.

Coté CJ, Lerman J, Anderson BJ. *Coté and Lerman's A Practice of Anesthesia for Infants and Children*, 5th edition. Philadelphia, PA: Elsevier, 2013; 987.

Society for Pediatric Anesthesia Quality and Safety Committee. (2013). Hypertension – Pediatric Critical Events Checklists (online). Available at www.pedsanesthesia.org/newnews/Critical_Event_Checklists.pdf (accessed September 18, 2013).

Part B **Cardiac**

Chapter 24

Hypotension

Catherine P. Seipel

1. Presentation
   Systolic blood pressure < 5th %ile for age. For patients > 1 year, 5th %ile systolic blood pressure = 70 mmHg + (2 × age in years).
2. Risk factors
   a) Trauma
   b) Critical illness
   c) Preexisting cardiac disease
   d) Prolonged fasting
   e) Inadequate fluid replacement
   f) Ongoing blood loss.
3. Differential diagnosis
   a) Decreased preload
      i) Hypovolemia (most common cause)
      ii) Impaired venous return (e.g., tension pneumothorax)
      iii) Cardiac tamponade
      iv) Pulmonary embolism
      v) Positive pressure ventilation.
   b) Decreased afterload
      i) Sepsis
      ii) Adrenal insufficiency
      iii) Drug-induced vasodilation (i.e., inhaled anesthetic agents)
      iv) Anaphylaxis.
   c) Decreased contractility
      i) Negative inotropic drugs
      ii) Myocardial ischemia
      iii) Heart failure.
   d) Heart rate
      i) Severe bradycardia
      ii) Severe tachycardia.
   e) Equipment malfunction
      Improper size or placement of blood pressure cuff.

Handbook of Critical Incidents and Essential Topics in Pediatric Anesthesiology, ed. David A. Young and Olutoyin A. Olutoye. Published by Cambridge University Press. © Cambridge University Press 2015.

4. Pathophysiology
   Pathophysiology depends on underlying etiology.
5. Management
   a) Decreased preload
      i) Secure adequate intravenous access
      ii) Volume resuscitation with isotonic crystalloids (initial bolus 10–20 mL/kg) or consider packed red blood cells if patient has low hematocrit
      iii) Place patient in level or Trendelenberg position
      iv) Pericardiocentesis if tamponade is suspected
      v) Needle decompression if tension pneumothorax is suspected
      vi) Consider administration of vasopressor medications (e.g., phenylephrine, norepinephrine, epinephrine).
   b) Decreased afterload
      i) Volume resuscitation
      ii) Initiate vasopressor therapy as indicated
      iii) Antibiotic therapy if sepsis is suspected
      iv) Administer steroids (hydrocortisone 1–2 mg/kg IV) if adrenal insufficiency is suspected
      v) Remove or discontinue suspected antigens (latex, medication)
      vi) Administer antihistamines for allergic reactions.
   c) Decreased contractility
      i) Discontinue negative inotropic drugs
      ii) Initiate inotropic support (epinephrine, dopamine, milrinone)
      iii) Increase oxygenation (relieve airway obstruction, place endotracheal tube, increase inspired concentration of oxygen).
   d) Heart rate
      i) Treat arrhythmias (check electrolytes, send arterial blood gas and correct abnormalities)
      ii) Consider pharmacologic (atropine, adenosine) and/or electrical therapy (pacing, synchronized cardioversion).
   e) Equipment
      Replace blood pressure cuff with appropriate size (width of the blood pressure cuff should be 40% of the circumference of the upper arm).
6. Prevention
   a) Assess volume status often; in trauma, maintain high index of suspicion for other undiagnosed injuries
   b) Review known allergies and preexisting illnesses
   c) Review patient's preexisting medications
   d) Review cardiac anatomy and function in patients with known congenital heart disease.

Further reading

Coté CJ, Lerman J, Anderson BJ. *Coté and Lerman's A Practice of Anesthesia for Infants and Children*, 5th edition. Philadelphia, PA: Elsevier, 2013; 987.

Society for Pediatric Anesthesia Quality and Safety Committee. (2013).

Hypotension – Pediatric Critical Events Checklists (online). Available at www.pedsanesthesia.org/newnews/Critical_Event_Checklists.pdf (accessed 18 September 2013).

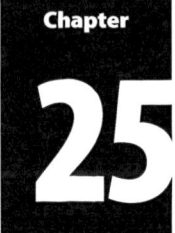

Part B Cardiac

Chapter 25

Inability to obtain vascular access

Graciela Argote-Romero and Jacquelyn Morillo-Delerme

1. Presentation
   Multiple failed attempts to secure vascular access.
2. Risk factors
   a) History of difficult vascular access
   b) Moderate to severe dehydration
   c) Prolonged fasting period prior to surgery
   d) Infants with moderate amount of fat pads on extremities
   e) Obesity
   f) Cardiovascular collapse.
3. Management
   a) Use of techniques to facilitate visibility of veins
      i) Transillumination techniques
      ii) Application of heat to extremities to vasodilate veins
      iii) Ultrasound guidance aids visibility of veins and prevents blind attempts.
   b) If unsuccessful with peripheral venous access, consider central venous access or for emergency situations: intraosseous route or medication administration via endotracheal tube (ETT)
   c) Central venous access: internal jugular, subclavian and femoral veins
      i) Ultrasound guidance facilitates success with first attempt and avoids multiple punctures and complications.
   d) Intraosseous (IO) route
      i) Rapid, reliable and safe approach to obtain vascular access via the bone marrow
      ii) Success rate of 80% on the first attempt
      iii) Sites: anterior tibia 1–3 cm below the tibial tuberosity (most common), distal radius, distal ulna, proximal humerus and the sternum (risk of cardiac laceration)
      iv) All medications, fluids and blood can be administered via the IO route at the same doses
      v) Preferred over the endotracheal route due to variable blood concentrations when compared to the endotracheal route
      vi) Common complications: subperiosteal infiltration and extravasation

Handbook of Critical Incidents and Essential Topics in Pediatric Anesthesiology, ed. David A. Young and Olutoyin A. Olutoye. Published by Cambridge University Press. © Cambridge University Press 2015.

vii) Rare complications: Bone fracture, compartment syndrome, osteomyelitis, and fat embolism.
 e) Intratracheal route via an endotracheal tube (ETT)
    i) Medications amenable to administration via the ETT: naloxone, atropine, vasopressin, epinephrine and lidocaine (NAVEL)
    ii) Doses: epinephrine dose is 10 times the intravascular dose.
 f) Expect lower concentrations and variable effects from doses via the ETT
 g) Following administration via the ETT, flush medication with 2–5 mL of normal saline and give five manual breaths to increase drug delivery to the alveoli.
4. Prevention
 a) Identify at-risk patients during the preoperative evaluation
 b) Consider awake, ultrasound-guided vascular access placement in at-risk patients.

Further reading

Coté CJ, Lerman J, Anderson BJ. *Coté and Lerman's A Practice of Anesthesia for Infants and Children*, 5th edition. Philadelphia, PA: Elsevier, 2013; 167.

Smith's Anesthesia for Infants and Children, 8th edition. Philadelphia: Elsevier, 2011; 320.

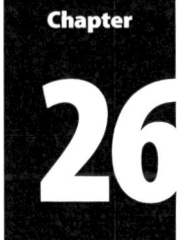

Part B Cardiac

Chapter 26

Local anesthetic toxicity

Smokey Clay and Senthilkumar Sadhasivam

1. Presentation
   a) The awake patient may report dizziness, tinnitus, drowsiness, or metallic taste momentarily after administration of local anesthetics
   b) Sedated or anesthetized patients may present with shivering, muscular twitching or tremors
   c) Toxicity may progress to arrhythmias, seizures, and cardiac arrest
   d) Neurologic symptoms typically precede cardiac symptoms.
2. Risk factors
   a) Anemia which reduces the buffering capacity of red blood cells for local anesthetics
   b) Malnutrition or low protein state
   c) Neonates and infants less than 6 months of age
      i) Reduced carrier proteins alpha-1-acid glycoprotein (AAG) and human serum albumin (HSA) allowing for an increased free fraction of local anesthetics
      ii) Immature cytochrome P450 (CYP450) system results in reduced local anesthetic metabolism.
   d) Low cardiac output states causing decreased liver blood flow and decreased drug metabolism
   e) Hepatocelluar disease causing reduced metabolism
   f) Acidosis allowing for high free fractions
   g) Abnormal anatomy or previous injury to neurons
   h) Choice of local anesthetic (e.g., lidocaine < bupivacaine in potential to cause toxicity)
   i) Total dose of local anesthetic exceeds recommendations (e.g., bupivacaine, ropivacaine, levobupivacaine: 3 mg/kg maximum dose, lidocaine with epinephrine: 7 mg/kg, lidocaine without epinephrine: 5 mg/kg)
   j) Site of local anesthetic administration (e.g., caudal > brachial plexus)
   k) Controversial if administration of a test dose or use of ultrasound reduces risk of toxicity.
3. Differential diagnosis
   a) Seizure disorder
   b) Primary cardiac arrhythmia
   c) Cerebrovascular accident

Handbook of Critical Incidents and Essential Topics in Pediatric Anesthesiology, ed. David A. Young and Olutoyin A. Olutoye. Published by Cambridge University Press. © Cambridge University Press 2015.

d) Organophosphate poisoning
  e) Hearing loss resulting in associated tinnitus
  f) Prior neuronal injury
  g) Vasovagal reaction
  h) Allergic reaction
  i) High spinal or epidural anesthesia.
4. Pathophysiology
  a) Central nervous system manifestations are due to the blockade of inhibitory pathways in the cerebral cortex
  b) Convulsions occur when facilitatory neurons are unopposed
  c) Arrhythmias occur when there is depression of the rapid phase of depolarization of cardiac action potential and a longer recovery phase
  d) Myotoxicity occurs due to disruption of calcium homeostasis at the mitochondrial level.
5. Management
  a) Be immediately prepared to institute resuscitation including tracheal intubation, epinephrine, defibrillation, and chest compressions
  b) Consider administration of benzodiazepine or propofol to manage seizures
  c) Consider hyperventilation to decrease acidosis and free fraction of local anesthetic
  d) Intralipid 20%
     i) 1.5 mL/kg over 1 minute
     ii) Follow immediately with an infusion at a rate of 0.25 mL/kg/min
     iii) Repeat boluses every 3–5 minutes up to 3 mL/kg total dose or until circulation is restored
     iv) Continue infusion until hemodynamic stability is restored
     v) Increase infusion rate to 0.5 mL/kg/min if blood pressure deteriorates
     vi) A maximum total dose of 8 mL/kg is recommended.
6. Prevention
  a) Aspiration prior to local anesthetic injection
  b) Utilization of a test dose and ultrasound is controversial
  c) Incremental fractionated dosing
  d) Dose reductions by 50% in infants < 6 months of age
  e) Administration of a total dose which is under the maximal allowable dose.

Further reading

Davis PJ, Cladis FP, Motoyama EK. *Smith's Anesthesia for Infants and Children*, 8th edition. Philadelphia: Elsevier Mosby, 2011; 457–8.

Guantenbein M, Attolini L, Bruguerolle B, et al. Oxidative metabolism of bupivacaine into pipecolylxylidine in humans is mainly catalyzed by CYP3A. *Drug Metab Dispos.* 2000;28:383–5.

Nouette-Gaulain K, Sirvent P, Canal-Raffin M, et al. Effects of intermittent femoral nerve injections of bupivacaine, levobupivacaine, and ropivacaine on mitochondrial energy metabolism and intracellular calcium homeostasis in rat psoas muscle. *Anesthesiology.* 2007; 106:1026–34.

Smith HS. ed. *Current Therapy in Pain.* Philadelphia: Saunders Elsevier, 2009.

Tucker GT, Boyes RN, Bridenbaugh PO, et al. Binding of anilide-type local anesthetics in human plasma: I. Relationships between binding, physiochemical properties, and anesthetic activity. *Anesthesiology*. 1970; 33:287–303.

Ved SA, Pinosky M, Nicodemus H. Ventricular tachycardia and brief cardiovascular collapse in two infants after caudal anesthesia using a bupivacaine-epinephrine solution. *Anesthesiology*. 1993; 79:1121–3.

Part B Cardiac

Chapter 27 Myocardial ischemia

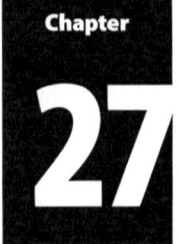

Stephen Robert Hays

1. Presentation
   a) Clinical: presentation may be nonspecific; myocardial ischemia occurs less commonly in children
      i) Cardiac: hypotension, severe bradycardia or tachycardia, arrhythmias, chest pain, diaphoresis
      ii) Respiratory: tachypnea, respiratory distress/failure
      iii) Other: poor feeding/failure to thrive, altered mental status.
   b) Electrocardiogram (EKG)
      i) Preexisting dysrhythmia, infarction, bundle branch block (from previous cardiac surgery), or pacemaker dependency can complicate EKG analysis and diagnosis
      ii) ST segment depression: subendocardial ischemia – coronary insufficiency
      iii) ST segment elevation: transmural ischemia – coronary occlusion
      iv) ST segment changes correlate anatomically with area(s) of ischemia
      v) Isolated T wave changes infrequently indicate ischemia
      vi) Infarction: pathologic Q waves, persistent T wave inversion.
   c) Echocardiogram (transthoracic, transesophageal)
      i) Regional wall motion abnormalities signify areas of focal ischemia
      ii) Global hypokinesis: diffuse ischemia
      iii) Visualizes cardiac filling and pump function
      iv) Interpretation can be challenging in complex congenital heart disease.
   d) Pulmonary artery catheter
      i) Decreased cardiac index, elevated filling pressures may suggest ischemia
      ii) Logistically challenging and rarely utilized in children.
   e) Elevated laboratory values
      i) Creatine kinase membrane band (CK-MB)
      ii) Troponin-I
      iii) B-type natriuretic peptide (BNP)
      iv) Lactate (acidosis).
2. Risk factors
   a) Coronary compromise: atherosclerosis less common in children

Handbook of Critical Incidents and Essential Topics in Pediatric Anesthesiology, ed. David A. Young and Olutoyin A. Olutoye. Published by Cambridge University Press. © Cambridge University Press 2015.

- i) Anomalous coronary artery
- ii) Kawasaki disease: coronary aneurysm, thrombosis
- iii) Immunosuppression after cardiac transplantation
- iv) Silent ischemia from long-standing diabetes mellitus.

b) Cardiomyopathy
- i) Myocarditis: infectious, auto-immune, idiopathic
- ii) Toxicity: chemotherapy, particularly of the anthracycline class (e.g., doxorubicin)
- iii) Neuromuscular: muscular dystrophy
- iv) Idiopathic: dilated, hypertrophic, and obstructive categories.

c) Conditions with impaired systemic perfusion
- i) Congenital heart disease (e.g., prostaglandin-dependent lesions prior to surgical repair)
- ii) Sepsis
- iii) Trauma
- iv) Surgical procedures with large, sudden fluid shifts/blood loss.

3. Differential diagnosis
   a) Primary cardiac disease (e.g., anomalous coronary artery)
   b) Systemic infection
   c) Pulmonary process
   d) Excessive intravascular volume
   e) Improper placement of EKG leads resulting in erroneous ST segment values
   f) Primary muscular or metabolic conditions resulting in falsely elevated nonspecific cardiac enzymes (e.g., total CK).

4. Pathophysiology
   a) Inadequate myocardial oxygen supply to meet overall demand
   - i) Coronary insufficiency: hemodymanic or pharmacologic stress
   - ii) Coronary occlusion: spasm, thrombosis, traumatic compromise.

5 Management
   a) Increase myocardial oxygen delivery
   - i) Optimize oxygenation; increase FiO_2
   - ii) If bradycardia is present: consider administration of vagolytic, adrenergic agent, or pacing
   - iii) If hypotension is present: consider supplemental intravascular volume, systemic vasoconstrictor, inotrope, consider transfusion of packed red blood cells.

   b) Decrease myocardial oxygen demand
   - i) If tachycardia is present: consider administration of β-blocker, anti-dysrhythmic, opioids, electrical cardioversion
   - ii) If hypertension is present consider afterload reduction: calcium channel blocker, angiotensin converting enzyme inhibitor.

   c) Consider obtaining diagnostic studies such as 12-lead EKG, echocardiogram, CK-MB, troponin, BNP

d) Prevent or treat coronary thrombosis: consider anticoagulant, thrombolytic
e) Consider extracorporeal support: balloon pump, assist device, extracorporeal membrane oxygenation (ECMO), cardiopulmonary bypass
f) Consult cardiology to determine if percutaneous intervention is indicated (e.g., angioplasty, stenting)
g) Consult cardiovascular surgery to determine if surgical intervention is indicated (e.g., coronary reimplantation, coronary artery bypass).

6. Prevention
   a) Recognition of risk factors
   b) Continuation of preoperative therapies (e.g., aspirin) for patients at risk
   c) Avoidance of extremes in heart rate, blood pressure, intravascular volume, oxygen carrying capacity.

Further reading

Coté CJ, Lerman J, Anderson BJ. *Coté and Lerman's A Practice of Anesthesia for Infants and Children*, 5th edition. Philadelphia, PA: Elsevier, 2013; 459.

Gregory GA, Andropoulos DB. *Gregory's Pediatric Anesthesia*, 5th edition. Chichester, UK: Wiley-Blackwell, 2012; 641–2.

Gui P, Wu Q, Wu J, et al. Protective effect of esmolol on myocardial ischemic injury during open heart surgery in children. *Paediatr Anaesth.* 2013; 23(3):217–21.

Miller RD. *Miller's Anesthesia*, 7th edition. Philadelphia: Churchill Livingstone-Elsevier, 2010; 1357–86; 1985–2044.

Rouine-Rapp K, Rouillard KP, Miller-Hance W, et al. Segmental wall-motion abnormalities after an arterial switch operation indicate ischemia. *Anesth Analg.* 2006; 103(5):1139–46.

Part B Cardiac

Chapter 28: Pericardial tamponade
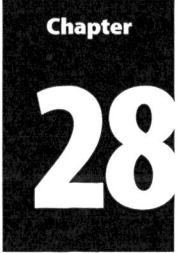
Lisa D. Heyden

1. Presentation
   a) Patients with tamponade physiology may present with dyspnea, tachycardia, distended neck veins, narrow pulse pressure, and pulsus paradoxus
   b) Characteristic findings include Beck's triad: hypotension, elevated systemic venous pressure, and muffled heart sounds on auscultation.

2. Risk factors
   There are numerous possible causes but they can be grouped into two main categories.
   a) Post-surgical/trauma
      i) Trauma
      ii) Post-surgical bleeding
      iii) Cardiac perforation from cardiac catheterization or central venous catheter placement
      iv) Pericardial effusion
      v) Post-pericardiotomy syndrome.
   b) Medical conditions
      i) Acute viral or bacterial infections
      ii) Malignancy
      iii) Congestive heart failure
      iv) Renal failure
      v) Inflammatory and autoimmune disorders
      vi) Pericardial cysts.

3. Differential diagnosis
   a) Acute myocardial infarction
   b) Tension pneumothorax
   c) Pulmonary embolism
   d) Cardiac arrhythmias.

4. Pathophysiology
   a) Cardiac tamponade occurs when fluid, blood, or blood clots fill the pericardial space and significantly reduce cardiac output

Handbook of Critical Incidents and Essential Topics in Pediatric Anesthesiology, ed. David A. Young and Olutoyin A. Olutoye. Published by Cambridge University Press. © Cambridge University Press 2015.

b) Tamponade physiology develops as the end diastolic pressure in all four chambers equalizes
　　c) Diastolic filling and thus stroke volume becomes restricted; the sympathetic nervous system compensates by increasing the contractile state, ejection fraction, and heart rate.
5. Management
　　a) Following diagnosis, personnel and equipment for immediate drainage and resuscitation must be immediately available
　　b) Drainage of a small amount of pericardial fluid under sedation (e.g., ketamine) and local anesthesia should be strongly considered
　　c) Induction of general anesthesia, tracheal intubation, and instituting positive pressure ventilation may all precipitate cardiovascular collapse
　　d) If general anesthesia must be induced, the patient should be preoxygenated, prepared and draped for possible emergent pericardiocentesis, and an intravascular fluid bolus should be administered, if feasible, to maximize venous return prior to induction
　　e) Etomidate is the preferred agent for rapid induction of anesthesia. Maintaining tachycardia along with normovolemia (to mild hypervolemia) should be the intraoperative goal
　　f) If possible, maintain spontaneous ventilation until some of the fluid is drained.
6. Prevention
Although prevention may not be possible in most cases, surveillance in patients who are at high risk of tamponade, such as post-surgical patients, may decrease morbidity and mortality.

Further reading

Andropoulos DB. *Anesthesia for Congenital Heart Disease*, 2nd edition. Chichester, UK: Wiley-Blackwell, 2010; 488–9.

Barash PG. *Clinical Anesthesia*, 5th edition. Philadephia: Lippincott Williams & Wilkins, 2006; 926.

Marino PL. *The ICU Book*, 2nd edition. Philadelphia: Lippincott Willams & Wilkins, 1998; 255.

Morgan GE, Mikhail MS, Murray MJ. *Clinical Anesthesiology*, 4th edition. New York: Lange Medical Books, 2006; 865, 1000.

Part B Cardiac

Chapter 29 Prolonged QT interval

Catherine P. Seipel

1. Presentation
   a) QTc interval greater than 460–480 milliseconds on EKG
   b) Congenital prolonged QT most often presents as syncope, cardiac arrest, sudden death
   c) Acquired prolonged QT may present as an isolated finding on an EKG
   d) Many patients are clinically asymptomatic and unaware of their diagnosis.
2. Risk factors
   a) Congenital syndromes (e.g., Romano-Ward, Jervell, Lange-Nielsen, Timothy syndromes)
   b) Medications (e.g., antiemetics, antidepressants, antipsychotics, antiarrhythmics, volatile anesthetics, methadone)
   c) Neurologic abnormalities (e.g., subarachnoid hemorrhage)
   d) Electrolyte abnormalities (e.g., hypokalemia, hypomagnesemia, hypocalcemia)
   e) Severe malnutrition
   f) Endocrine abnormalities.
3. Differential diagnosis
   Other abnormal rhythms.
4. Pathophysiology
   a) Congenital syndromes: several genetic defects alter sodium and potassium membrane channels within the myocardium
      i) Prolonged repolarization allows later depolarization to trigger premature ventricular contractions
      ii) Altered homeostasis places patients at risk for unstable arrhythmias including prolonged QT syndrome, torsades de pointes, ventricular tachycardia, ventricular fibrillation and bradyarrhythmias.
   b) In acquired forms of prolonged QT syndrome, metabolic abnormalities or medications affect normal cardiac conduction.
5. Management
   a) Beta-blockers are the mainstay of therapy
   b) Implantable cardioverter defibrillators are indicated in patients with previous symptomatic events (e.g., ventricular tachycardia)

Handbook of Critical Incidents and Essential Topics in Pediatric Anesthesiology, ed. David A. Young and Olutoyin A. Olutoye. Published by Cambridge University Press. © Cambridge University Press 2015.

c) Correct electrolyte abnormalities (potassium, calcium, magnesium)
   d) Minimize sympathetic stimulation. Provide generous anxiolysis and analgesia; consider regional anesthesia and deep extubation techniques
   e) Consider placement of defibrillator pads empirically
   f) Continue beta-blockade therapy
   g) Avoid medications associated with prolongation of the QT interval (e.g., ondansetron, methadone).
6. Prevention
   a) There is no available prevention for congenital forms
   b) Prompt correction of electrolyte abnormalities, optimal beta-blockade, minimal sympathetic stimulation and avoidance of QT prolonging drugs can help decrease the risk of unstable arrhythmias in both congenital and acquired forms.

Further reading

Coté CJ, Lerman J, Anderson BJ. *Coté and Lerman's A Practice of Anesthesia for Infants and Children*, 5th edition. Philadelphia, PA: Elsevier, 2013; 314.

Watson TW. *Stoelting's Anesthesia and Co-existing Disease*, 5th edition. Philadelphia: Churchill Livingstone, 2008; 73.

Part B Cardiac

Chapter 30
Pulmonary hypertensive crisis

Stephen Robert Hays

1. Presentation
   Patients with severe pulmonary hypertension have significantly increased perioperative risk regardless of the surgical procedure. Patients may present suddenly with the following:
   a) Systemic hypotension
   b) Bradycardia
   c) Hypoxemia
   d) Cardiac arrest.

2. Risk factors
   Several factors increase pulmonary vascular resistance and can result in the development of pulmonary hypertensive crisis (Table 30.1).

3. Differential diagnosis
   a) Systemic infection (e.g., sepsis)
   b) Primary pulmonary process (e.g., laryngospasm, bronchospasm)
   c) Cardiac process (e.g., tachycardia, heart failure)
   d) Anaphylactic / anaphylactoid reaction
   e) Hypovolemia.

4. Pathophysiology
   a) Acute increase in pulmonary vascular resistance (Table 30.1) results in decreased oxygenated blood to the systemic circulation, compromised right ventricular function, reduced cardiac output, myocardial ischemia, and ultimately cardiac arrest
   b) Many conditions can result in the development of pulmonary hypertension; these conditions may result in the development of increased pulmonary vascular resistance (Table 30.2).

Handbook of Critical Incidents and Essential Topics in Pediatric Anesthesiology, ed. David A. Young and Olutoyin A. Olutoye. Published by Cambridge University Press. © Cambridge University Press 2015.

Table 30.1 Factors increasing pulmonary vascular resistance.

Acidosis: metabolic, respiratory
Hypercarbia
Hypoxemia
Hypothermia

Mechanical factors
  Intrinsic: atelectasis, pneumonia, pneumothorax, surgical manipulation
  Transmitted: positive airway pressure

Increased sympathetic tone: pain, anxiety, light anesthesia, surgical stress response

Table 30.2 Updated clinical classification of pulmonary hypertension.

Group 1: Pulmonary arterial hypertension
  Idiopathic
  Heritable
  Drug/toxin induced
  Associated with specific diseases
  Persistent pulmonary hypertension of the newborn
  Pulmonary veno-occlusive disease/pulmonary capillary hemangiomatosis

Group 2: Pulmonary hypertension owing to left heart disease
  Systolic dysfunction
  Diastolic dysfunction
  Valvular disease

Group 3: Pulmonary hypertension owing to lung diseases/hypoxia
  Chronic obstructive pulmonary disease
  Interstitial lung disease
  Other pulmonary diseases with mixed restrictive/obstructive pattern
  Sleep-disordered breathing
  Alveolar hypoventilation disorders
  Chronic exposure to high altitude
  Developmental abnormalities

Group 4: Chronic thromboembolic pulmonary hypertension

Group 5: Pulmonary hypertension with unclear/multifactorial mechanisms
  Hematologic disorders
  Systemic disorders
  Metabolic disorders
  Other

Modified from Simonneau G, Robbins IM, Beghetti M, et al. Updated clinical classification of pulmonary hypertension. *J Am Coll Cardiol.* 2009;54(1 Suppl):S43–54 with permission from Elsevier.

5. Management
    a) Notify surgeon and staff of intraoperative emergency
    b) Call for code cart if not already present
    c) Hyperventilate with 100% FiO_2 to goal of $ETCO_2$ of 30 mmHg
    d) Administer nitric oxide starting at 20 ppm
    e) Consider administration of sodium bicarbonate (1–2 mEq/kg) to treat metabolic acidosis
    f) Consider administration of analgesics (e.g., fentanyl) to deepen anesthesia

g) Administer epinephrine 1 µg/kg for severe hemodynamic compromise
h) Consider inotropic infusions, particularly for right ventricular support
i) Reduce peak ventilatory pressures if feasible
j) Request echocardiogram, cardiology consult, and ICU bed
k) Consider extracorporeal support: assist device, extracorporeal membrane oxygenation (ECMO), cardiopulmonary bypass.

6. Prevention
   a) Recognition of preoperative risk factors
   b) Continuation of preoperative therapies for patients at risk (e.g., preoperative pulmonary vasodilator medications such as epoprostenol (Flolan) should not be discontinued due to the risk of rebound pulmonary hypertension)
   c) Avoidance of conditions that produce increased pulmonary vascular tone: acidosis, hypercarbia, hypoxemia, hypothermia, mechanical stress, increased sympathetic tone.

Further reading

Coté CJ, Lerman J, Anderson BJ. *Coté and Lerman's A Practice of Anesthesia for Infants and Children*, 5th edition. Philadelphia, PA: Elsevier, 2013; 459.

Davis PJ, Cladis FP, Motoyama EK. *Smith's Anesthesia for Infants and Children*, 8th edition. Philadelphia: Elsevier Mosby, 2011; 678–9.

Friesen RH, Williams GD. Anesthetic management of children with pulmonary arterial hypertension. *Paediatr Anaesth*. 2008; 18(3):208–16.

Gregory GA, Andropoulos DB. *Gregory's Pediatric Anesthesia*, 5th edition. Chichester, UK: Wiley-Blackwell, 2012; 103, 707–8.

Simonneau G, Robbins IM, Beghetti M, et al. Updated clinical classification of pulmonary hypertension. *J Am Coll Cardiol*. 2009; 54(1 Suppl):S43–54.

van der Griend BF, Lister NA, McKenzie IM, et al. Postoperative mortality in children after 101,885 anesthetics at a tertiary pediatric hospital. *Anesth Analg*. 2011; 112(6):1440–7.

Part B **Cardiac**

Chapter

31 Pulseless electrical activity

Julia Chen

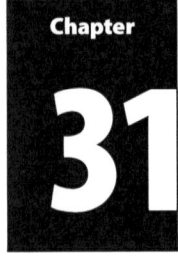

1. Presentation
   Pulseless electrical activity (PEA) is a type of electrocardiographic (EKG) rhythm consisting of an organized rhythm (e.g., sinus rhythm) that is associated with no palpable pulses or cardiac output.

2. Risk factors
   a) Reversible causes of cardiac arrest include (H's and T's)
      i) H's: hypovolemia, hypoxia, hydrogen ion (acidosis), hypo/hyperkalemia, hypoglycemia, hypothermia
      ii) T's: toxins, cardiac tamponade, tension pneumothorax, thrombosis (coronary or pulmonary), and trauma.
   b) Special circumstances increasing the risk for the development of cardiac arrest include: trauma, drowning, anaphylaxis, poisoning, congenital heart disease, and pulmonary hypertension
   c) PEA is most associated with conditions resulting from lack of preload (e.g., tension pneumothorax, severe hypovolemia) which do not involve primary defects of the cardiac electrical framework.

3. Differential diagnosis
   Other rhythms associated with cardiac arrest:
   a) Asystole
   b) Pulseless ventricular tachycardia
   c) Ventricular fibrillation.

4. Pathophysiology
   Absence of cardiac contractions/ineffective cardiac output in the presence of coordinated electrical activity.

5. Management
   The American Academy of Pediatrics and American Heart Association Pediatric Advanced Life Support (PALS) guidelines for pediatric resuscitation includes the management of PEA as outlined in the Pediatric Pulseless Arrest Algorithm.
   a) Declare an intraoperative emergency, notify the operating room surgeon/staff, and call for additional help

---

Handbook of Critical Incidents and Essential Topics in Pediatric Anesthesiology, ed. David A. Young and Olutoyin A. Olutoye. Published by Cambridge University Press. © Cambridge University Press 2015.

b) Immediately start high-quality cardiopulmonary resuscitation (CPR), chest compressions, and attach defibrillator
c) If the rhythm is not shockable (PEA is a non-shockable rhythm), follow the PALS algorithm for asystole/PEA
d) Continue high-quality cardiopulmonary resuscitation (CPR)
e) Verify that vascular access is present: intravenous (IV) and intraosseous (IO) routes are preferable to the endotracheal route for administration of medications
f) Consider placement of tracheal tube if not present
g) Once vascular access is established, administer epinephrine
   i) Epinephrine IO/IV dose: 10 μg/kg
   ii) If IV access is not present, administer epinephrine in endotracheal dose: 100 μg/kg
   iii) Repeat epinephrine administration every 3–5 minutes if arrest persists.
h) Treat potentially reversible causes of cardiac arrest (i.e., perform needle decompression for tension pneumothorax, give volume bolus)
i) Every 2 minutes (after five cycles of chest compressions) recheck the rhythm
   i) If the rhythm check reveals a non-shockable rhythm, resume CPR
   ii) If a shockable rhythm is present at any time, move to management of ventricular tachycardia/ventricular fibrillation as outlined in the PALS algorithm
   iii) If the rhythm is organized, check for a pulse. If a pulse is present, proceed with post-resuscitation care.

6. Prevention
   a) Maintain vigilance for the reversible causes of cardiac arrest (H's and T's) especially during higher risk cases
   b) Verify pulsatile flow (pulse check) is present when pulse oximetry signifies no reading.

Further reading

Barash PG. *Clinical Anesthesia*, 7th edition. Philadelphia: Lippincott Williams & Wilkins, 2013; 1690, 1693.

Chameides L, Samson R, Schexnayder S, et al. *PALS Provider Manual*. Dallas, TX: American Academy of Pediatrics, American Heart Association, 2010; 141–67.

Coté CJ, Lerman J, Anderson BJ. *Coté and Lerman's A Practice of Anesthesia for Infants and Children*, 5th edition. Philadelphia, PA: Elsevier, 2013; 815.

Gregory GA, Andropoulos DB. *Gregory's Pediatric Anesthesia*, 5th edition. Hoboken: Wiley-Blackwell, 2012; 255–69.

Part B Cardiac

Chapter 32 Sinus tachycardia

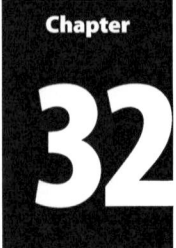

Amanda K. Brown and Rhonda A. Alexis

1. Presentation
   a) Heart rate is greater than expected for the patient's age; infants: heart rate < 220 beat/min; children < 180 BPM
   b) EKG morphology: narrow QRS axis with a P wave which precedes every QRS complex
   c) Presentation is usually benign unless associated with conditions such as hypoxemia, hypovolemia, anemia, shock, myocardial ischemia, or pulmonary edema.
2. Risk factors
   a) Physiologic
      i) Preoperative
         (1) Fever
         (2) Anxiety/stress
         (3) Pain.
      ii) Intraoperative
         (1) Surgical stimulus
         (2) Inadequate anesthesia
         (3) Hyperthermia
         (4) Medications which augment heart rate (e.g., glycopyrrolate)
         (5) Hypovolemia.
   b) Pathologic
      i) Preoperative
         (1) Hyperthyroidism
         (2) Illicit drug use
         (3) Underlying cardiac disease.
      ii) Intraoperative
         (1) Hypovolemia
         (2) Malignant hyperthermia.
3. Differential diagnosis
   a) Hypoxemia

Handbook of Critical Incidents and Essential Topics in Pediatric Anesthesiology, ed. David A. Young and Olutoyin A. Olutoye. Published by Cambridge University Press. © Cambridge University Press 2015.

b) Hypovolemia
   c) Myocardial ischemia
   d) Pulmonary edema
   e) Malignant hyperthermia
   f) Pain
   g) Supraventricular tachycardia
   h) Ventricular tachycardia.
4. Pathophysiology
   a) Most patients are hemodynamically stable with this condition
   b) For every 1° Celsius rise in temperature, there is a corresponding increase in heart rate by an average of 9.6 BPM
   c) Prolonged sinus tachycardia may impair diastolic filling time, limit ventricular preload and diminish cardiac output in susceptible children (e.g., children with ventricular hypertrophy or diastolic dysfunction).
5. Management
   a) Goal is to determine and treat the specific etiology of the tachycardia
   b) Obtain detailed history and evaluate current medications
   c) Once etiology is established, provide supportive care and treat the underlying cause (e.g., acetaminophen for fever, morphine for pain, parental presence for anxiety, clear fluids for hunger, dantrolene for malignant hyperthermia).
6. Prevention
   Maintain increased vigilance for preoperative, intraoperative, and postoperative factors known to precipitate tachycardia and treat expeditiously.

Further reading

Coté CJ, Lerman J, Anderson BJ. *Coté and Lerman's A Practice of Anesthesia for Infants and Children*, 5th edition. Philadelphia, PA: Elsevier, 2013; 311.

Doniger SJ, Sharieff GQ. Pediatric dysrhythmias. *Pediatr Clin North Am.* 2006; 53(1):85–105.

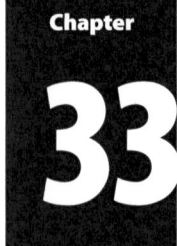

Part B **Cardiac**

Chapter 33

Supraventricular tachycardia

Catherine P. Seipel

1. Presentation
   a) Infants: poor feeding, rapid breathing, irritability, hypotension, and cyanosis
   b) Older children: palpitations, shortness of breath, chest pain, altered mental status and hypotension
   c) EKG:
      i) Heart rate > 220 BPM (infants)
      ii) Heart rate > 180 BPM (children)
      iii) P waves are not detectable
      iv) Regular rhythm with a narrow complex QRS.
   d) Supraventricuar tachycardia (SVT) with aberrant conduction and wide QRS is possible, but less common (< 10%).
2. Risk factors
   a) Congenital heart disease
   b) Fever
   c) Inotropic medications or medications with vagolytic properties
   d) Electrolyte disturbances.
3. Differential diagnosis
   a) Normal sinus rhythm
   b) Sinus tachycardia
   c) Ventricular arrhythmia.
4. Pathophysiology
   a) Cardiac conduction through a reentry circuit involving the atrioventricular node
   b) Cardiac conduction through a reentry circuit involving an accessory pathway (e.g., Wolff–Parkinson–White syndrome)
   c) Cardiac conduction originates from an ectopic focus in the atria that depolarizes faster than the sino-atrial node
      i) Can occur following cardiac surgical repair due to cardiac irritability.
5. Management
   a) Check for pulse; if no pulse is present, proceed with the Pediatric Advanced Life Support (PALS) Pulseless Arrest algorithm

---

Handbook of Critical Incidents and Essential Topics in Pediatric Anesthesiology, ed. David A. Young and Olutoyin A. Olutoye. Published by Cambridge University Press. © Cambridge University Press 2015.

b) Assess perfusion (blood pressure, mental status)
   c) If pulse is present, use the PALS Tachycardia algorithm
   d) Stable patient:
      i) Attempt vagal maneuvers (ice to forehead, blow through obstructed straw, Valsalva maneuver)
      ii) Adenosine is the pharmacologic treatment of choice:
         (1) Initial dose is 0.1 mg/kg rapid IV bolus (maximum dose is 6 mg)
         (2) If SVT persists, administer second dose 0.2 mg/kg (max dose 12 mg) within 1–2 minutes
         (3) Rapid flush of medication after administration is strongly recommended.
   e) Unstable patient: use synchronized cardioversion; do not delay for vagal maneuvers or peripheral intravenous catheter placement
      i) 1st attempt: 0.5–1 J/kg
      ii) 2nd attempt: 2 J/kg
      iii) Treat or discontinue other contributing factors: fever, electrolyte abnormalities, and inotropic medications
      iv) Consider administration of procainamide (15 mg/kg IV over 30–60 minutes) *or* amiodarone (5 mg/kg IV over 20–60 minutes).

6. Prevention
   a) Correct underlying electrolyte abnormalities
   b) Review indications and need for inotropic medications
   c) Review preoperative status of patients with congenital heart disease.

Further reading

Coté CJ, Lerman J, Anderson BJ. *Coté and Lerman's A Practice of Anesthesia for Infants and Children*, 5th edition. Philadelphia, PA: Elsevier, 2013; 316, 14–815.

Recognition and Management of Bradyarrhythmias and Tachyarrhythmias. *Pediatric Advanced Life Support Provider Manual*. Dallas, TX: American Heart Association, 2006; 128–132.

Part B Cardiac

Chapter 34

Tetralogy of Fallot spell

Lisa D. Heyden

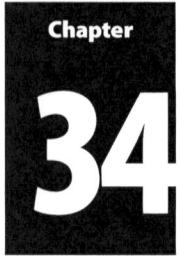

1. Presentation
   a) Echocardiogram findings of: ventricular septal defect (VSD), right ventricular outflow tract obstruction (RVOTO), overriding aorta, and right ventricular hypertrophy
   b) Cyanosis (occurs in 20–70% of affected patients) may be observed during crying, feeding
   c) Desaturation during anesthesia following noxious stimuli or inadequate anesthesia.
2. Risk factors
   a) Increased right ventricular outflow tract obstruction due to pain, inadequate anesthesia, and anatomic defect
   b) Decreased systemic vascular resistance.
3. Differential diagnosis
   There are a variety of causes for cyanosis in children.
   a) Life-threatening causes
      i) Respiratory – upper airway obstruction, impairment of chest wall or lung expansion, intrinsic lung disease
      ii) Circulatory – congenital heart disease, pulmonary edema, pulmonary hypertension, pulmonary embolism, pulmonary hemorrhage, shock
      iii) Severe methemoglobinemia
      iv) Neurologic conditions resulting in disordered breathing – major head trauma, poisoning, seizures.
   b) Other causes
      i) Cyanotic breath-holding spells
      ii) Cold exposure
      iii) Acrocyanosis.
4. Pathophysiology
   a) The ventricular septal defect and RVOTO results in a right-to-left shunt
   b) Dynamic narrowing of the subpulmonary infundibulum (right ventricular outflow tract obstruction) results in increased right-to-left shunting and the development of hypercyanotic "tet spells"

Handbook of Critical Incidents and Essential Topics in Pediatric Anesthesiology, ed. David A. Young and Olutoyin A. Olutoye. Published by Cambridge University Press. © Cambridge University Press 2015.

c) Metabolic acidosis, increased $PaCO_2$, circulating catecholamines, and surgical stimulation result in pulmonary vasoconstriction, right ventricular outflow tract obstruction and increased right-to-left shunting of blood
  d) The degree of hypoxemia depends on the relationship between the RVOTO and systemic vascular resistance.
5. Management
   a) 100% oxygen
   b) Hyperventilation
   c) Intravenous fluid administration to increase cardiac preload
   d) Sedation with benzodiazepines (e.g., midazolam) or analgesia with opioids (e.g., fentanyl)
   e) Consider sodium bicarbonate to treat acidosis
   f) Vasoconstriction
      i) Phenylephrine, 0.5 µg/kg bolus then 1–5 µg/kg/min
      ii) Norepinephrine, 0.5 µg/kg bolus then 0.1–0.5 µg/kg/min.
   g) Beta-blockers to relax infundibular spasm and reduce heart rate: propranolol 0.1–0.3 mg/kg.
6. Prevention
   a) Avoid conditions that will exacerbate infindibular spasm (increased sympathetic stimulation)
   b) Palliation surgery followed by surgical repair of cardiac defects.

Further reading

Andropoulos DB. *Anesthesia for Congenital Heart Disease*, 2nd edition. Chichester, UK: Wiley-Blackwell, 2010; 427–32.

Coté CJ, Lerman J, Anderson BJ. *Coté and Lerman's A Practice of Anesthesia for Infants and Children*, 5th edition. Philadelphia, PA: Elsevier, 2013; 342–3.

Gregory GA, Andropoulos DB. *Gregory's Pediatric Anesthesia*, 5th edition. Chichester, UK: Wiley-Blackwell, 2012; 633–7.

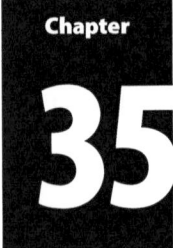

Part B **Cardiac**

Chapter 35

Thrombotic pulmonary embolism

Lisa D. Heyden

1. Presentation
   a) Mild cases of pulmonary embolism (PE) are frequently asymptomatic
   b) Presentation may be acute or chronic
      i) Acute PE
         (1) Symptoms include dyspnea, pleuritic pain, cough, orthopnea, calf or thigh pain or swelling, and wheezing
         (2) Signs include hypotension, tachypnea, tachycardia, rales, decreased breath sounds, jugular venous distension, hemoptysis, hypoxemia, elevated central venous pressure (or neck vein distension), acute right ventricular failure and/or cardiac arrest.
      ii) Chronic PE: progressive dyspnea over an extended time period due to pulmonary hypertension.
2. Risk factors
   a) Prolonged immobility or bed rest
   b) Prior history of thromboembolism
   c) Cancer and nephrotic syndrome
   d) Preexisting hypercoagulable state
   e) Major surgery
   f) Central venous instrumentation
   g) Venous stasis or vascular injury
   h) Generalized hypercoagulable state (caused by thromboplastin release and depressed levels of antithrombin III).
   i) Oral contraceptive use.
3. Differential diagnosis
   a) Acute myocardial infarction
   b) Tension pneumothorax
   c) Pericardial tamponade
   d) New onset arrhythmia.

Handbook of Critical Incidents and Essential Topics in Pediatric Anesthesiology, ed. David A. Young and Olutoyin A. Olutoye. Published by Cambridge University Press. © Cambridge University Press 2015.

4. Pathophysiology
   a) Most pulmonary emboli arise from thrombi in the deep venous system of the lower extremities. However, they may also originate in the right heart, pelvic, or upper extremities
   b) Emboli lodge in pulmonary artery causing severe pulmonary hypertension, right heart failure, and cardiovascular collapse.
5. Management
   a) Stabilize the patient with respiratory and hemodynamic support as needed
   b) Anticoagulation is the primary treatment
   c) Low molecular weight heparin is the treatment of choice in children
   d) Thrombolysis
   e) Surgical intervention: embolectomy and consideration for placement of inferior vena cava filters to prevent further PE.
6. Prevention
   a) Graded compression stockings to promote venous flow in the legs
   b) Intermittent pneumatic compression boots are more effective than compression stockings
   c) Routine thromboprophylaxis is recommended for all moderate to high-risk patients
   d) Low-dose heparin can inhibit thrombus formation without risk of hemorrhage
      i) Heparin activates antithrombin III
      ii) Antithrombin III inhibits the conversion of prothrombin to thrombin
      iii) Low-dose heparin does not provide optimal prophylaxis in high-risk patients.
   e) Low molecular weight heparin (enoxaparin)
   f) Low-dose warfarin – requires dose titration and monitoring
   g) Placement of vena cava filter, this is indicated in the following scenarios
      i) Presence of thrombus
         (1) Documented iliofemoral vein thrombosis
         (2) Contraindication to anticoagulation
         (3) Occurrence of pulmonary embolism during anticoagulation
         (4) Free-floating thrombus.
      ii) Absence of thrombus
         (1) Long-term prophylaxis is necessary
         (2) High risk for both thromboembolism and hemorrhage
         (3) High-risk condition for fatal PE.

Further reading

Barash PG. *Clinical Anesthesia*, 5th edition. Philadephia: Lippincott Williams & Wilkins, 2006; 1125.

Marino PL. *The ICU Book*, 2nd edition. Philadelphia: Lippincott Willams & Wilkins, 1998; 106–19.

Sharma M, Carpenter SL. Thromboprophylaxis in a pediatric hospital. *Curr Probl Pediatr Adolesc Health Care*. 2013; 43(7):178–83.

Part B Cardiac

Chapter 36

Venous air embolism

Amanda K. Brown and Rhonda A. Alexis

1. Presentation
   a) Many cases are subclinical; most cases are during general anesthesia
   b) Decreased end-tidal carbon dioxide (EtCO$_2$)
   c) More severe cases are characterized by cardiovascular collapse (e.g., hypotension, cardiac arrest)
   d) Presentation varies with the rate and volume of air entrained.
2. Risk factors
   a) Any condition where a pressure gradient exits between the operative site and the heart (increasing risk of entrainment of air into the central circulation)
      i) Intracranial procedures where air entry occurs via venous sinuses, bone, or bridging veins
      ii) Craniofacial procedures
      iii) Patients with intracardiac shunts
      iv) Surgical procedures performed in the sitting position
      v) Inadvertent delivery of air from mechanical intravenous pumps or fluid infusers.
3. Differential diagnosis
   a) Acute coronary syndrome
   b) Severe bronchospasm
   c) Cerebral hypoperfusion
   d) Intracranial hemorrhage
   e) Pulmonary thromboembolism
   f) Hypovolemia
   g) Cardiac arrest from other causes.
4. Pathophysiology
   a) Rapid entry of air into the systemic circulation causes right heart strain and subsequent increase in pulmonary artery pressure
   b) Right ventricular outflow obstruction and decreased pulmonary venous return results in decreased left ventricular preload and decreased cardiac output.

Handbook of Critical Incidents and Essential Topics in Pediatric Anesthesiology, ed. David A. Young and Olutoyin A. Olutoye. Published by Cambridge University Press. © Cambridge University Press 2015.

5. Management
   a) Urgent notification of the surgical team
   b) Immediate flooding of operative field with saline and application of bone wax to exposed bone edges
   c) Discontinue nitrous oxide and reduce other anesthetic agents based on hemodynamic status
   d) Strongly consider placing patient in the Trendelenburg position (increases cerebral venous pressure, stops air entrainment and increases systemic blood pressure)
   e) Consider aspiration of air through multi-orifice catheter if present
   f) Resuscitation
      i) Perform chest compressions if cardiac arrest occurs
      ii) Consider administration of vasopressors to maintain cardiac output.
6. Prevention
   a) Identify patients who are at increased risk before surgery
   b) Increased vigilance may allow for early detection and effective management
   c) Monitoring for signs of venous air embolism: precordial Doppler (mill-wheel murmur), capnograph (abrupt decrease in end-tidal carbon dioxide), most sensitive is transthoracic echocardiography.

Further reading

Butterworth JF. *Morgan and Mikhail's Clinical Anesthesiology*, 5th edition. New York: McGraw-Hill Company, Inc,, 2013; 333.

Coté CJ, Lerman J, Anderson BJ. *Coté and Lerman's A Practice of Anesthesia for Infants and Children*, 5th edition. Philadelphia, PA: Elsevier, 2013; 519–20.

Part B Cardiac

Chapter 37
Ventricular fibrillation

Kha M. Tran

1. Presentation
   a) Pulseless cardiac arrest
   b) Loss of end-tidal carbon dioxide ($EtCO_2$)
   c) Loss of pulse oximeter wave form
   d) Classic appearance on EKG: chaotic, asynchronous ventricular activity that does not generate cardiac output
   e) Apnea.
2. Risk factors
   a) Preexisting cardiac disease, structural or conduction problems
   b) Previous history of ventricular fibrillation
   c) Cocaine or methamphetamine use
   d) Long QT syndrome
   e) Conditions which lower cardiac threshold for fibrillation
      i) Electrolyte abnormalities (high or low levels) affecting potassium, calcium, sodium, and magnesium)
      ii) Hydrogen ions (respiratory or metabolic acidosis)
      iii) Hypovolemia
      iv) Hypoxia
      v) Hypothermia.
   f) Toxins (digoxin, beta blockers, etc.)
   g) Tamponade
   h) Tension pneumothorax
   i) Thrombosis (pulmonary or cardiac)
   j) Trauma.
3. Differential diagnosis
   a) EKG lead malfunction
   b) Artifact from the electrosurgical unit
   c) In magnetic resonance imaging scanner, some scanning sequences will cause dramatic artifact to both the EKG and pulse oximeter.

Handbook of Critical Incidents and Essential Topics in Pediatric Anesthesiology, ed. David A. Young and Olutoyin A. Olutoye. Published by Cambridge University Press. © Cambridge University Press 2015.

4. Pathophysiology
   Uncoordinated depolarization and ineffective contraction of regions of the myocardium results in a lack of forward flow of blood and decreased or no cardiac output.
5. Management
   a) Call for help and initiate cardiopulmonary resuscitation (CPR)
   b) Discontinue anesthetic agents, open IV fluids, and administer 100% oxygen
   c) Prompt defibrillation is the priority
   d) Initial defibrillation of 2 J/kg, followed by chest compressions for 2 minutes
   e) Increase energy to 4 J/kg for persistent ventricular fibrillation (VF):
      i) Gel pads are more commonly utilized than paddles
      ii) Gel should not be continuous between paddles
      iii) Paddle size: infant paddles for patients < 10 kg; adult paddles > 10 kg
      iv) Ensure firm placement of pads and paddles on chest wall.
   f) Continue CPR
   g) Intravenous medications to consider while continuing CPR and defibrillation:
      i) Epinephrine 10 μg/kg (should be administered every 3 minutes)
      ii) Amiodarone 5 mg/kg (one-time bolus).
   h) Search for etiology, obtain laboratory values and blood gas analysis: treat abnormal labs values during resuscitation
   i) Place definitive airway if not present
   j) Consider placement of invasive monitors
   k) Arrange for intensive care unit disposition.
6. Prevention
   a) Avoid conditions that may lower cardiac threshold for fibrillation
   b) Maintain increased vigilance in children with previous history of cardiac arrhythmias or previous cardiac surgery
   c) If previous history of fibrillation exists, ensure recent consultation with cardiologist to ensure patient is medically optimized
   d) Prophylactic placement of defibrillation pads should be considered in high-risk patients prior to surgery.

Further reading

Coté CJ, Lerman J, Anderson BJ. *Coté and Lerman's A Practice of Anesthesia for Infants and Children*, 5th edition. Philadelphia, PA: Elsevier, 2013; 316.

Davis PJ. *Smith's Anesthesia for Infants and Children*, 8th edition. Philadelphia: Elsevier, 2011; 1240–2.

Part B **Cardiac**

Chapter
Ventricular tachycardia

Matthew Mitchell and Jacquelyn Morillo-Delerme

1. Presentation
   a) Uncommon phenomenon in children with structurally normal hearts
   b) Three or more consecutive ventricular beats occurring at a heart rate greater than 120 BPM
   c) Non-sustained ventricular tachycardia (VT): lasts > 30 seconds and terminates spontaneously without therapeutic intervention
   d) Sustained rhythm: VT lasting > 30 seconds and requires intervention
   e) Prolonged and wide QRS complex. P waves may or may not be recognizable, depending on the ventricular rate, and T waves are opposite in polarization to the QRS
   f) Most VT is monomorphic; however, polymorphic VT can occur when the QRS complexes vary in their appearance (e.g., torsade de pointes)
   g) Torsades de pointes: a subtype of VT in which the QRS complexes increase and decrease in amplitude, undulating around the EKG isoelectric line
      i) Associated with congenital long QT syndrome, hypomagnesemia, and drug toxicities.
   h) Majority of children are asymptomatic but symptoms such as pallor, fatigue, and chest palpitations may be present
   i) Patients may initially present with sudden death/cardiac arrest.
2. Risk factors
   a) Cardiac conditions: underlying cardiac disease, depressed myocardial function, poor hemodynamics, prior surgical interventions, cardiomyopathies, myocardial tumors, acute injury, history of cardiac dysrhythmias (prolonged QT syndromes)
   b) Electrolyte or metabolic abnormalities
   c) Hypoxemia, acidosis
   d) Electrolyte abnormalities: hypo- or hyperkalemia, hypomagnesemia (predisposes to torsades de pointes), hypocalcemia
   e) Drug toxicity.
3. Differential diagnosis
   a) Other wide complex tachyarrhythmias
   b) Supraventricular tachycardia with aberrant conduction of the QRS complex

Handbook of Critical Incidents and Essential Topics in Pediatric Anesthesiology, ed. David A. Young and Olutoyin A. Olutoye. Published by Cambridge University Press. © Cambridge University Press 2015.

c) Torsades de pointes.
4. Pathophysiology
   a) Origin of the tachycardia is below the bifurcation of the bundle of His
   b) VT is characterized by reentrant phenomenon or increased automaticity.
5. Management
   a) Detect etiology and optimize by:
      i) Providing adequate oxygenation/ventilation
      ii) Correcting existing electrolyte or metabolic abnormalities
      iii) Treating drug intoxication if present.
   b) Specific treatment should be instituted in parallel with the American Heart Association, Pediatric Advanced Life Support (PALS) algorithms
   c) First check for a pulse: If pulse is present use PALS Tachycardia algorithm; if no pulse, use PALS Pulseless Arrest algorithm
   d) VT with palpable pulse: use synchronized cardioversion: 0.5–1 J/kg, increase to 2 J/kg for further attempts if initially ineffective
   e) Pulseless VT: immediate defibrillation: 2 J/kg, repeat at 4 J/kg after 2 minutes of chest compressions if first dose ineffective
   f) Initiation of chest compressions and initiation of medical treatment for persistent pulseless VT
   g) Chest compressions followed by
      i) IV epinephrine 10 μg/kg given every 3 minutes
      ii) IV amiodarone 5 mg/kg (maximum dose of 300 mg); given as bolus if pulseless or over 20–60 minutes if pulse is present
      iii) IV procainamide 15 mg/kg over 30–60 minutes.
   h) IV magnesium therapy (25–50 mg/kg) for torsade de pointes.
6. Prevention
   a) Maintain increased vigilance of cardiac rhythm disorders, especially for at-risk patients
   b) Maintain high suspicion for close monitoring of electrolyte levels to avoid severe derangements and promote early detection
   c) Regular cardiology follow-up visits for children with structurally abnormal hearts.

Further reading

Biondi EA. Focus on diagnosis: cardiac arrhythmias in children. *Pediatr Rev.* 2010; 31(9):375–9.

Coté CJ, Lerman J, Anderson BJ. *Coté and Lerman's A Practice of Anesthesia for Infants and Children*, 5th edition. Philadelphia, PA: Elsevier, 2013; 314–16.

Davis PJ, Cladis FP, Motoyama EK. *Smith's Anesthesia for Infants and Children*, 8th edition. Philadelphia: Mosby, Inc., 2011; 1128.

Gregory GA, Andropoulos DB. *Gregory's Pediatric Anesthesia*, 5th edition. Hoboken: Wiley-Blackwell, 2012; 954.

Part C Metabolic

Chapter 39

Acute adrenal insufficiency

Julia Chen

1. Presentation
    a) Primary manifestation is refractory hypotension
    b) Other manifestations include abdominal pain, severe vomiting, diarrhea, weakness, confusion, lethargy, and electrolyte abnormalities (hyponatremia, hyperkalemia, hypoglycemia)
    c) Classical symptoms of adrenal insufficiency may not be present in critically ill patients.
2. Risk factors
    a) Acute adrenal insufficiency may occur in the following:
        i) Undiagnosed adrenal insufficiency during severe physiologic stress
        ii) Diagnosed adrenal insufficiency without adequate steroid replacement therapy or during additional physiologic stress
        iii) Patients receiving high-dose steroid therapy during additional physiologic stress
        iv) Patients abruptly withdrawn from chronic steroid therapy
        v) Adrenal, pituitary, or hypothalamic injury
        vi) Congenital disorders: congenital adrenal hyperplasia, adrenoleukodystrophy, X-linked adrenal hypoplasia congenita, and ACTH receptor defects.
3. Differential diagnosis
    See Risk factors.
4. Pathophysiology
    a) In the hypothalamic–pituitary–adrenal (HPA) axis, hypothalamic corticotropin-releasing hormone (CRH) regulates secretion of pituitary adrenocorticotropic hormone (ACTH) and subsequently the downstream production of the adrenocortical steroids (mineralocorticoids, glucocorticoids, and androgens)
    b) The end-product of the glucocorticoid pathway is cortisol, the primary regulator of the HPA axis
    c) Primary adrenal insufficiency is related to disease intrinsic to the adrenal cortex and is associated with glucocorticoid and mineralocorticoid deficiency
    d) Secondary and tertiary adrenal insufficiency is related to the impaired release of ACTH and CRH, respectively, and is associated with glucocorticoid deficiency.

Handbook of Critical Incidents and Essential Topics in Pediatric Anesthesiology, ed. David A. Young and Olutoyin A. Olutoye. Published by Cambridge University Press. © Cambridge University Press 2015.

5. Management
   a) Patients presumed to have acute adrenal insufficiency should receive immediate therapy prior to diagnostic testing
      i) Fluid resuscitation as guided by vital signs, assessment of volume status and urine output
      ii) Glucocorticoid replacement with hydrocortisone (2 mg/kg); alternative glucocorticoid preparations (prednisolone, prednisone, and dexamethasone) have minimal or no mineralocorticoid activity
      iii) Correct electrolyte abnormalities
      iv) Precipitating causes should be sought and treated.
   b) Future diagnostic testing may include determination of the patient's pituitary-adrenal responsiveness (measurement of serum ACTH or by stimulating the adrenal gland with exogenous ACTH)
   c) Consultation with an endocrinologist may be helpful to coordinate long-term management.
6. Prevention
   a) Patients with known adrenal insufficiency require additional doses of glucocorticoids when subjected to physiologic stress
      i) Additional steroid dosing should originate in the preoperative phase and continue as needed throughout the perioperative period.
   b) Patients receiving high-dose steroid therapy are at risk for iatrogenic HPA axis suppression and may require additional doses of glucocorticoids when subjected to physiologic stress
      i) Recovery of full HPA function may take 6–9 months following discontinuation of long-term high-dose steroid therapy.

Further reading

Barash PG. *Clinical Anesthesia*, 7th edition. Philadelphia: Lippincott Williams & Wilkins, 2013; 597–8, 1597.

Coté CJ, Lerman J, Anderson BJ. *Coté and Lerman's A Practice of Anesthesia for Infants and Children*, 5th edition. Philadelphia, PA: Elsevier, 2013; 551–3.

Davis PJ, Cladis FP, Motoyama EK. *Smith's Anesthesia for Infants and Children*, 8th edition. Philadelphia: Elsevier Mosby, 2011; 1104–5.

Gregory GA, Andropoulos. *Gregory's Pediatric Anesthesia*, 5th edition. Hoboken: Wiley-Blackwell, 2012; 957, 986.

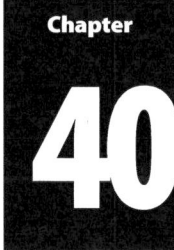

Part C Metabolic

Chapter 40: Hypercalcemia

Julia Chen

1. Presentation
   a) Commonly defined as serum ionized calcium level > 1.35 mmol/L or total calcium > 10.5 mg/dL
   b) Symptoms related to degree of hypercalcemia and rate of rise of serum calcium
   c) A total serum calcium level above 15 mg/dL is considered a medical emergency
   d) Nonspecific signs and symptoms: nausea, vomiting, anorexia, polyuria, pain due to nephrolithiasis
   e) Severe hypercalcemia
      i) Neuromyopathic symptoms: muscle weakness, lethargy, stupor, seizures, and coma
      ii) Cardiac
         (1) Bradycardia
         (2) Shortened QT interval
         (3) Hypertension.
2. Risk factors
   a) Primary hyperparathyroidism
      i) Adenoma
      ii) Parathyroid hyperplasia (multiple endocrine neoplasia, MEN1 and less commonly MEN 2A)
      iii) Parathyroid carcinoma.
   b) Malignancy
      i) Direct bone resorption
      ii) Ectopic production of parathyroid hormone-related protein (PTHrP)
      iii) Osteoclast-activating factors (leukemia, lymphoma).
   c) Vitamin D related
      i) Increased conversion of calcidiol to calcitriol in granulomatous disorders
      ii) Vitamin D intoxication.

Handbook of Critical Incidents and Essential Topics in Pediatric Anesthesiology, ed. David A. Young and Olutoyin A. Olutoye. Published by Cambridge University Press. © Cambridge University Press 2015.

d) Medications
     i) Vitamin A intoxication
     ii) Thiazide diuretics
     iii) Lithium.
  e) Genetic disorders
     i) Williams syndrome.
3. Differential diagnosis
   See Risk factors.
4. Pathophysiology
   a) Calcium homeostasis
      i) Parathyroid hormone (PTH) is released from parathyroid glands in response to a decrease in serum ionized calcium concentration
      ii) PTH increases serum calcium by:
          (1) Calcium reabsorption in the distal tubule
          (2) Upregulation of osteoclast mediated calcium and phosphate release from bone
          (3) Renal synthesis of calcitriol
          (4) Intestinal absorption of calcium.
5. Management
   a) Initial laboratory evaluation
      i) Total serum calcium (corrected for albumin), ionized calcium, PTH
      ii) Additional laboratory data may guide diagnosis: phosphate, magnesium, alkaline phosphatase, calcidiol, calcitriol, urine calcium.
   b) Treatment for acute hypercalcemia – urgency of therapy determined by degree of hypercalcemia and rate of rise of serum calcium
   c) Serum calcium concentration greater than 13–15 mg/dL typically requires treatment regardless of symptoms. Strategies effective in lowering the serum calcium level include:
      i) Isotonic rehydration
      ii) Furosemide to enhance calcium excretion by kidney
      iii) Osteoclast-inhibiting agents
           (1) Calcitonin (efficacy limited to first 24 hours due to tachyphylaxis)
           (2) Bisphosphonates (maximum effect 2–4 days, usually used in conjunction with other agents).
      iv) Glucocorticoids – minimally effective in improving hypercalcemia related to malignancy or hyperparathyroidism.
   d) Dialysis for resistant, life-threatening hypercalcemia
   e) Correction of underlying causes (e.g., parathyroid carcinoma resection).
6. Prevention
   a) Identification and treatment of risk factors
   b) Treatment for chronic hypercalcemia

i) Bisphosphonates
ii) Surgical excision of pathologic sources of excessive PTH in cases of primary hyperparathyroidism.

Further reading

Barash PG. *Clinical Anesthesia*, 7th edition. Philadelphia: Lippincott Williams & Wilkins, 2013; 354–355, 1332–4.

Coté CJ, Lerman J, Anderson BJ. *Coté and Lerman's A Practice of Anesthesia for Infants and Children*, 5th edition. Philadelphia, PA: Elsevier, 2013; 551.

Davis PJ, Cladis FP, Motoyama EK. *Smith's Anesthesia for Infants and Children*, 8th edition. Philadelphia: Elsevier Mosby, 2011; 149–51.

Gregory GA, Andropoulous DB. *Gregory's Pediatric Anesthesia*, 5th edition. Hoboken: Wiley-Blackwell, 2012; 1304.

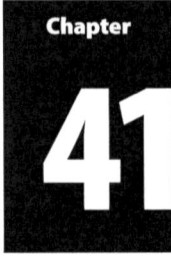

Part C Metabolic

Chapter 41 Hyperglycemia

Mary A. Felberg

1. Presentation
   a) Definition: serum glucose > 150 mg/dL
   b) Temporary and mildly elevated values are typically asymptomatic and inconsequential
   c) Signs and symptoms:
      i) General: polyuria, polydipsia, nausea, vomiting, fruity breath
      ii) Central nervous system: altered mental status, lethargy, coma, or seizures
      iii) Cardiopulmonary: tachypnea, tachycardia.
   d) Associated laboratory findings: hypokalemia, hyponatremia, lactic acidosis, ketouria
   e) Signs and symptoms may be nonspecific and undetectable during general anesthesia.

2. Risk factors
   a) Increased serum glucose
      i) Stress response to trauma, surgery, or inadequate level of anesthesia
      ii) Infection
      iii) Glucose infusions or medications (e.g., total parenteral nutrition, steroids).
   b) Insulin deficiency
      i) Lack of insulin production (e.g., diabetes mellitus, cystic fibrosis)
      ii) Epinephrine inhibition of insulin release
      iii) Hypothermia-induced decreased insulin response (e.g., cardiac surgery).
   c) Insulin resistance – type II diabetes mellitus.

3. Differential diagnosis
   a) Diabetic ketoacidosis
   b) Hyperglycemic, hyperosmotic, nonketotic syndrome
   c) Excessive exogenous glucose
   d) Increased sympathetic response from a variety of causes
   e) Laboratory error.

Handbook of Critical Incidents and Essential Topics in Pediatric Anesthesiology, ed. David A. Young and Olutoyin A. Olutoye. Published by Cambridge University Press. © Cambridge University Press 2015.

4. Pathophysiology
   a) Increased serum glucose with deficiency of intracellular glucose for energy (ATP) production
   b) Decrease in ATP production leads to central nervous system disorders
   c) Alternate mechanisms of energy substrate production are initiated: glycogenolysis, gluconeogenesis, lipolysis and ketogenesis. Byproducts of the latter two processes are organic acids. Respiratory patterns are compensatory responses to metabolic acidosis
   d) Increased serum glucose leads to osmotic diuresis, increased urine output, electrolyte abnormalities and intravascular volume depletion.
5. Management
   a) Consider ordering arterial blood gas, electrolytes, ketones
   b) Check for adequate level of anesthesia
   c) Verify lack of glucose containing intraoperative fluids
   d) Isotonic crystalloid 10–20 mL/kg to restore intravascular volume; may repeat as indicated
   e) Treat glucose > 250 mg/dL with regular insulin
      i) Avoid rapid overcorrection (risk for development of hypoglycemia)
      ii) Intraoperative glucose goal of 100–200 mg/dL (excluding neonates)
      iii) Administer regular insulin 0.1 unit/kg
      iv) Consider insulin infusion 0.1 unit/kg/hr, titrate hourly according to glucose response
      v) Co-administer maintenance fluids that contain glucose (e.g., D5LR, D10)
      vi) Consider adding KCl to maintenance fluids based on serum K^+ and established urine output.
   f) Monitor serum glucose levels every hour until stabilized.
6. Prevention
   a) Identification of patients at risk for hyperglycemia
   b) Perioperative glucose monitoring for at-risk patients
   c) Diabetics: preoperative consultation, develop management plan prior to surgery
   d) Emergency cases may preclude optimization of glucose control
   e) Consider volume replacement prior to induction with 10–20 mL/kg crystalloid
   f) Ensure adequate level of anesthesia
   g) Avoid dextrose-containing fluids for replacing intraoperative losses.

Further reading

Coté CJ, Lerman J, Anderson BJ. *Coté and Lerman's A Practice of Anesthesia for Infants and Children*, 5th edition. Philadelphia, PA: Elsevier, 2013; 18.

Gregory GA, Andropoulos DB. *Gregory's Pediatric Anesthesia*, 5th edition. Hoboken: Wiley-Blackwell, 2012; 220–221, 984–6.

Kliegman RM. *Nelson Textbook of Pediatrics*, 19th edition. Philadelphia: Elsevier, Saunders, 2011; 1979–80.

Part C Metabolic

Chapter 42 Hyperkalemia

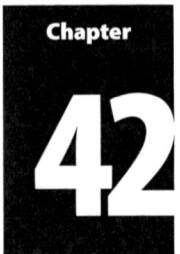

Luigi Viola and Senthilkumar Sadhasivam

1. Presentation
   a) Plasma potassium concentration (K$^+$) above 5.5 mmol/L; many patients are clinically asymptomatic but may display overall weakness
   b) EKG changes are typically the first signs and are progressive:
      i) K$^+$ at approximately 7 mmol/L: PR prolongation, tent-shaped (peaked) T waves
      ii) K$^+$ at approximately 9 mmol/L: Short QT, QRS widening, ST depression
      iii) K$^+$ at approximately 11 mmol/L: Loss of P wave and progressive QRS widening progressing to ventricular fibrillation.

2. Risk factors
   a) Decreased excretion: impaired renal function can be associated with hyperkalemia
   b) Transcellular shift: acidosis from many causes exacerbates the shift of potassium from intracellular space to extracellular space
   c) Increased administration: massive transfusion, especially with old and irradiated packed red cells, can cause severe hyperkalemia.

3. Differential diagnosis
   a) Redistribution (elevation of plasma K$^+$ without increase in total body content):
      i) Acidosis (metabolic more than respiratory); K$^+$ is exchanged with H$^+$
      ii) Diabetic ketoacidosis
      iii) Tissue damage (trauma, burns, hemolysis, rhabdomyolysis, tumor lysis, acute graft rejection)
      iv) Succinylcholine: acute/transient rise of K$^+$ secondary to increased K$^+$ permeability (exacerbated in patients with upregulated extrajunctional acetylcholine receptors (e.g., burns, spinal cord injuries).
   b) Increased intake
      i) Intravenous fluid administration
      ii) Total parenteral nutrition
      iii) Rapid transfusion of large volumes of old or irradiated blood.
   c) Decreased renal excretion
      i) Acute renal failure
      ii) Aldosterone deficiency

Handbook of Critical Incidents and Essential Topics in Pediatric Anesthesiology, ed. David A. Young and Olutoyin A. Olutoye. Published by Cambridge University Press. © Cambridge University Press 2015.

iii) Adrenal insufficiency
iv) Drugs (that interfere with renin–angiotensin–aldosterone system): non steroidal anti-inflammatory drugs, angiotensin converting enzyme inhibitors, heparin, spironolactone
v) Obstructive uropathy.

d) Pseudohyperkalemia: artifactual elevation in the measured plasma potassium
   i) Thrombocytosis
   ii) Leukocytosis
   iii) Prolonged tourniquet application
   iv) Hemolysis.

4. Pathophysiology
   a) Muscle weakness occurs due to sustained depolarization and inactivation of muscle membrane sodium channels
   b) EKG changes are secondary to delayed depolarization.

5. Management
   a) Emergency treatment required for hyperkalemia > 7 mmol/L; be prepared to perform cardiopulmonary resuscitation
   b) Discontinue all potassium-containing fluids
   c) Administer intravenous calcium gluconate (100 mg/kg) to stabilize myocardial cell membrane
   d) Increase minute ventilation to induce alkalosis (intracellular K^+ shift)
   e) Administer sodium bicarbonate (1–2 mEq/kg)
   f) Consider administration of regular insulin (0.1 units/kg) with 2–5 mL/kg dextrose 10.
   g) Consider administration of albuterol or low-dose epinephrine infusion (0.02 µg/kg/min) to promote intracellular shifting of potassium
   h) Consider administration of polystyrene sulfonate either orally or via enema; this method removes K^+ over many hours and may result in hyperosmolality
   i) Consider administration of furosemide IV (1 mg/kg)
   j) Consider dialysis for refractory and severe hyperkalemia.

6. Prevention
   a) Avoid succinylcholine in patients with renal failure, trauma, burns, muscle or spinal cord lesions
   b) Avoid potassium-containing solutions in patients with hyperkalemia and renal dysfunction
   c) Use fresh or washed packed red cells in high-risk patients requiring massive transfusion
   d) Screen for acidosis and hyperkalemia in high-risk patients.

Further reading

Bissonnette B. *Pediatric Anesthesia*. Shelton, CT: People's Medical Publishing House, 2011; 10: 163–4.

Davis PJ, Cladis FP, Motoyama EK. *Smith's Anesthesia for Infants and Children*, 8th edition. Philadelphia: Mosby, 2011; 140–4.

Part C Metabolic

Chapter 43 Hypernatremia

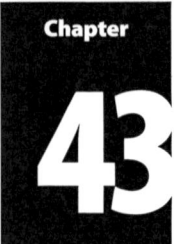

Andrew J. Costandi and Senthilkumar Sadhasivam

1. Definition
   a) Normal plasma sodium: 135–145 mEq/L
   b) Mild hypernatremia: 145–150 mEq/L
   c) Moderate hypernatremia: 150–160 mEq/L
   d) Severe hypernatremia: > 160 mEq/L.

2. Presentation

   Acute hypernatremia is more common in children than in adults, with mortality rates for severe hypernatremia > 40% if acute and 10% if a chronic presentation.

   a) Clinically asymptomatic, particularly in less severe forms
   b) Dehydration and thirst
   c) CNS symptoms: irritability, restlessness, hyperpnea, apnea, lethargy, confusion, seizures, and coma.

3. Risk factors
   a) Hypernatremia caused by free water loss
      i) Renal losses
         (1) Central diabetes insipidus – deficiency of antidiuretic hormone (ADH): divided into (a) congenital: thalamic and pituitary disorders; (b) acquired: trauma or tumor to the thalamic or pituitary axis
         (2) Nephrogenic diabetes insipidus (high ADH): renal unresponsiveness to ADH
         (3) Drug-induced: (e.g., mannitol, furosemide).
      ii) Extrarenal losses
         (1) Diarrhea and vomiting
         (2) Neonates receiving phototherapy
         (3) High protein intake
         (4) Hyperosmolar nonketotic coma (HONK)
         (5) Diabetic ketoacidosis
         (6) Sepsis
         (7) Heat stroke
         (8) Massive hemorrhage
         (9) Lactic acidosis.

Handbook of Critical Incidents and Essential Topics in Pediatric Anesthesiology, ed. David A. Young and Olutoyin A. Olutoye. Published by Cambridge University Press. © Cambridge University Press 2015.

iii) Inadequate water replacement
- (1) No access to water
- (2) Iatrogenic.

b) Hypernatremia caused by excess sodium
  i) Excessive administration of saline (NaCl), hypertonic saline, or $NaHCO_3$
  ii) Endocrine causes: Cushing syndrome
  iii) Neonates due to immature renal function.

4. Differential diagnosis
   a) Laboratory error
   b) See Risk factors.

5. Pathophysiology
   Relative sodium excess to water leads to cell dehydration due to a shift of the intracellular fluid into the extracellular compartment. Severe sodium excess (from dehydration or hydration with hypotonic fluids) may result in brain shrinkage, subarachnoid hemorrhage, and permanent brain injury.

6. Management
   a) Assess vitals and fluid status to manage accordingly
   b) Prepare for possible resuscitation including tracheal intubation in severe cases
   c) Check serum glucose: hyperglycemia occurs in 25% of patients
   d) Check serum calcium: hypocalcemia occurs in 10–20% of patients
      i) Hypovolemic hypernatremia
         (1) Fluid resuscitation with isotonic fluids to restore vitals and correct sodium over 24–48 hours.
      ii) Normovolemic hypernatremia
         (1) Hypotonic fluid as free water or D5W to correct sodium: administer at a rate that decreases plasma osmolality by no more than 2 mOsmol/kg/hr
         (2) Correct underlying cause (e.g., administer DDAVP for diabetes insipidus).
      iii) Hypervolemic hypernatremia
         (1) Discontinue sodium containing solutions
         (2) Consider furosemide (1 mg/kg) with adequate replacement of urine with 5% dextrose in water (D5W).

7. Prevention
   a) Follow plasma sodium levels when administering large quantities of fluids
   b) Consider hypernatremia as a cause of altered mental status
   c) Evaluate for hypernatremia when significant hypovolemia is present.

Further reading

Coté CJ, Lerman J, Anderson BJ. *Coté and Lerman's A Practice of Anesthesia for Infants and Children*, 5th edition. Philadelphia, PA: Elsevier, 2013; 173.

Davis PJ, Cladis FP, Motoyama EK. *Smith's Anesthesia for Infants and Children*, 8th edition. Philadelphia: Elsevier Mosby, 2011; 134–6.

Ruskin KJ, Rosenbaum SH. *Anesthesia Emergencies*. Oxford: Oxford University Press, 2011.

Part C **Metabolic**

Chapter

44 Hyperthermia

Lisa D. Heyden

1. Presentation
    a) Temperature above 38°C (100.4°F)
    b) Vasodilation – skin flushing, sweating, tachycardia.
2. Risk factors
    a) Iatrogenic
        i) Aggressive warming
        ii) Transfusion reaction
        iii) Medication-associated fever.
    b) Disease based
        i) Underlying viral or bacterial infection
        ii) Arthrogryposis multiplex
        iii) Osteogenesis imperfecta
        iv) Central nervous system abnormalities (Riley-Day syndrome)
        v) Thyroid storm
        vi) Pheochromocytoma
        vii) Neuroleptic malignant syndrome
        viii) Monoamine oxidase inhibitors and meperidine
        ix) Cocaine toxicity
        x) Malignant hyperthermia (see section on malignant hyperthermia).
3. Differential diagnosis
    See Risk factors.
4. Pathophysiology
    a) Hyperthermia is a manifestation of cytokine release in response to a variety of stimuli. Fever-associated cytokines are released by tissue trauma and do not necessarily signal infection
    b) Children with genetic disorders, such as osteogenesis imperfecta, may have greater cytokine release and a more sustained febrile response
    c) Hyperthermia may also develop as a result of hypermetabolism such as in malignant hyperthermia or thyroid storm.

5. Management
   a) Management depends on the cause of the hyperthermia (e.g., dantrolene for malignant hyperthermia, beta antagonists for thyroid storm, removal of blankets for iatrogenic causes)
   b) Nonsteroidal anti-inflammatory agents such as ibuprofen or ketorolac (NSAIDs) as well as glucocorticoids suppress cytokine release, thus reducing the magnitude of the febrile response
   c) Acetaminophen (10–15 mg/kg IV or PO) is a very effective antipyretic agent
   d) Aspirin should not be used to treat hyperthermia as it interferes with platelet function and is associated with Reye syndrome
   e) Consider removal of unnecessary linens and blankets along with cooling measures (ambient forced air, placement of damp towels)
   f) Consider ingestion of cool, clear liquids.
6. Prevention
   a) Continuous temperature monitoring intraoperatively
   b) Prevention depends on individual patient history and etiology.

Further reading

Coté CJ, Lerman J, Anderson BJ. *Coté and Lerman's A Practice of Anesthesia for Infants and Children*, 5th edition. Philadelphia, PA: Elsevier, 2013; 59.

Morgan GE, Mikhail MS, Murray MJ. *Clinical Anesthesiology*, 4th edition. New York: Lange Medical Books, 2006; 949.

Part C Metabolic

Chapter 45

Hypocalcemia

Kha M. Tran

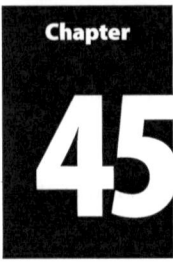

1. Presentation
   a) Serum calcium levels < 8.5 mg/dL or ionized calcium levels < 4.5 mg/dL (or < 1–1.3 mmol/L)
   b) Presentation may vary widely from clinically asymptomatic (common) to hemodynamically unstable
   c) Presentation varies with age:
      i) Neonates: jitteriness, twitching, apnea, and seizures
      ii) Infants: may be very nonspecific – lethargy, poor feeding, vomiting
      iii) Older children: above symptoms in addition to cramping, numbness and tingling of the hands, toes, and lips; irritability, anxiety, and depression.

2. General findings
   a) EKG findings: prolonged QT interval, cardiac arrhythmias
   b) Congestive heart failure
   c) Chvostek sign – ipsilateral twitching of face after tapping facial nerve
   d) Trousseau sign – spasm of muscle and hand after a blood pressure cuff is inflated on the arm and remains inflated for several minutes
   e) Laryngospasm
   f) Hypotension and cardiovascular collapse.

3. Risk factors
   a) Preoperative
      i) Prematurity
      ii) DiGeorge syndrome
      iii) Renal failure
      iv) Low levels of vitamin D
      v) High levels of phosphate
      vi) Hypomagnesemia
      vii) Drugs: calcitonin, phosphate, and bisphosphonates.
   b) Intraoperative
      i) Transfusion of blood products
      ii) Parathyroidectomy.

Handbook of Critical Incidents and Essential Topics in Pediatric Anesthesiology, ed. David A. Young and Olutoyin A. Olutoye. Published by Cambridge University Press. © Cambridge University Press 2015.

4. Pathophysiology
   a) Low calcium levels increases central nervous system irritability by decreasing excitation threshold for neurons; this may result in seizures
   b) Calcium is required for muscular contractions and low levels will cause weakness and possibly decreased myocardial contractility resulting in hypotension
   c) Citrate present in packed blood components binds calcium and lowers serum calcium levels.
5. Management
   a) Diagnose and treat primary cause of the hypocalcemia
      i) Repletion of calcium levels with either intravenous (IV) calcium chloride 10 mg/kg or IV calcium gluconate 30 mg/kg
      ii) Calcium chloride can irritate veins and is best administered via a central line.
   b) Recheck calcium levels to assess adequacy of therapy
   c) Repeat therapy as needed depending on the severity.
6. Prevention
   a) Increased vigilance for clinical symptoms for at-risk patients
   b) Low threshold to check calcium levels for at-risk patients.

Further reading

Cote CJ. *A Practice of Anesthesia for Infants and Children*, 4th edition. Philadelphia: Saunders, 2009; 550–1.

Davis PJ. *Smith's Anesthesia for Infants and Children*, 8th edition. Philadelphia: Elsevier, 2011; 148–9.

Umpaichitra V, Bastian W, Castells S. Hypocalcemia in children: pathogenesis and management, *Clin Pediatr.* 2001; 40(6):305–12.

Part C Metabolic

Chapter 46 Hypoglycemia

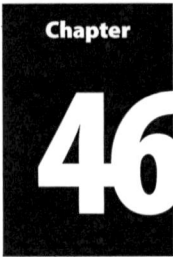

Mary A. Felberg

1. Presentation
   a) Decreased serum glucose level is age dependent:
      i) Full-term neonate during first day of life: < 30–40 mg/dL
      ii) All other patients: < 50 mg/dL.
   b) Nonspecific signs and symptoms are divided into two categories:
      i) Neurologic:
         (1) Reflects decreased cerebral energy substrates
         (2) Progressive from altered mental status, anxiety, seizures, to coma.
      ii) Sympathomimetic:
         (1) Reflects activation of mechanisms to maintain glucose homeostasis
         (2) Tachycardia, pallor, palpitations, diaphoresis.
   c) Patients on β-blockers may be asymptomatic despite significant hypoglycemia
   d) Signs and symptoms may be nonspecific and undetectable during general anesthesia.
2. Risk factors
   a) Age: Small for gestational age, prematurity, neonates < 24 hours old
   b) Decreased substrate availability
      i) Prematurity
      ii) Inborn errors of metabolism
      iii) Glycogen storage diseases
      iv) Acquired liver disease
      v) Prolonged fasting.
   c) Hyperinsulinemia
      i) Neonates especially during first day of life
      ii) Infant of a diabetic mother
      iii) Beckwith–Weidemann syndrome
      iv) Insulinoma
      v) Diabetic patient receiving insulin or oral sulfonamides preoperatively without glucose-containing intravenous solutions
      vi) Abrupt discontinuation of glucose-containing solutions (e.g total parenteral nutrition).

Handbook of Critical Incidents and Essential Topics in Pediatric Anesthesiology, ed. David A. Young and Olutoyin A. Olutoye. Published by Cambridge University Press. © Cambridge University Press 2015.

d) Increased glucose utilization
   i) Sepsis
   ii) Stress: surgical or hypothermia-induced.
3. Differential diagnosis
   a) Delayed emergence
   b) Hypopituitarism or insulinoma
   c) Severe hepatic disease
   d) Neurologic and cardiac disorders (e.g., altered mental status from intracranial pressure, tachycardia from pain)
   e) Pseudohypoglycemia (e.g., leukemia, polycythemia vera).
4. Pathophysiology
   a) Glucose is the preferred substrate for cerebral energy metabolism
   b) Inadequate glucose levels trigger the release of epinephrine and other hormones in attempt to restore glucose homeostasis
   c) Long-term consequences of untreated hypoglycemia are severe and include developmental delay.
5. Management
   a) Severe hypoglycemia is considered a medical emergency
   b) Infants and children require glucose 3–8 mg/kg/min to maintain cerebral metabolism and growth
   c) Initial treatment: administer 2.5 mL/kg bolus of dextrose 10%
   d) Recheck glucose level after interventions and at regular intervals
   e) Consider addition of glucose-containing solutions to perioperative fluid plan.
6. Prevention
   a) Preoperative identification of at-risk patients
   b) Consider perioperative glucose monitoring
   c) Minimize fasting times and provide exogenous glucose to at-risk patients
   d) Consider glucose-containing intravenous fluids for maintenance replacement.

Further reading

Cornblath M, Hawdon JM, Williams AF. Controversies regarding definition of neonatal hypoglycemia: suggested operational thresholds. *Pediatrics*. 2000; 10(5):1141–5.

Coté CJ, Lerman J, Anderson BJ. *Coté and Lerman's A Practice of Anesthesia for Infants and Children*, 5th edition. Philadelphia, PA: Elsevier, 2013; 18.

Gregory GA, Andropoulos DB. *Gregory's Pediatric Anesthesia*, 5th edition. Hoboken: Wiley-Blackwell, 2012; 211–23.

Kliegman RM. *Nelson Textbook of Pediatrics*, 19th edition. Philadelphia: Elsevier, Saunders, 2011; 517–31.

Part C Metabolic

Chapter 47 Hypokalemia

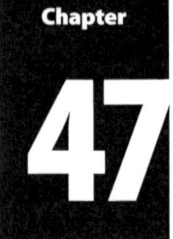

Amanda K. Brown and Rhonda A. Alexis

1. Presentation
   a) Serum potassium values < 3 mEq/L
   b) Physical examination may be normal; however, multi-system involvement may occur in severe cases:
      i) Neuromuscular system: muscle weakness, tetany
      ii) Cardiovascular system: cardiac arrhythmias (prolonged QT interval, ST segment depression, T wave flattening and appearance of U waves), palpitations, bradycardia
      iii) Gastrointestinal system: ileus
      iv) Renal system: polyuria due to inability to concentrate urine.
2. Risk factors
   a) Decreased potassium intake:
      i) Malnutrition
      ii) Anorexia nervosa
   b) Total body potassium depletion:
      i) Extrarenal losses: diarrhea, vomiting, sweating
      ii) Renal losses: Fanconi and Bartter syndromes
      iii) Other causes of acute potassium loss:
         (1) Diabetic ketoacidosis
         (2) Dialysis therapy.
   c) Medications (due to increased excretion):
      i) Laxatives
      ii) Diuretics
      iii) Cisplatin
      iv) Amphotericin B
      v) Corticosteroids.
   d) Transcellular shifts of potassium from extracellular to intracellular space:
      i) Alkalosis
      ii) Insulin therapy in hyperglycemia

Handbook of Critical Incidents and Essential Topics in Pediatric Anesthesiology, ed. David A. Young and Olutoyin A. Olutoye. Published by Cambridge University Press. © Cambridge University Press 2015.

iii) Sympathomimetic agents (i.e., β-agonists)
iv) Hypomagnesemia.
3. Differential diagnosis
   a) Other causes of cardiac arrhythmias (hyperthyroidism, hypertrophic cardiomyopathy, anemia, and other electrolyte anomalies)
   b) Other causes of muscle weakness such as inherited or acquired muscular disorders.
4. Pathophysiology
   a) Acute onset of hypokalemia is more significant
   b) Hypokalemia induces hyperpolarization and delays repolarization, resulting in atrial and ventricular dysrhythmias.
5. Management
   Depends on renal function and severity of symptoms.
   a) Slow replacement is strongly recommended, especially in the presence of renal failure or renal dysfunction
   b) Oral K$^+$ replacement can be administered over a number of days
   c) Intravenous replacement is indicated for symptomatic patients with very low levels (< 3 mEq/L)
      i) Central access is recommended due to venous irritation
      ii) EKG monitoring is recommended during intravenous potassium replacement
      iii) Administer potassium chloride at 0.5 mEq/kg/dose. Rate for replacement should not exceed 9 mEq/hr.
6. Prevention
   Identify patients at risk and consider obtaining a serum potassium level.

Further reading

Coté CJ, Lerman J, Anderson BJ. *Coté and Lerman's A Practice of Anesthesia for Infants and Children*, 5th edition. Philadelphia, PA: Elsevier, 2013; 175.

Unwin RJ, Friedrich CL, Shirley DG. Pathophysiology and management of hypokalemia: a clinical perspective. *Nat Rev Nephrol.* 2011; 7(2):75–84.

Part C **Metabolic**

Chapter 48 Hypomagnesemia

Amanda K. Brown and Rhonda A. Alexis

1. Presentation
   a) Serum levels < 1.7 mg/dL or < 0.7 mmol/L
   b) Most cases are asymptomatic
   c) Symptoms include:
      i) Anorexia
      ii) Weakness
      iii) Fasciculation
      iv) Paresthesias
      v) Confusion
      vi) Ataxia
      vii) Seizures.
   d) Cardiac manifestations include:
      Electrical irritability (EKG changes), ventricular (torsade de pointes) and supraventricular arrhythmias.

2. Risk factors
   Acquired conditions.
   a) Inadequate intake due to reduced gastrointestinal absorption:
      i) Malabsorption
      ii) Small bowel fistulas
      iii) Prolonged nasogastric suctioning
      iv) Severe diarrhea.
   b) Increased renal losses:
      i) Acute renal failure
      ii) Diuresis
      iii) Primary renal tubular magnesium wasting
      iv) Diabetic ketoacidosis
      v) Hyperparathyroidism
      vi) Hyperaldosteronism
      vii) Hypophosphatemia
      viii) Medications (e.g., diuretics).

Handbook of Critical Incidents and Essential Topics in Pediatric Anesthesiology, ed. David A. Young and Olutoyin A. Olutoye. Published by Cambridge University Press. © Cambridge University Press 2015.

c) Miscellaneous:
   i) Pancreatitis
   ii) Burns
   iii) Critically ill or malnourished children
   iv) Chronic alcoholism.
3. Differential diagnosis

   Magnesium is predominately an intracellular cation; the differential diagnosis relates to manifestations of decreased serum concentrations of other intracellular cations.
4. Pathophysiology

   Hypomagnesemia is frequently associated with enhanced effects of hypocalcemia and hypokalemia (prolonged QT interval).
5. Management
   a) Commonly an asymptomatic or incidental finding; oral replacement with magnesium sulfate or oxide is typically sufficient
   b) Severe symptoms: intravenous replacement with magnesium sulfate (25 mg/kg IV)
   c) Evaluate and treat other electrolyte deficiencies since concomitant hypokalemia and hypocalcemia may also be present.
6. Prevention
   a) Replace magnesium in high-risk groups such as the critically ill and malnourished
   b) Prompt treatment of hypocalcemia and hypokalemia.

Further reading

Coté CJ, Lerman J, Anderson BJ. *Coté and Lerman's A Practice of Anesthesia for Infants and Children*, 5th edition. Philadelphia, PA: Elsevier, 2013; 309.

Davis PJ. *Smith's Anesthesia for Infants and Children*, 8th edition. Philadelphia: Mosby Inc., 2011; 152–3.

Morgan M et al. *Clinical Anesthesiology*, 4th edition. New York: Lange, 2006.

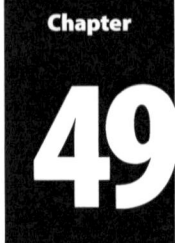

Part C Metabolic

Chapter 49

Hyponatremia

Andrew J. Costandi and Senthilkumar Sadhasivam

1. Presentation
   a) Definition: plasma Na⁺ < 135 mEq/L
   b) Mild forms of hyponatremia are common among post-surgical patients; most patients do not require therapy
   c) Patients may be asymptomatic, particularly in less severe forms
   d) Initial symptoms may include headache, ataxia, nausea, and vomiting
   e) Plasma Na⁺ levels < 125 mEq/L: obtundation, altered mental status, and seizures
   f) Plasma Na⁺ levels < 110 mEq/L: coma, cerebral edema, brainstem herniation.

2. Risk factors
   a) Excessive free water or electrolyte-free fluid administration
      i) Hypotonic intravenous fluids.
   b) Endocrine causes:
      i) SIADH (syndrome of inappropriate antidiuretic hormone)
      ii) Adrenal insufficiency
      iii) Hypothyroidism.
   c) Edema-forming conditions:
      i) Liver failure, renal failure, congestive heart failure, and burns.
   d) Neurologic causes:
      i) Cerebral salt wasting syndrome.
   e) Gastrointestinal causes:
      i) Vomiting, diarrhea, protein-losing enteropathy.
   f) Renal causes:
      i) Nephrotic syndrome
      ii) Acute and chronic renal failure.
   g) Drugs (e.g., thiazide diuretics, mannitol)
   h) Pain (e.g., postoperative pain)
   i) Pseudo-hyponatremia (e.g., hyperglycemia, hyperlipidemia, and hypoproteinemia).

Handbook of Critical Incidents and Essential Topics in Pediatric Anesthesiology, ed. David A. Young and Olutoyin A. Olutoye. Published by Cambridge University Press. © Cambridge University Press 2015.

3. Differential diagnosis
   a) Laboratory error
   b) Sample dilution
   c) Hyperglycemia/hyperlipidemia.
4. Pathophysiology
   a) Total body Na$^+$ deficiency (negative Na$^+$ balance as occurs with diuretics)
   b) Dilutional (positive water balance): due to relative excess of free water with low, normal, or high plasma Na$^+$
   c) Pseudohyponatremia.
5. Management
   a) Review vital signs and assess mental status
   b) Prepare for possible resuscitation including tracheal intubation in severe cases
   c) Check glucose levels to exclude pseudohyponatremia due to hyperglycemia
   d) Depending on the fluid status and presentation:
      i) Asymptomatic pseudohyponatremia: correct hyperglycemia
      ii) Asymptomatic dilutional hyponatremia: free water restriction, consider furosemide (1 mg/kg) if patient is hypervolemic
      iii) Symptomatic hyponatremia: 3–5 mL/kg of 3% hypertonic saline (514 mEq/L) over an hour is adequate to raise the plasma Na$^+$ to 125 mEq/L. Full correction may be estimated using the following formula:
      Na$^+$ deficit (mEq) = 0.6 × total body weight (kg) × (desired−actual plasma Na$^+$)
      iv) Corrections should be limited to 0.3–0.5 mEq/L/hr as rapid corrections lead to irreversible demyelinating disorder that may lead to permanent neurologic injury (central pontine myelinolysis)
      v) Chronic hyponatremia (over 48 hours): Usually clinically asymptomatic. Treatment is focused on correcting primary disorder, discontinuing any offending agents (diuretic), and free water restriction.
6. Prevention
   a) Use isotonic intravenous fluids perioperatively
   b) Follow plasma sodium levels when administering large quantities of fluids
   c) Consider hyponatremia as a cause of altered mental status.

Further reading

Coté CJ, Lerman J, Anderson BJ. *Coté and Lerman's A Practice of Anesthesia for Infants and Children*, 5th edition. Philadelphia, PA: Elsevier, 2013; 173–4.

Davis PJ, Cladis FP, Motoyama EK. *Smith's Anesthesia for Infants and Children*, 8th edition. Philadelphia: Elsevier Mosby, 2011; 132–4.

Ruskin KJ, Rosenbaum SH. *Anesthesia Emergencies*. Oxford: Oxford University Press, 2011.

Part C Metabolic

Chapter 50 Hypothermia

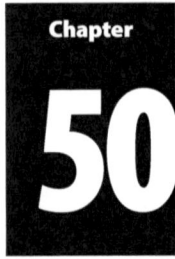

Paul A. Stricker

1. Presentation

   Hypothermia is a common perioperative occurrence, especially in children, who are at increased risk due to higher body surface area to mass ratios. Neonates and infants are the most vulnerable populations.

2. Risk factors

   a) Decreased age: infants and neonates
   b) Decreasing weight: patients with failure to thrive and poor nutrition
   c) Large surface areas exposed intraoperatively (e.g., abdominal surgery with bowel exposure to environment)
   d) Inadequate hypothermia preventive measures.

3. Pathophysiology

   a) General anesthetic inhibition of normal thermoregulatory processes promotes intraoperative hypothermia, both through effects on central hypothalamic control and through alterations in normal heat distribution between the core and periphery mediated by general anesthetic-induced vasodilation
   b) Mechanisms of heat loss (in decreasing order of contribution to typical heat loss):
      i) Radiation: heat loss through infrared electromagnetic radiation. Responsible for the majority of heat loss in the operating room. Minimized by preoperative warming of operating room and covering the patient
      ii) Convection: heat loss through cooler airflow next to the body. Minimized by insulation (covering the patient with blankets, etc.)
      iii) Evaporation: heat loss through latent heat of vaporization. Occurs with large open cavities, exposed wet body surfaces, during use of skin preparation solutions, and when dry inspired gases are used. Minimized by warmed irrigation solutions, and use of a heat-moisture exchanger on the anesthesia machine breathing circuit
      iv) Conduction: direct heat transfer through surface contact, as with a cold gel pad on the bed (minimized with heating devices placed against the body).

Handbook of Critical Incidents and Essential Topics in Pediatric Anesthesiology, ed. David A. Young and Olutoyin A. Olutoye. Published by Cambridge University Press. © Cambridge University Press 2015.

c) Effects:
   i) Cardiovascular: peripheral vasoconstriction, sensitization of myocardium to dysrhythmias/conduction abnormalities, increased oxygen consumption and development of shivering (except in newborns)
   ii) Neurologic: delayed emergence from anesthesia and prolonged recovery period
   iii) Coagulation: impaired platelet function and coagulation functions
   iv) Pharmacokinetic: decreased drug metabolism and clearance, resulting in prolonged effects (e.g., muscle relaxants, opioids).
4. Management
   a) Employ active measures to achieve and maintain normothermia (warm operating room, use forced air warming devices, use warmed intravenous fluids).
5. Prevention
   a) Most effective strategy to avoid hypothermia is to preoperatively increase the ambient temperature in operating room
   b) Covering the patient with blankets/plastic sheets reduces radiant and convective heat loss
   c) Warming operating room prior to patient's arrival: Reduces radiation and convection losses
   d) Overhead radiant warming lights direct radiant warming to patient but maintain vigilance to avoid thermal injuries.

Further reading

Davis PJ, Cladis FP, Motoyama EK. *Smith's Anesthesia for Infants and Children*, 8th edition. Philadelphia: Elsevier Mosby, 2011; 167–70.

Pabelick C, Harrison T, Flick RP. Clinical complications in pediatric anesthesia. In: Gregory GA, Andropoulos DB, ed. *Gregory's Pediatric Anesthesia*, 5th edition. Hoboken: Wiley-Blackwell, 2012.

Rajagopalan S, Mascha E, Na J et al. The effects of mild perioperative hypothermia on blood loss and transfusion requirement. *Anesthesiology* 2008; 108:71–7.

Part C Metabolic

Chapter 51: Malignant hyperthermia

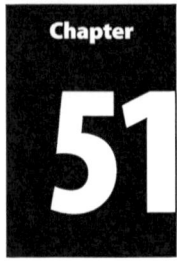

Tae W. Kim

1. Presentation
   Increase in end-tidal CO_2, diffuse skeletal muscle rigidity, hyperthermia, tachycardia, tachypnea, combined respiratory and metabolic acidosis, brown colored urine.

2. Risk factors
   a) Exposure to halogenated volatile anesthetics or succinylcholine
   b) Genetic predisposition: *RYR1* gene defect on chromosome 19q13.1
   c) Comorbidity: neuromuscular disorders especially Central core disease and King–Denborough syndrome
   d) Controversial if there is increased susceptibility from masseter muscle rigidity and muscular dystrophy.

3. Differential diagnosis
   a) Sepsis
   b) Thyrotoxicosis
   c) Neuroleptic malignant syndrome
   d) Serotonin syndrome
   e) Inadequate depth of anesthesia
   f) Exhausted CO_2 absorbent
   g) Equipment malfunction (e.g., faulty expiratory valve).

4. Pathophysiology
   a) Triggering agent signals ryanodine receptor protein to release calcium from the sarcoplasmic reticulum into myoplasm
   b) Unregulated calcium activation of actin and myosin results in sustained and generalized skeletal muscle contractions
   c) Aerobic metabolism switches to anaerobic metabolism after exhaustion of available substrates and oxygen; this results in acidosis development
   d) Cellular integrity is eventually compromised resulting in release of intracellular potassium, myoglobin, and creatine kinase
   e) Hyperkalemia as well as mixed metabolic and respiratory acidosis may contribute to the development of cardiac dysrhythmias
   f) Myoglobinuria and renal failure from myoglobin toxicity to renal tubules may also occur.

5. Management
   a) Declare MH crisis, alert surgeon and staff, call for help and MH cart
   b) Discontinue halogenated volatile anesthetic agents
   c) Switch to non-triggering technique and hyperventilate with 100% oxygen using high fresh gas flow rates
   d) It is not necessary to change the anesthesia machine or breathing circuit
   e) Imperative to administer dantrolene with initial bolus 2.5 mg/kg, repeat as necessary, no maximum limit but typically effective response observed with doses < 10 mg/kg
   f) Actively cool patient using IV solutions, forced air devices set at cooling, ice packs, lavage of body cavities
   g) Place arterial line for continuous hemodynamic monitoring and frequent arterial blood sampling as clinically indicated
   h) Correct metabolic acidosis with sodium bicarbonate (starting dose 1–2 mEq/kg)
   i) Reduce cardiac irritability with calcium gluconate (30 mg/kg) or calcium chloride (10 mg/kg)
   j) Correct hyperkalemia with regular insulin (0.1 units/kg) and glucose (D50 1 mL/kg)
   k) Place urinary catheter to monitor urine output and renal function; goal to maintain urine output of 2 mL/kg/hr
   l) Do not administer calcium channel blockers; they are associated with cardiovascular collapse and hyperkalemia
   m) Prepare for ICU care and continuation of dantrolene for 24–48 hours (1 mg/kg every 4–6 hours given as an infusion); recrudescence may occur up to 36 hours after event
   n) Call the MH Hotline for further assistance at 1-800-MH-HYPER.

6. Prevention
   a) Rare disease; many patients unaware of status until MH crisis occurs
   b) Known or suspected MH susceptible patients should have a non-triggering anesthetic technique, (i.e., TIVA technique)
   c) Patients experiencing severe masseter muscle rigidity or "jaws of steel" should have anesthesia aborted if elective and observed for possible rhabdomyolysis and MH development
   d) Use a decontaminated anesthesia machine or an anesthesia machine dedicated to caring for only MH patients. Develop an institutional protocol for managing patients with MH
   e) Obtain a dedicated MH cart stocked with 36 vials of dantrolene and the supplies necessary to treat MH (e.g., sterile water) for all anesthetizing locations.

Further reading

Coté CJ, Lerman J, Anderson BJ. *Coté and Lerman's A Practice of Anesthesia for Infants and Children*, 5th edition. Philadelphia, PA: Elsevier, 2013; 817–34.

Kim TW, Nemergut ME. Preparation of modern anesthesia workstations for malignant hyperthermia-susceptible patients: a review of past and present practice. *Anesthesiology*. 2011; 114(1):205–12.

www.mhaus.org/healthcare-professionals/mhaus-recommendations/anesthesia-workstation-preparation (accessed October 21, 2013).

Part C   Metabolic

Chapter 52

Metabolic acidosis

Paul A. Stricker

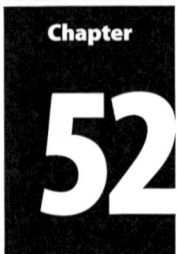

1. Presentation
   Metabolic acidosis refers to a process in which the plasma bicarbonate (HCO_3^-) concentration is reduced, resulting in a lowered pH. In non-anesthetized individuals, respiratory compensation occurs whereby minute ventilation increases (compensatory respiratory alkalosis) to reduce $PaCO_2$. Patients can also present with complex mixed acid–base disorders (combined metabolic and respiratory acidosis, etc.) as well as a compensatory response to primary respiratory alkalosis.

2. Risk factors
   Risk factors relate to the specific etiology for metabolic acidosis.

3. Differential diagnosis
   The anion gap is the difference between the normally measured cations and anions: $[Na^+] - ([Cl^-] + [HCO_3^-])$. The normal anion gap is 5–11.

   a) High anion gap acidosis
      i) Lactic acidosis
      ii) Ketoacidosis
      iii) Renal failure (retained organic acids)
      iv) Rhabdomyolysis
      v) Toxic ingestions (e.g., salicylates, methanol).

   b) Normal anion gap acidosis (hyperchloremic acidosis)
      i) Fluid resuscitation with 0.9% saline
      ii) HCO_3^- loss through diarrhea
      iii) Renal HCO_3^- loss (renal tubular acidosis), pathologic or acetazolamide-induced
      iv) Hypoaldosteronism (type 4 renal tubular acidosis).

4. Pathophysiology
   Plasma $[HCO_3^-]$ can be lowered either by loss of HCO_3^- or by buffering of an acid.

   a) HCO_3^- loss: diarrhea, renal HCO_3^- loss
   b) Buffering of acids: $HA + NaHCO_3 \rightarrow NaA + H_2CO_3 \rightarrow CO_2 + H_2O$ (HA represents an acid/hydrogen donor).

Handbook of Critical Incidents and Essential Topics in Pediatric Anesthesiology, ed. David A. Young and Olutoyin A. Olutoye. Published by Cambridge University Press. © Cambridge University Press 2015.

5. Management
   a) Determine etiology (see above)
      Most common intraoperative cause is lactic acidosis from inadequate tissue perfusion (low cardiac output, hypovolemia, reduced oxygen carrying capacity, alone or in combination).
   b) Determine chronicity
      Patients on acetazolamide will have compensatory respiratory alkalosis and may develop reduced apneic threshold; targeting a "normal" $ETCO_2$ of approximately 35 mmHg may result in acidosis.
   c) Direct therapy at underlying cause
      i) Lactic acidosis with circulatory failure – correct hypovolemia, restore adequate cardiac output
      ii) Decreased HCO_3^- and pH < 7.2: correction with bicarbonate
         1. Formula for correction: mEq $NaHCO_3$ administered = (weight in kg × base excess) × 1/3
         2. Must have effective ventilation to eliminate CO_2 that forms following bicarbonate administration. If ventilation cannot be increased to eliminate additional CO_2 produced, respiratory acidosis will worsen and further decrease the pH.
6. Prevention
   a) Maintain cardiac output, euvolemia, and tissue oxygen delivery to reduce lactic acidosis
   b) Maintain low threshold to send electrolytes and blood gas to evaluate for acidosis development in high-risk situations (large fluid shifts, suspected poisoning).

Further reading

Coté CJ, Lerman J, Anderson BJ. *Coté and Lerman's A Practice of Anesthesia for Infants and Children*, 5th edition. Philadelphia, PA: Elsevier, 2013; 212–13.

Rose B. *Clinical Physiology of Acid-Base and Electrolyte Disorders*. New York: McGraw-Hill, Inc., 1994.

Part C Metabolic

Chapter 53: Metabolic alkalosis

Lisa D. Heyden

1. Presentation
   a) Typically asymptomatic – symptoms are usually related to the underlying etiology or accompanying electrolyte abnormalities:
      i) Volume depletion (easy fatigability, muscle cramps, postural dizziness)
      ii) Hypokalemia (muscle weakness, cardiac arrhythmias, and possibly polyuria and polydipsia).
   b) Severe metabolic alkalosis can cause agitation, disorientation, seizures and coma.
2. Risk factors
   a) Prolonged vomiting or nasogastric suction – loss of hydrogen chloride (e.g., pyloric stenosis)
   b) Diuretic therapy (e.g., loop diuretics)
   c) Hypovolemia
   d) Compensation from respiratory acidosis
   e) Diarrhea:
      i) Laxative abuse
      ii) Villous adenoma
      iii) Chloridorrhea.
   f) Mineralocorticoid excess/primary aldosteronism
      i) Licorice (glycyrrhizic acid) ingestion
      ii) Genetic disorders involving renal tubular transport (such as Bartter, Gitelman, or Liddle syndromes).
3. Differential diagnosis

   Measurement of urine chloride, urine sodium and urine pH may help to detect the etiology of alkalosis.

   a) Low urine chloride concentration (< 20 mEq/L and often < 10 mEq/L)
      i) Vomiting or nasogastric suctioning
      ii) Diuretics
      iii) Extracellular fluid volume contraction
      iv) Laxative abuse.

Handbook of Critical Incidents and Essential Topics in Pediatric Anesthesiology, ed. David A. Young and Olutoyin A. Olutoye. Published by Cambridge University Press. © Cambridge University Press 2015.

b) Urine chloride not low (usually > 40 mEq/L)
     i) Primary aldosteronism
     ii) Liddle syndrome
     iii) Excess licorice ingestion
     iv) Apparent mineralocorticoid excess syndrome.
4. Pathophysiology
   a) Hypovolemia stimulates the renin–angiotensin–aldosterone axis resulting in release of aldosterone; this promotes loss of potassium and hydrogen ions in the distal tubule
   b) Loss of free water during hypovolemia concentrates the existing bicarbonate stores
   c) Diuretic use inhibits renal tubular reabsorption of sodium and potassium, resulting in hypokalemia and an associated alkalosis
   d) Metabolic alkalosis may persist due to inability to excrete the excess bicarbonate in the urine as a result of intravascular volume depletion, reduced effective arterial blood volume (i.e., heart failure), chloride depletion, hypokalemia, or renal impairment
   e) Loss of chloride ions as occurs in diarrhea is associated with an accompanying loss of hydrogen ions
   f) Hypoventilation and increase in $PaCO_2$ occurs to compensate for metabolic alkalosis ($PaCO_2$ increases by 0.7 mmHg for every 1 mEq/L elevation in plasma bicarbonate concentration). Respiratory compensation is most effective acutely and then becomes inconsequential after 12–24 hours).
5. Management
   a) Most cases of metabolic alkalosis are chloride responsive
      i) Isotonic saline is the most common initial therapy
      ii) Correct hypokalemia with potassium chloride
      iii) Dilute hydrogen chloride produces the most rapid correction but may be irritating to the veins during administration
      iv) Consider use of diuretics such as a carbonic anhydrase inhibitor (e.g., acetazolamide) or a potassium-sparing diuretic (e.g., spironolactone) if edema is present.
   b) Chloride-resistant alkalosis. Treat the underlying mineralocorticoid excess and correct potassium deficits.
6. Prevention
   Maintain increased vigilance for this condition in at-risk patients, which includes consideration for arterial blood gas sampling in symptomatic patients.

Further reading

Gregory GA, Andropoulos DB. *Gregory's Pediatric Anesthesia*, 5th edition. Hoboken: Wiley-Blackwell, 2012; 709–10.

Marino PL. *The ICU Book*, 2nd edition. Philadelphia: Lippincott Willams & Wilkins, 1998; 608–16.

Marston N, Kehl D, Copp J, Nourbakhsh N. Alkalotics anonymous: severe metabolic alkalosis *Am J Med.* 2014;127(1):25–7.

Part C Metabolic

Chapter 54 Thyrotoxicosis

Julia Chen

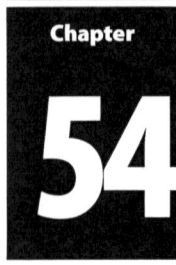

1. Presentation
    a) Clinical symptoms may vary depending on severity and disease duration
    b) Hyperthyroidism
        i) Nonspecific manifestations: heat intolerance, weakness, sweating, weight loss with normal/increased appetite
        ii) Cardiovascular: tachycardia, palpitations, arrhythmias, increased systolic blood pressure, increased cardiac output
        iii) Central nervous system: nervousness, restlessness, tremors, behavioral disturbances
        iv) Large-sized goiters can potentially cause tracheo-esophageal compression leading to respiratory distress and a difficult airway.
    c) Thyroid storm
        i) Hyperthermia
        ii) Exaggeration of hyperthyroidism presentation
        iii) Cardiovascular: tachycardia, arrhythmias, cardiovascular collapse
        iv) Central nervous system symptoms: delirium, stupor, coma.
    d) Laboratory testing would be expected to reveal increased triiodothyronine (T_3) and thyroxine (T_4) levels and as well as a decreased thyroid stimulating hormone (TSH) level.
2. Risk factors
    a) Graves disease – most common cause of hyperthyroidism in children
    b) Thyroiditis
        i) Autoimmune thyroiditis
        ii) Infectious thyroiditis.
    c) Iodine-induced hyperthyroidism
    d) Toxic multinodular goiter
    e) Solitary thyroid nodule
    f) McCune–Albright syndrome
    g) Thyroid hormone ingestion
    h) Noncompliance with antithyroid and cardiovascular (e.g., propranolol) medications.

Handbook of Critical Incidents and Essential Topics in Pediatric Anesthesiology, ed. David A. Young and Olutoyin A. Olutoye. Published by Cambridge University Press. © Cambridge University Press 2015.

3. Differential diagnosis
   a) Malignant hyperthermia
   b) Pheochromocytoma
   c) Carcinoid crisis
   d) Neuroleptic malignant syndrome.
4. Pathophysiology
   a) Thyroid hormone production is regulated by the hypothalamic–pituitary–thyroid axis:
      i) Most of the clinical effects of thyroid hormones are due to T_3 which is secreted directly from the thyroid gland and produced from the conversion of T_4 to T_3 in peripheral tissues.
   b) Pathophysiology of hyperthyroidism related to an underlying cause:
      i) Graves disease is caused by thyrotropin receptor antibodies which activates the receptors thereby increasing thyroid hormone synthesis and secretion
      ii) Hashimoto thyroiditis is an autoimmune thyroiditis that is associated with hypothyroidism but may occasionally produce hyperthyroidism.
   c) Thyroid storm – precipitated by conditions that lead to an acute increase in thyroid hormone levels in an uncompensated state (e.g., surgery, trauma, infection, acute iodine load).
5. Management
   a) Thyroid storm
      i) Priority is to control the cardiovascular effects from the thyroid hormones.
         (1) Beta-blockers: (propranolol, esmolol)
         (2) Iodine-containing solutions (potassium iodide, Lugol solution): these are administered orally and may take several weeks for a clinical response.
      ii) Supportive treatment
         (1) Intravenous fluids
         (2) Active cooling
            - Acetaminophen
            - Cold lavage
            - Cooling blankets.
         (3) Glucocorticoids – decreases conversion of T_4 to T_3, promotes vasomotor stability, treatment for associated adrenal insufficiency.
      iii) Treat precipitating event (i.e., sepsis).
   b) Treatment of hyperthyroidism
      i) Antithyroid medications: propylthiouracil, methimazole
      ii) Radioactive iodine
      iii) Thyroidectomy.
6. Prevention
   a) Patients should be clinically and biochemically euthyroid prior to elective surgery.

Further reading

Barash PG. *Clinical Anesthesia*, 7th edition. Philadelphia: Lippincott Williams & Wilkins, 2013; 1328–30.

Coté CJ, Lerman J, Anderson BJ. *Coté and Lerman's A Practice of Anesthesia for Infants and Children*, 5th edition. Philadelphia, PA: Elsevier, 2013; 549–50.

Davis PJ, Cladis FP, Motoyama EK. *Smith's Anesthesia for Infants and Children*, 8th edition. Philadelphia: Elsevier Mosby, 2011; 1108.

Gregory GA, Andropoulos DB. *Gregory's Pediatric Anesthesia*, 5th edition. Hoboken: Wiley-Blackwell, 2012; 87–8.

Part D: Neurologic

Chapter 55: Altered mental status

Normidaris Jimenez and Jacquelyn Morillo-Delerme

1. Presentation
   Change is observed in:
   a) Behavior (e.g., new onset combativeness)
   b) Level of consciousness or altered awareness of self (e.g., new onset somnolence)
   c) Impaired cognitive function
   d) Decreased attention span.
2. Risk factors
   a) Cardiovascular
      i) Hypotension or severe hypertension
      ii) Tachycardia/bradycardia
      iii) Cardiac arrhythmias.
   b) Pharmacologic (effects of certain drugs)
      i) Opiates, benzodiazepines or other anesthetic agents
      ii) Anticholinergics
      iii) Local anesthetic toxicity
      iv) Antidopaminergic drugs
      v) Steroids
      vi) Recreational drug intoxication
      vii) Drug withdrawal.
   c) Neurologic
      i) Epilepsy or postictal state
      ii) Stroke
      iii) Cerebral ischemia
      iv) Intracranial bleed secondary to arteriovenous malformation or tumor
      v) Increased intracranial pressure
      vi) Underlying psychogenic or psychiatric condition
      vii) Cerebral edema
      viii) Blindness.
   d) Metabolic
      i) Hypo- or hyperglycemia

Handbook of Critical Incidents and Essential Topics in Pediatric Anesthesiology, ed. David A. Young and Olutoyin A. Olutoye. Published by Cambridge University Press. © Cambridge University Press 2015.

ii) Poisoning
iii) Acidosis or alkalosis
iv) Hypo/hypernatremia
v) Other electrolyte abnormalities
vi) Hypo/hyperthermia
vii) Hypo/hyperthyroidism
viii) Alcohol intoxication or withdrawal
ix) Hepatic encephalopathy
x) Uremia
xi) Inborn errors of metabolism (neonates or infants with undiagnosed conditions).

e) Infectious
i) Central nervous system infection
ii) Sepsis.

3. Differential diagnosis
   a) Preexisting psychiatric conditions
   b) Preexisting neurologic conditions
   c) Emergence delirium (see Chapter 58, Emergence agitation)
   d) Drug reactions
   e) Emergence following prolonged surgery (especially cerebrovascular, neurosurgical and cardiac surgeries).

4. Pathophysiology
   The pathophysiology depends on the specific etiology.

5. Management
   a) Evaluate patient's airway and hemodynamic status: consider securing airway if moderate to severe degree of somnolence is present, treat abnormal vital signs as needed
   b) Check electrolytes (glucose, sodium, and other electrolytes) and obtain arterial blood gas
   c) Identify medications that may have been recently administered and consider antidotes (i.e., flumazenil)
   d) Consider computed tomography (CT) scan and/or magnetic resonance imaging (MRI) of head if no causes have been identified with previous steps and no improvement is observed
   e) Once etiology has been identified, treat accordingly.

6. Prevention
   a) Obtain thorough preoperative history; this may highlight the need to modify perioperative medications
   b) Strict monitoring of blood glucose in diabetic patients presenting for surgery.

Further reading

Davis PJ, Cladis FP, Motoyama EK. *Smith's Anesthesia for Infants and Children*, 8th edition. Philadelphia: Mosby, Inc., 2011.

Miller RD. *Miller's Anesthesia*, 7th edition. Philadelphia: Churchill Livingstone, 2009.

Part D Neurologic

Chapter 56 Blindness and perioperative vision loss

Yang Liu

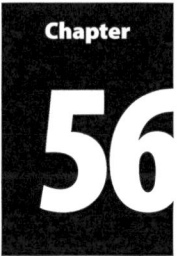

1. Presentation
   a) Postoperative visual loss
   b) Most cases are associated with prone position during spine surgeries.

2. Risk factors
   a) Prone positioning
   b) Intraoperative hemodynamic compromise:
      i) Decreased systemic blood pressure
      ii) Significant blood loss
      iii) Anemia
      iv) Massive fluid replacement.
   c) Surgery of prolonged duration
   d) Undiagnosed congenital heart disease and paradoxical embolism
   e) Direct external ocular injury or compression
   f) Newborns and infants are at increased risk if they are positioned on inappropriately sized horseshoe headrests – potential for direct ocular pressure.

3. Differential diagnosis
   a) Ischemic optic neuropathy – most common cause of visual loss
   b) External ocular injury – corneal abrasion or sclera injury (usually accompanied by pain in affected eye)
   c) Cortical blindness – usually accompanied by signs of stroke in parietal-occipital region. Pupillary reflexes are preserved
   d) Retinal ischemia – branch or central retinal artery occlusion accompanied by unilateral painless visual loss and abnormal pupil reactivity
   e) Acute angle-closure glaucoma – characterized by painful red eyes, blurred vision, headache, nausea and vomiting.

4. Pathophysiology
   a) Direct ocular pressure, systemic emboli or decreased perfusion pressure results in retinal artery occlusion
   b) Prolonged hypotension is believed to be associated with ischemic optic neuropathy.

Handbook of Critical Incidents and Essential Topics in Pediatric Anesthesiology, ed. David A. Young and Olutoyin A. Olutoye. Published by Cambridge University Press. © Cambridge University Press 2015.

5. Management
   a) Obtain urgent ophthalmologic consultation for potential visual loss
   b) Consider magnetic resonance imaging to rule out intracranial causes of blindness
   c) Optimize hemoglobin level
   d) Optimize arterial oxygen saturation
   e) Optimize hemodynamic status
   f) Provide supportive care.
6. Prevention
   a) Identify high-risk population
   b) Patient positioning
      i) Apply eye lubricant and tape eyes closed after induction
      ii) Avoid direct ocular pressure
      iii) Consider positioning head in pinhead holder if patient's head does not adequately fit in headrest.
   c) Early administration of volume expanders to maintain adequate intravascular volume
   d) Maintain adequate hematocrit
   e) Consider staging of lengthy procedures with potential for large volume blood loss
   f) Avoid entrainment of air in patients with congenital heart disease.

Further reading

Apfelbaum JL, Roth S, Connis RT. Practice advisory for perioperative visual loss associated with spine surgery: An Updated Report by the American Society of Anesthesiologists Task Force on Perioperative Visual Loss. *Anesthesiology.* 2012; 116(2):274–85.

Gregory GA, Andropoulos DB. *Gregory's Pediatric Anesthesia*, 5th edition. Hoboken: Wiley-Blackwell, 2012; 666, 1175–6.

Grover VK, Jangra K. Perioperative vision loss: A complication to watch out. *J Anaesthesiol Clin Pharmacol.* 2012; 28(1):11–16.

Part D **Neurologic**

Chapter 57

Delayed emergence

David A. Young

1. Presentation
   a) Lack of return to the preoperative level of consciousness within the expected time period
   b) There is no established definition or time period for delayed emergence; however, high suspicion occurs after 20–45 minutes of discontinuing all anesthetic agents
   c) Presenting features may be nonspecific and include unresponsiveness, apnea, flaccid extremities, pupillary constriction and/or irregularity.
2. Risk factors
   a) Preoperative altered level of consciousness
   b) Recently received pharmacologic agents (e.g., inhaled anesthetic agents, neuromuscular blocking agents)
   c) Preexisting neurologic conditions (e.g., seizure disorder, developmental delay)
   d) Preexisting metabolic conditions (e.g., diabetes mellitus, hypothyroidism)
   e) Recently completed neurosurgical procedure (e.g., brain tumor resection).
3. Differential diagnosis
   There are numerous possible causes but they can grouped into three main categories.
   a) Pharmacologic
      i) Inhaled anesthetic agents
      ii) Opioids
      iii) Neuromuscular blocking agents
      iv) Intravenous agents (e.g., propofol, dexmedetomidine)
      v) Other agents (e.g., midazolam, scopolamine).
   b) Metabolic
      i) Hypoxemia
      ii) Hypercarbia
      iii) Hypothermia
      iv) Hyper- and hypoglycemia
      v) Hyper- and hyponatremia
      vi) Hypocalcemia

Handbook of Critical Incidents and Essential Topics in Pediatric Anesthesiology, ed. David A. Young and Olutoyin A. Olutoye. Published by Cambridge University Press. © Cambridge University Press 2015.

vii) Hypermagnesemia
viii) Acidosis.
   c) Neurologic
       i) Postictal from intraoperative seizure
       ii) Intracranial hemorrhage
       iii) Thromboembolic event
       iv) Increased intracranial pressure
       v) Cerebral edema.
4. Pathophysiology

   The pathophysiology may be initially unknown until a specific etiology has been determined.

5. Management
   a) Initially evaluate airway, breathing, pupils, and vital signs
   b) Review recently administered medications
       i) Consider administration of naloxone or flumazenil if indicated (dose 10 µg/kg; may repeat as needed)
       ii) Consider possibility of a medication administration error.
   c) Evaluate the degree of neuromuscular blockade – consider administration of neostigmine and glycopyrrolate if not previously administered
   d) Review past medical history for possible causes (e.g., diabetes mellitus, hypothyroidism, epilepsy, coagulopathies, neurologic conditions)
   e) Obtain an arterial blood gas, glucose, and electrolytes (sodium, calcium, magnesium) if a metabolic cause is suspected
   f) Perform a focused neurologic examination concentrating on level of consciousness, pupils, strength, and detection of lateralizing signs
   g) Consider emergent imaging (e.g., CT of brain without contrast) if a neurologic etiology is suspected
   h) Once the etiology is determined, provide supportive care and treat the underlying cause (e.g., administer glucose, warm the patient, etc.).
6. Prevention
   a) Consider utilizing reduced dosages of anesthetic agents in patients with a history of delayed emergence, developmental delay, hepatic, or renal insufficiency
   b) Consider intraoperative evaluation of metabolic conditions (e.g., serum glucose)
   c) Frequently evaluate the degree of neuromuscular blockade
   d) Have an increased vigilance for neurologic conditions in high-risk patients.

Further reading

Atlee JL. *Complications in Anesthesia*, 2nd edition. Philadelphia: Saunders, 2006; 885–6.

Bready JL. *Decision Making in Anesthesiology: An Algorithmic Approach*, 4th edition. Philadelphia: Mosby, 2007; 582–5.

Cottrell JE. *Cottrell and Young's Neuroanesthesia*, 5th edition. Philadelphia: Mosby, 2010; 195–6.

Gregory GA, Andropoulos DB. *Gregory's Pediatric Anesthesia*, 5th edition. Hoboken: Wiley-Blackwell, 2012; 344.

Part D: Neurologic

Chapter 58: Emergence agitation

David Moore and Senthilkumar Sadhasivam

1. Presentation
   a) Definition: a dissociative state of consciousness noted during recovery from general anesthesia characterized by lack of coherence, restlessness, and inconsolability
   b) Patients with emergence agitation (EA) are often noted to have the triad of consciousness, altered mental status, and perceived noxious stimuli.

2. Risk factors
   a) Age < 5 years
   b) Surgical procedure – ophthalmology and otolaryngology greater than other types of surgery
   c) Use of insoluble volatile anesthetics (i.e., sevoflurane)
   d) Prior history of emergence agitation
   e) Preoperative anxiety/poor socialization/low adaptability scores.

3. Differential diagnosis
   a) Postoperative pain
   b) Postoperative anxiety
   c) Hypoxemia/hypercarbia
   e) Anticholinergic agitation
   f) Metabolic disorders (i.e., hypoglycemia).

4. Pathophysiology
   Pathophysiology unknown but related to the triad of consciousness, altered mental status, and perceived noxious stimuli. EA is characteristically self-limited, lasting approximately 5–20 minutes after cessation of general anesthesia, and typically requires no medical therapy.

5. Management
   a) Initially exclude hypoxemia and hypercarbia. Evaluate for adequate ventilation and absence of airway obstruction. Exclude postoperative pain/anxiety versus emergence delirium by determining coherence
   b) Priority is to maintain physical safety of patient; patient may require additional caregivers and protective items such as pillows to prevent patient injury

---

Handbook of Critical Incidents and Essential Topics in Pediatric Anesthesiology, ed. David A. Young and Olutoyin A. Olutoye. Published by Cambridge University Press. © Cambridge University Press 2015.

c) Treatment focused on one or more aspects of the triad of consciousness, altered mental status, and perceived noxious stimuli. Pharmacologic therapy may be considered if increased concern for patient safety is present or if an appropriate amount of time has passed without clinical improvement
d) Consciousness has been treated by inducing sleep with various medications such as propofol
e) Consider administering flumazenil for suspected paradoxical reactions after midazolam use
f) Real or perceived noxious stimuli has been treated with opioids such as fentanyl due to its rapid onset
g) Consider physostigmine if suspected anticholinergic administration
h) Consider laboratory testing to exclude metabolic disorders in refractory cases.

6. Prevention

   a) Consider avoiding insoluble volatile anesthetics such as sevoflurane in patients with a previous history of significant EA. For long cases, consider transitioning to non-volatile anesthetic agents prior to emergence
   b) Consider avoiding oral midazolam in patients with a previous history of significant EA. Oral midazolam has been shown to increase EA
   c) Reduce postoperative pain by implementing regional anesthesia and/or judicious usage of opioids. Fentanyl, clonidine, and dexmedetomidine have all been associated with reducing EA
   d) Reduce postoperative or separation anxiety in young children by having parents present in the post-anesthesia care unit promptly after conclusion of surgery
   e) Administration of single doses of propofol, fentanyl, and dexmedetomidine has been equivocal in the literature with regards to reducing EA.

Further reading

Cole JW, Murray DJ, McAllister JD, Hirshberg GE. Emergence behavior in children: defining the incidence of excitement and agitation following anaesthesia. *Paediatr Anaesth*. 2002; 12:442–7.

Coté CJ, Lerman J, Anderson BJ. *Coté and Lerman's A Practice of Anesthesia for Infants and Children*, 5th edition. Philadelphia, PA: Elsevier, 2013; 983–4.

Eckenhoff JE, Kneale DH, Dripps RD. The incidence and etiology of postanesthetic excitement: a clinical survey. *Anesthesiology*. 1961; 22:667.

Fronapfel PJ. Prevention of emergence delirium. *Paediatr Anaesth*. 2008; 18:1113–14.

Uezono S, Goto T, Terui K, et al. Emergence agitation after sevoflurane versus propofol in pediatric patients. *Anesth Analg*. 2000; 91(3):563–6.

Part D Neurologic

Chapter 59: Increased intracranial pressure

Yang Liu

1. Presentation
   a) Headache
   b) Vomiting
   c) Papilledema
   d) Seizures
   e) Behavior changes
   f) Altered level of consciousness
      i) Irritability
      ii) Lethargy
      iii) Obtundation
      iv) Coma.
   g) Focal neurologic findings
   h) Cushing's triad – constellation of systemic hypertension, bradycardia, and irregular respirations
   i) Specific presentation in infants:
      i) Drowsiness
      ii) Bulging fontanelle, cranial suture separation, and macrocephaly.
2. Risk factors
   a) Neurocutaneous syndromes (tuberous sclerosis, neurofibromatosis, Sturge–Weber disease)
   b) Malfunctioning ventriculo-peritoneal shunts
   c) Traumatic brain injury (TBI).
3. Differential diagnosis
   a) Traumatic brain injury
   b) Intracranial hemorrhage
      i) Ruptured aneurysm
      ii) Arteriovenous malformation or other vascular anomalies.
   c) Hydrocephalus
   d) Brain tumors

Handbook of Critical Incidents and Essential Topics in Pediatric Anesthesiology, ed. David A. Young and Olutoyin A. Olutoye. Published by Cambridge University Press. © Cambridge University Press 2015.

e) Central nervous system infections
      i) Encephalitis
      ii) Meningitis
      iii) Abscess.
  f) Idiopathic intracranial hypertension (pseudotumor cerebri)
  g) Hypoxic brain swelling.
4. Pathophysiology
  a) Normal range of intracranial pressure (ICP) varies with age. Values in the pediatric population are not well established but an ICP of > 20–25 mmHg is considered increased
  b) If the fontanelles are closed, ICP depends on the relationship between the skull volume and its contents (brain tissue, cerebrospinal fluid, and blood)
  c) Obstruction to drainage of flow or pathologic contents (brain tumor, foreign body) can result in increased ICP
  d) In normal conditions, a small increase in volume of intracranial contents causes only a mild increase in ICP
  e) In pathologic conditions that increase the volume of intracranial contents, a small increase in volume causes a marked increase in ICP
  f) Elevation of ICP may fluctuate depending on blood pressure changes, ventilation, oxygenation status, change in head position, temperature, and cerebrovascular stability
  g) Arterial carbon dioxide levels ($PaCO_2$) have a significant effect on cerebral blood flow (CBF)
  h) Increased ICP and decreased cerebral perfusion pressure (CPP) may cause ischemic injury to the brain
  i) A pressure gradient between the intracranial compartments may result in herniation of brain tissue.
5. Management
  a) Early recognition of elevated ICP may reduce neurologic sequelae and/or death
  b) Maintain adequate oxygenation
  c) Maintain adequate ventilation
      i) Secure the airway with an endotracheal tube
      ii) Maintain $PaCO_2$ between 35 and 40 mmHg
      iii) Hyperventilation to a $PaCO_2$ of 30–35 mmHg should be reserved for patients with signs of herniation
      iv) Avoid high peak inspiratory pressures and peak end – expiratory pressures.
  d) Maintain adequate blood pressure to prevent secondary ischemic injury
  e) Consider elevation of the head of the bed
  f) Consider administration of the following medications:
      i) Mannitol (0.5–1 g/kg)
      ii) Hypertonic saline
      iii) Barbiturates (to induce a barbiturate coma)
      iv) Corticosteroids.

g) Consider administration of prophylactic anticonvulsants
   h) Maintain adequate analgesia and sedation
   i) Consider placement of an ICP monitor
   j) Drainage of cerebrospinal fluid via surgical insertion of an external ventricular drain, lumbar drain or ventriculo-peritoneal shunt
   k) Hypothermia
   l) Decompressive craniectomy.
6. Prevention
   a) Prevention of increased ICP depends on the etiology of underlying disease
   b) Maintain increased vigilance for signs/symptoms of increased ICP in at-risk patients (TBI, brain tumor).

Further reading

Brasher WK, Tasker RC. Elevated intracranial pressure (ICP) in children. Retrieved from www.uptodate.com/contents/elevated-intracranial-pressure-icp-in-children (accessed September 15, 2013).

Gregory GA, Andropoulos DB. *Gregory's Pediatric Anesthesia*, 5th edition. Hoboken: Wiley-Blackwell, 2012; 974–6.

Part D Neurologic

Chapter 60 Intraoperative awareness

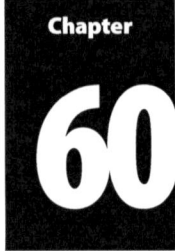

Carlos Rodriguez

1. Presentation
   a) A patient having explicit recall of events that occurred during the intraoperative period but not taking place during awake extubation or prior to administration of induction agents
   b) Intraoperative portions associated with tachycardia, tachypnea, hypertension, and patient movement
   c) Development of significant postoperative psychological symptoms including post-traumatic stress disorder
   d) Most studies report an incidence of awareness for children just under 1%; this is higher than for adults
   e) The reporting of intraoperative awareness may be delayed and not easily ascertained.
2. Risk factors
   a) Inadequate amount of anesthetic agents administered to a patient with normal requirements (e.g., vaporizer malfunction or unintentionally turned off)
      i) Patients receiving neuromuscular blocking agents.
   b) Patients with repeated airway manipulations
   c) Excessively reduced doses of anesthetic agents delivered to a patient with decreased requirements
      i) Patients with limited cardiovascular reserve (e.g., cardiac failure, sepsis, trauma).
   d) Appropriate doses of anesthetic agents delivered to a patient with relatively increased requirements
      i) Patients may have preexisting tolerance to medications (i.e., opioids).
3. Differential diagnosis
   a) Confusion with other events such as during awake extubation and being present in the post-anesthesia care unit
   b) Implicit memory formation under anesthesia; these are unconscious memories and would not be reported by the patient.

4. Management

   Supportive therapy:

   a) A thorough and sympathetic discussion should occur with the patient and family
   b) The patient and family should be given a complete explanation of how awareness may have occurred (e.g., low blood pressure due to hemodynamic instability)
   c) Psychological counseling should be offered
   d) System-level processes should be addressed when appropriate (e.g., anesthesia machine maintenance).

5. Prevention

   a) Identify high-risk patients in advance (i.e., high-risk procedures, previous awareness history)
   b) Perform preoperative equipment checks to assure appropriate delivery of anesthetic agents
   c) Consider administration of supplemental medications (e.g., midazolam)
   d) Minimize the use of neuromuscular blocking agents
   e) Consider the use of processed EEG monitors
   f) Consider discussing the risk for awareness during the preoperative evaluation
   g) Consider the use of vasoactive medications (e.g., dopamine) when necessary to increase the dosing of anesthetic medications (i.e., to deliver > 1 MAC of volatile agent).

Further reading

Gregory GA, Andropoulos DB. *Gregory's Pediatric Anesthesia*, 5th edition. Hoboken: Wiley-Blackwell, 2012; 290–4.

Miller RD. *Miller's Anesthesia*, 7th edition. Philadelphia: Churchill Livingstone, 2010; 2809–18.

Part D Neurologic

Chapter 61

Peripheral nerve injury

Vidya Chidambaran and Senthilkumar Sadhasivam

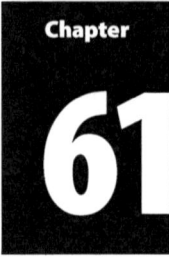

1. Presentation

   Peripheral nerve injury (PNI) has an incidence of 0.03 to 1.4% and is the second most common reason for litigation against anesthetists. Commonly injured nerves include the ulnar nerve (28%), brachial plexus (20%), and the lumbosacral roots (16%). Characteristics suggestive of an anesthesia-associated PNI include:

   a) Presentation immediately after recovery from anesthesia or perhaps several days later
   b) Sensory deficits include loss of tactile, pain, thermal, vibration
   c) Reports of anesthesia, hypoesthesia, paresthesia, hyperesthesia, allodynia, neuralgia
   d) Motor symptoms including paresis or even paralysis
   e) Autonomic dysfunction and sympathetic dystrophy including muscle wasting, joint stiffening, and bone demineralization.

2. Risk factors

   a) Nerve injury: preoperative chemotherapy with vinca alkaloids, methotrexate or cisplatin, systemic diseases such as diabetes mellitus, rheumatoid arthritis, collagen vascular diseases and presence of tumor surrounding the nerve
   b) Intraoperative: prolonged duration of tourniquet use, positioning with nerve compression or stretching
   c) Perioperative hypovolemia or hypotension
   d) Regional anesthesia procedures such as epidurals and peripheral nerve blocks.

3. Differential diagnosis

   a) Neurologic events (thromboembolic events)
   b) Electrolyte disturbances (hypocalcemia, hypermagnesemia)
   c) Psychiatric disorders (conversion disorders)
   d) Musculoskeletal disorders (contusion, sprain).

4. Pathophysiology

   a) Three stages of PNI have been described: initial demyelination, paranodal demyelination, and eventually axonal degeneration
   b) Neurapraxia involves only local myelin injury which results in temporary loss of sensory and motor function

---

Handbook of Critical Incidents and Essential Topics in Pediatric Anesthesiology, ed. David A. Young and Olutoyin A. Olutoye. Published by Cambridge University Press. © Cambridge University Press 2015.

c) Axonotmesis is disruption of axonal continuity and Wallerian degeneration, but the epineurium is preserved
   d) Neurotmesis is severance of the entire nerve
   e) Sunderland classified nerve injury as types 1 to 5, based on functional loss. While type 1 and type 5 correspond to neurapraxia and neurotmesis stages of Seddon respectively, types 2–4 represent worsening function within axonotmesis.
5. Management
   a) Review preoperative evaluation for preexisting neurologic injuries and associated conditions (diabetes mellitus, sickle cell disease)
   b) Review intraoperative records for positioning notes, development of intraoperative hypotension, use of a tourniquet, and for the performance of regional anesthesia
   c) Perform a detailed neurovascular examination
   d) Identify actionable factors, (e.g., bivalving a tight cast, evacuation of hematoma, positioning to reduce edema, and padding at pressure sites)
   e) In case of severe injury, consult neurologist/neurosurgeon, and possibly consult physical medicine and rehabilitation services
   f) Nerve conduction velocity tests and electromyography can be considered to differentiate demyelinating from degenerative disorders, and to monitor progress of recovery of nerve function. These studies are recommended a few weeks after surgery as the degenerative process takes about 14 days and studies done too early would be misleading (or suggest a preexisting injury)
   g) Prognosis is generally good for types 1 and 2; significant recovery typically occurs over weeks or months. Disruption of endoneurium, axonal misdirection, and intraneural scarring in types 3 and 4 may necessitate surgery, while nerve repair is necessary with guarded prognosis for type 5 nerve injuries. The rate of regeneration varies from 1 to 4 mm/day followed by remyelination. If no regeneration occurs by 1.5 years, the prognosis is poor since the Schwann cells have most likely been replaced by fibrous tissue
   h) Provide supportive care; consider use of nerve stabilizers such as gabapentin, and chronic pain consult for neuropathy.
6. Prevention
   a) Diligent preoperative risk assessment
   b) Avoid intraoperative detrimental factors such as hypotension and prolonged tourniquet times. Recommended tourniquet guidelines – inflation pressure 100 mmHg above systolic blood pressure, inflation time ≤ 120 minutes, deflation time ≥ 30 minutes
   c) Careful positioning of every patient, utilizing proper padding and prevention of stretching to the nerves
   d) Vigilant postoperative monitoring of neurological function especially after regional analgesia.

Further reading

Chidambaran V, Mahmoud M, Sadhasivam S. Risk for peroneal nerve injury after femur osteosarcoma resection: is regional analgesia safe? *J Clin Anesth*. 2013; 25(1):76–8. Epub 2012/12/19.

Davis PJ, Cladis FP, Motoyama EK. *Smith's Anesthesia for Infants and Children*, 8th edition. Philadelphia: Elsevier Mosby, 2011; 458–60.

Jacob AK, Mantilla CB, Sviggum HP, Schroeder DR, Pagnano MW, Hebl JR. Perioperative nerve injury after total knee arthroplasty: regional anesthesia risk during a 20-year cohort study. *Anesthesiology*. 2011; 114(2):311–17. Epub 2011/01/18.

Lalkhen AG, Bhatia K. Perioperative peripheral nerve injuries. *Contin Educ Anesth Crit Care Pain*. 2012; 12:38–42.

Pollock M. Nerve regeneration. *Curr Opin Neurol*. 1995; 8(5):354–8. Epub 1995/10/01.

Seddon HJ. A classification of nerve injuries. *Br Med J*. 1942; 2(4260):237–9. Epub 1942/08/29.

Part D Neurologic

Chapter 62 Seizure

Yang Liu

1. Presentation
   a) Most common neurologic disorder of childhood
   b) Paroxysmal electrical discharge of neurons resulting in altered function or behavior
   c) Status epilepticus: continuous seizure activity lasting > 5–30 minutes or multiple seizures without a return to a baseline level of consciousness lasting > 5 minutes
   d) Focal or partial seizures
      i) Simple partial seizure: abnormal motor activity but consciousness not impaired
      ii) Complex partial seizure: abnormal motor activity accompanied by aura (abnormal perception or hallucination).
   e) Generalized seizures: consciousness is always impaired
      i) Generalized tonic-clonic seizure: succession of muscle contractions followed by sudden relaxation
      ii) Absence seizure: sudden interruption of activities with blank stare and unresponsiveness (< 30 seconds)
      iii) Atonic seizures: a sudden loss of muscle activity (drop attacks)
      iv) Myoclonic seizures: rapid, jerking contractions of isolated muscles or group of muscles
      v) Clinical constellation of one or more seizure types may be observed
      vi) Febrile seizures.
2. Risk factors
   a) Low birth weight infants
   b) Birth asphyxia
   c) Intracranial hemorrhage
   d) Brain infections
   e) Traumatic brain injury
   f) Brain tumors
   g) Metabolic conditions (hypoglycemia, hypoxia, hypomagnesemia, hypocalcemia, hypercarbia, inborn errors of metabolism)
   h) Poisoning/drug toxicity
   i) Drugs which lower the seizure threshold (meperidine)

Handbook of Critical Incidents and Essential Topics in Pediatric Anesthesiology, ed. David A. Young and Olutoyin A. Olutoye. Published by Cambridge University Press. © Cambridge University Press 2015.

j) Interruption in usual epileptic medication regimen
   k) Syndromes: Lennox–Gastaut syndrome, West syndrome.
3. Differential diagnosis
   See Risk factors.
4. Pathophysiology
   a) Disruption in the balance between excitatory and inhibitory currents in the brain produces abnormal and increased neuronal discharges which results in seizures, tachycardia, hypertension and hyperglycemia
   b) Convulsions result in difficulty maintaining a patent airway, hypoxemia, hypercarbia, and potential for patient injury
   c) Prolonged seizure activity may cause lactic acidosis, rhabdomyolysis, hyperkalemia, hyperthermia and hypoglycemia.
5. Management
   a) Acute management
      i) Support airway and breathing; positive pressure ventilation and tracheal intubation may be required
      ii) Termination of seizure activity: intravenous propofol (1–2 mg/kg), benzodiazepines (midazolam or diazepam), anticonvulsant medications
      iii) Physically support patients during event to reduce occurrence of self-injury.
   b) Long-term management
      i) Medical antiepileptic therapy
      ii) Surgical interventions (reserved for patients with intractable seizures)
         (1) Implantation of vagus nerve stimulator
         (2) Surgical resection of epileptic foci
         (3) MRI-guided stereotactic laser ablation (SLA).
5. Prevention
   a) Consider prophylactic antiepileptic medications following head injury or brain surgery
   b) Continue all anticonvulsant therapy in the perioperative period
   c) Prompt correction of abnormal electrolytes or metabolic conditions
   d) Avoid administration of glucose-containing solutions to children on ketogenic diet (lowers ketone levels and reduces seizure threshold).

Further reading

Blumstein MD, Fredman MJ. Childhood seizures. *Emerg Med Clin North Am.* 2007; 25(4):1061–86.

Friedman MJ, Sharieff GQ. Seizures in children. *Pediatr Clin North Am.* 2006; 53: 257–77.

Gregory GA, Andropoulos DB. *Gregory's Pediatric Anesthesia*, 5th edition. Hoboken: Wiley-Blackwell, 2012; 280–1, 560.

Part D Neurologic

Chapter 63

Stroke

Yang Liu

1. Presentation
    a) The risk of stroke (cerebrovascular accident) in children is greatest in the first year of life
    b) Mortality in children is 10–25%; 25% will have a recurrence
    c) Sixty percent of pediatric survivors will suffer permanent neurologic deficits (commonly hemiparesis or hemiplegia)
    d) Majority of signs and symptoms are nonspecific:
        i) Hemiparesis or focal neurological deficit
        ii) Change in mental status
        iii) Seizure
        iv) Headaches
        v) Speech disorder
        vi) Vision impairment
        vii) Behavior and personality changes.
2. Risk factors
    a) Congenital or acquired heart disorders
    b) Hematologic conditions:
        i) Sickle cell disease (SCD)
        ii) Prothrombotic disorders (e.g., deficiency of protein C and S)
        iii) Factor VII and VIII deficiencies causing hemorrhagic stroke.
    c) Infections (e.g., meningitis and encephalitis)
    d) Head trauma
    e) Vascular disorders (e.g., arteriovenous malformations, Moyamoya disease and vasculitis)
    f) Maternal related disease (e.g., infection, premature rupture of membranes and preeclampsia)
    g) Syndromic and metabolic disorders (Marfan syndrome, tuberous sclerosis, familial lipoprotein disorders).

3. Differential diagnosis
   a) Migraines
   b) Focal seizures
   c) Intracranial tumor
   d) Central nervous system infection
   e) Metabolic abnormalities
      i) Hypoglycemia
      ii) Mitochondrial encephalomyopathy, lactic acidosis, and stroke-like episodes (MELAS syndrome).
4. Pathophysiology
   The pathophysiology is dependent on the specific etiology of the stroke.
5. Management
   a) Specific treatment of the precipitating cause
   b) Supportive care:
      i) Maintain adequate hydration and normal body temperature
      ii) Maintain blood glucose within normal levels
      iii) Employ maneuvers to decrease intracranial pressure: head elevation, hyperventilation, diuresis
      iv) Consider anticonvulsant therapy
      v) Control high blood pressure (gradual decrease of elevated blood pressure is recommended).
   c) Hemorrhagic stroke:
      i) Correct coagulation deficiencies
      ii) Consider surgical evacuation which may prevent deterioration from increased mass effect.
   d) Acute ischemic stroke: consider anticoagulation with low molecular weight heparin or heparin infusion
   e) Sickle cell induced cerebral ischemic infarction:
      i) Hydration
      ii) Emergency exchange transfusion to reduce the level of circulating hemoglobin S to < 30% and to maintain a hemoglobin value > 10 g/dL.
   f) Anesthetic management for patients with stroke or risk factors will vary on a case-by-case basis according to the etiology and patient's clinical status
   g) Thrombolytic therapy with t-PA (tissue plasminogen activator) is generally not recommended for treating young children with stroke
   h) Avoidance of succinylcholine is recommended
   i) Meticulous care to avoid entrainment of air into intravenous lines is strongly recommended especially in patients with congenital heart disease.
6. Prevention
   a) Preventing a first stroke may be difficult due to undiagnosed at-risk conditions
   b) Identification of risk factors is important in reducing the development of stroke in at-risk patients

c) Acute ischemic stroke: anticoagulation with low molecular weight heparin may reduce subsequent events
d) Sickle cell disease:
   i) Maintain adequate hydration, normothermia, and oxygenation
   ii) Consider preoperative red blood cell transfusion or exchange blood transfusion.
e) Coagulation defects: ensure adequate factor replacement
f) Cardiac defects: ensure adequate anticoagulation when indicated to prevent thrombosis or embolic events.

Further reading

American Heart Association and American Stroke Association. Knowing No Bounds: Stroke in infants, children, and youth. Retrieved from www.strokeassociation.org/idc/groups/heart-public/@wcm/@adv/documents/downloadable/ucm_302255.pdf (accessed September 15, 2013).

Gregory GA, Andropoulos DB. *Gregory's Pediatric Anesthesia*, 5th edition. Hoboken: Wiley-Blackwell, 2012; 238, 984.

Stroke Association. Childhood stroke. Retrieved from www.stroke.org.uk/sites/default/files/Childhood%20stroke.pdf (accessed September 15, 2013).

Tsze DS, Valente JH. Pediatric stroke: A review. *Emerg Med Int.* 2011; 2011:734506.

Part E: Equipment

Chapter 64: Anesthesia machine failure

Carlos Rodriguez

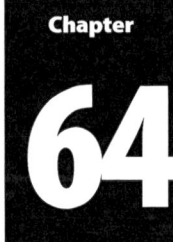

1. Presentation
   a) Unable to adequately ventilate and provide general anesthesia. Chest rise does not occur despite the ventilator being powered on
      i) With an ascending bellows, the bellows will not rise. Low pressure alarm monitors may be activated.
   b) Complete electrical failure of the machine. The machine cannot be turned on or suddenly turns off during the intraoperative phase.
2. Differential diagnosis
   a) Disconnection distal to the anesthesia machine
   b) Large leak located within the anesthesia machine or distal to the anesthesia machine
   c) Occlusion or obstruction distal to the anesthesia machine
   d) Malfunctioning ventilator relief valve (closed or partially closed)
   e) Incompetent ventilator relief valve
   f) Complete power failure to individual operating room or entire hospital
   g) Electrical failure to anesthesia machine such as activated circuit breaker or failure of anesthesia machine backup battery
   h) Inappropriate ventilator settings selected.
3. Management
   a) If unable to ventilate the patient, call for help and immediately provide ventilation from an external source such as a portable oxygen tank
   b) Verify that the monitoring of vital signs is possible; if not, transition to a battery-powered monitor
   c) Examine the breathing circuit to detect any disconnections from the anesthesia machine to the circuit and circuit to the airway device
   d) Confirm that airway device is appropriated placed and that a large airway leak from low cuff volumes is not present
   e) Examine the airway device and breathing circuit to confirm lack of kinking
   f) Pass a suction catheter to confirm patency of the airway device
   g) Verify appropriate mechanical ventilator settings are programmed into the anesthesia machine

---

Handbook of Critical Incidents and Essential Topics in Pediatric Anesthesiology, ed. David A. Young and Olutoyin A. Olutoye. Published by Cambridge University Press. © Cambridge University Press 2015.

h) Consider changing the breathing circuit and reevaluate for leaks
i) If power is present in the operating room, consider rebooting the anesthesia machine and plugging the machine into a different outlet
j) If power is not present in the operating room, continue to use battery-powered monitor and external sources of ventilation until surgical procedure can be promptly completed.

4. Prevention
   a) Perform a thorough anesthesia machine check daily
   b) Verify that appropriate backup equipment is immediately available (battery-powered monitor, external oxygen source)
   c) Perform an appropriate machine check before starting every case
   d) Vigilance by the anesthesiologist to detect audible alarms, excessive leaks, and requirement for anesthesia machine to utilize backup battery
   e) Regularly check the breathing circuit to verify that all connections are tight and secure
   f) Routinely activate low pressure alarms to appropriately alert the user to a possible disconnect
   g) Utilize the exhaled carbon dioxide monitor to have additional redundancy in the detection of a possible system leak
   h) Ensure that the anesthesia machine has a charged backup battery system.

Further reading

Davis PJ, Cladis FP, Motoyama EK. *Smith's Anesthesia for Infants and Children*, 8th edition. Philadelphia: Elsevier Mosby, 2011; 297–302.

Miller RD. *Miller's Anesthesia*, 7th edition. Philadelphia: Churchill Livingstone, 2010; 1578–82.

Part E Equipment

Chapter 65

Line isolation monitor activation

Stephen Robert Hays

1. Presentation
   a) Electrical shock
      i) Macroshock: high voltage/current anywhere in body
      ii) Microshock: low voltage/current directly delivered to the heart
      iii) Line isolation monitor does not protect against microshock.
   b) Electrical power
      i) Grounded circuit: single contact may shock
      ii) Isolated circuit: single contact will not shock.
   c) Electrical equipment
      i) Non-grounded: potential for significant shock with fault
      ii) Grounded: reduced severity of shock with fault.
2. Risk factors
   a) Electrical power supplied to the operating room (OR) is typically isolated and not grounded (isolated power supply, IPS)
   b) Electrical equipment in the OR is typically grounded
   c) Line isolation monitor (LIM) detects potential leakage current from IPS to ground
   d) Non-grounded equipment will not activate LIM
   e) LIM activation does not interrupt circuit: equipment remains powered; activation only alerts that leakage threshold has been exceeded.
3. Differential diagnosis
   a) First-generation (static) LIM
      i) Cannot detect balanced fault (equal in both lines of IPS)
      ii) Cannot detect loss of ground to monitor
      iii) Alarm activation at 2 mA: results in frequent false alarms.
   b) Second-generation (dynamic) LIM
      i) Detect balanced fault, possible interference with physiologic monitoring
      ii) Cannot detect loss of ground to monitor
      iii) Alarm activation at 2 mA: results in frequent false alarms.
   c) Third-generation (current) LIM
      i) Detects balanced fault, no interference with physiologic monitoring

---

Handbook of Critical Incidents and Essential Topics in Pediatric Anesthesiology, ed. David A. Young and Olutoyin A. Olutoye. Published by Cambridge University Press. © Cambridge University Press 2015.

ii) Detects loss of ground to monitor
iii) Alarm activation at 5 mA: results in fewer false alarms.
4. Pathophysiology
   a) Single equipment fault
      i) Grounded electrical equipment develops fault
      ii) Increased potential current from IPS to ground, generally > 5 mA
      iii) LIM activation: IPS no longer isolated, potential for shock only with second fault.
   b) Excessive equipment
      i) All electrical equipment generates small amounts of leakage current
      ii) Excessive electrical equipment causes total excessive leakage current, generally < 5 mA
      iii) LIM activation: IPS no longer isolated, potential for shock with additional fault.
5. Management
   a) Verify current
      i) < 2 mA: likely false alarm
      ii) 2–5 mA: likely total excessive equipment
      iii) > 5 mA: likely single equipment fault.
   b) Identify equipment causing activation
      i) Usually last item connected causes LIM to activate
      ii) May require sequential disconnection until alarm ceases (and total leakage current reduced under threshold).
   d) Rearrange/repair/replace
      i) Excessive equipment: rearrange outlet selection
      ii) Single equipment fault: repair or replace
      iii) May continue to use equipment: IPS no longer isolated, potential for shock only with additional fault.
6. Prevention
   a) Understand types of electric shock, electric power, electrical equipment
   b) Maintain electrical equipment appropriately
   c) Avoid environmental electrical hazards
   d) Avoid plugging multiple devices into outlets.

Further reading

Courtney NM, McCoy EP, Scolaro RJ, et al. A serious and repeatable electrical hazard--compressed electrical cord and an operating table. *Anaesth Intensive Care.* 2006; 34(3):392–6.

Ehrenwerth J, Eisenkraft JB, Berry JM. *Anesthesia Equipment: Principles and Applications*, 2nd edition. Philadelphia: Saunders Elsevier, 2013; 621–52.

Gregory GA, Andropoulos DB. *Gregory's Pediatric Anesthesia*, 5th edition. Chichester, UK: Wiley-Blackwell, 2012; 934.

Miller RD. *Miller's Anesthesia*, 7th edition. Philadelphia: Churchill Livingstone Elsevier, 2010; 3041–51.

Wills JH, Ehrenwerth J, Rogers D. Electrical injury to a nurse due to conductive fluid in an operating room designated as a dry location. *Anesth Analg.* 2010; 110(6):1647–9.

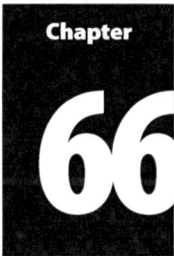

Part E Equipment

Chapter 66

Power failure

Stephen Robert Hays

1. Presentation
   a) In the United States medical facilities generally have two types of power outlets
      i) Conventionally colored (typically white) outlet covers: supplied by external main power
      ii) Red colored outlet covers: supplied by external main power with emergency generator backup.
   b) Partial power failure is more common and typically temporary
      i) Main power failure: emergency generator backup active supplying power to only red outlets.
   c) Complete power failure to all outlets.
2. Risk factors
   a) Localized power failure
      i) Circuit overload, construction, scheduled outage for maintenance
      ii) Affected areas are generally limited
      iii) Power generally available from unaffected areas.
   b) Outside (external to hospital) main power failure
      i) Adverse weather, industrial accident, construction mishap, natural disaster
      ii) Affected areas are typically widespread
      iii) Red outlets are functional only if emergency generator backup active.
   c) Backup emergency generator failure
      i) Scheduled outage, construction mishap, unexpected malfunction to backup generator
      ii) Affected areas potentially widespread, particularly with external main power failure
      iii) All conventional outlets powered if main outside power preserved despite back-up generator failure.
3. Differential diagnosis
   a) Failure of equipment (i.e., faulty power cable, software, fuse)
   b) Failure of structural components in building (i.e., power outlet, circuit breaker).
4. Management
   a) Clear, concise, open communication is essential

Handbook of Critical Incidents and Essential Topics in Pediatric Anesthesiology, ed. David A. Young and Olutoyin A. Olutoye. Published by Cambridge University Press. © Cambridge University Press 2015.

b) Activate local emergency response plan, including specific plan for power failure if available
c) Determine extent and etiology of power failure (i.e., isolated power failure vs. building fire requiring evacuation)
d) Attempt to obtain light: open doors and windows, flashlight, laryngoscope, cell phone, emergency lighting
e) Verify which outlets are still powered (determine if backup power is functional): connect critical equipment to powered outlets
f) Ensure backup battery function is present on anesthesia machine and critical devices (i.e., medication infusion pumps)
g) Employ portable battery-powered, non-electric/manual alternatives as necessary
h) Transport patient elsewhere if feasible and if power failure likely to be prolonged.

5. Management of general anesthesia during a total power failure
   a) Ensure safety of patient
      i) Manual ventilation if ventilator inoperative
      ii) Convert to tanked oxygen if wall supply compromised or nonfunctional; be vigilant for tank supply exhaustion
      iii) Convert monitoring to battery-powered devices if available including use of code cart monitor
      iv) If no devices available, monitor by observation (chest rise, detection of cyanosis), auscultation (breath and heart sounds), and palpation (peripheral and central pulses).
   b) Determine surgical plan options
      i) Wait until power restored
      ii) Abort non-emergent procedure
      iii) Continue surgery
      iv) Transport elsewhere.

6. Prevention
   a) Perform anesthesia machine check prior to initiating every anesthetic
   b) Keep vigilant for institution-wide construction and maintenance
   c) Be aware of impending natural disasters (i.e., hurricane, tornado warning)
   d) Regularly review your institutional emergency response plans
   e) Ensure availability and know location of appropriate emergency supplies and equipment.

Further reading

Carpenter T, Robinson ST. Case reports: response to a partial power failure in the operating room. *Anesth Analg.* 2010; 110(6):1644–6.

Ehrenwerth J, Eisenkraft JB, Berry JM. *Anesthesia Equipment: Principles and Applications*, 2nd edition. Philadelphia: Saunders Elsevier, 2013; 621–52.

Eichhorn JH, Hessel EA 2nd. Electrical power failure in the operating room: a neglected topic in anesthesia safety. *Anesth Analg.* 2010; 110(6):1519–21.

Ivani G, Walker I, Enright A, et al. Safe perioperative pediatric care around the world. *Paediatr Anaesth.* 2012; 22(10):947–51.

Miller RD. *Miller's Anesthesia*, 7th edition. Philadelphia: Churchill Livingstone Elsevier, 2010; 3041–51.

Part F Hematology

Chapter 67: Coagulopathy

Paul A. Stricker

1. Presentation
   a) Abnormal bleeding from a variety of etiologies
   b) May present as abnormal bleeding or bruising associated with apparently minor injuries
   c) May be asymptomatic and first present as abnormal bleeding intraoperatively, or preoperative laboratory testing may give isolated abnormal test results
   d) Diffuse microvascular bleeding in a patient with massive blood loss.
2. Risk factors
   a) Family history of bleeding diathesis
   b) Massive hemorrhage
   c) Anticoagulant administration
   d) Hypothermia
   e) Medications (e.g., ketorolac, aspirin).
3. Differential diagnosis
   a) Congenital coagulopathy
      i) Von Willebrand disesase
      ii) Hemophilia.
   b) Acquired coagulopathy
      i) Anticoagulants
      ii) Dilutional coagulopathy following massive hemorrhage.
   c) Etiology
      i) Abnormal platelet function or quantity
      ii) Abnormal coagulation factor quantity or function
      iii) Complex disturbances involving one or more of the following:
         (1) Hyperfibrinolysis
         (2) Dilution
         (3) Hypothermia
         (4) Disseminated intravascular coagulation.
4. Pathophysiology
   a) Von Willebrand disease
      i) One of the most common bleeding disorders (incidence approximately 1 in 1,000)

Handbook of Critical Incidents and Essential Topics in Pediatric Anesthesiology, ed. David A. Young and Olutoyin A. Olutoye. Published by Cambridge University Press. © Cambridge University Press 2015.

ii) Clinical presentation is that of impaired platelet function
iii) Three variants:
- (1) Type 1: most common; heterozygotic – moderate quantitative von Willebrand factor (vWF) deficiency; typically responsive to Desmopressin acetate (DDAVP)
- (2) Type 2: qualitatively abnormal vWF; DDVAP contraindicated
- (3) Type 3: homozygotic – severe quantitative vWF deficiency.

b) Hemophilia
   i) Hemophilia A: congenital factor VIII deficiency
   ii) Hemophilia B: congenital factor IX deficiency.

c) Acquired bleeding disorders
   i) Anticoagulants: heparin, coumadin, low molecular weight heparin
   ii) Vitamin K defiency: nutritional/fat absorption disorders
   iii) Acquired inhibitors/hemophilia: due to development of antibodies against coagulation factors.

d) Thrombocytopenia
   i) Congenital: rare; most common is Wiscott–Aldrich syndrome
   ii) Acquired: secondary to disease states, sequestration, or dilution
   iii) Platelet function defects.

e) Acute dilutional coagulopathy with massive hemorrhage
   i) Soluble factor based coagulopathy develops at losses of 1–2 blood volumes; treatment is fresh frozen plasma (FFP)
   ii) Thrombocytopenia develops at losses of 2 blood volumes; treatment is platelet transfusion
   iii) Hypofibrinognemia – current ASA guidelines recommend maintaining fibrinogen at ≥ 80–100 mg/dL.

5. Management
   a) Von Willebrand disease/hemophilia: consultation with hematology, replacement of deficient items (e.g., DDAVP, synthetic factor VIII)
   b) Vitamin K administration for vitamin K deficiency
   c) Platelet, FFP, or cryoprecipitate therapy per indications above.

6. Prevention
   a) Identify patients at increased risk for surgical bleeding in the preoperative period
   b) Develop perioperative plan for product administration; patients may require preoperative and postoperative administration of factors.

Further reading

Davis PJ, Cladis FP, Motoyama EK. *Smith's Anesthesia for Infants and Children*, 8th edition. Philadelphia: Elsevier Mosby, 2011; 1150–3.

Hiippala ST, Myllyla GJ, Vahtera EM. Hemostatic factors and replacement of major blood loss with plasma-poor red cell concentrates. *Anesth Analg.* 1995; 81:360–5.

Practice guidelines for perioperative blood transfusion and adjuvant therapies: an updated report by the American Society of Anesthesiologists Task Force on Perioperative Blood Transfusion and Adjuvant Therapies. *Anesthesiology* 2006; 105:198–208.

Part F Hematology

Chapter 68

Massive hemorrhage

Paul A. Stricker

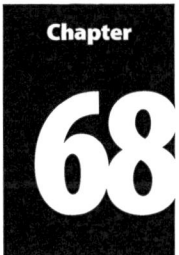

1. Presentation

   Replacement of one or more blood volumes of blood loss. In children, the most common cause of intraoperative cardiac arrest from cardiovascular causes is hypovolemia, usually from massive hemorrhage.

   a) Immediate concerns
      i) Hypovolemia
      ii) Hypotension
      iii) Inadequate oxygen delivery with end-organ dysfunction
      iv) Cardiovascular collapse/cardiac arrest.

   b) Secondary sequelae
      i) Dilutional coagulopathy: develops at losses > 1–2 blood volumes when losses are replaced with crystalloid/colloid
      ii) Thrombocytopenia: typically develops at losses > 2 blood volumes
      iii) Hypofibrinogenemia (< 100 mg/dL): develops at losses > 1–2 blood volumes
      iv) Hyperkalemia due to rapid transfusion of stored packed red blood cells (PRBC)
         (1) Potassium content of stored PRBCs increases in a linear fashion over time
         (2) Irradiation drastically accelerates this process
         (3) Risk factors include rapid administration of large volumes of older PRBCs.
      v) Hypocalcemia (due to citrate toxicity), is more likely to occur during rapid transfusion in the setting of impaired hepatic perfusion or function
      vi) Hypothermia from multiple factors further impairs coagulation.

2. Risk factors

   a) Trauma
   b) Specific operations:
      i) Craniosynostosis
      ii) Spine surgery
      iii) Craniotomy/Neurosurgery
      iv) Cardiac surgery
      v) Liver transplant
      vi) Abdominal procedures (e.g., Wilms tumor).

Handbook of Critical Incidents and Essential Topics in Pediatric Anesthesiology, ed. David A. Young and Olutoyin A. Olutoye. Published by Cambridge University Press. © Cambridge University Press 2015.

c) Preexisting coagulopathy.
3. Pathophysiology

    Ineffective replacement of blood loss results in deficient intravascular volume, coagulation factors, oxygen carrying capacity, and platelets. These events result in the production of lactic acidosis, cardiovascular depression, and coagulopathy which can ultimately result in cardiac arrest.

4. Management

    General guidelines for blood component therapy administration:

    a) PRBCs: Maintain hemoglobin > 7 based on patient and clinical scenario; transfusion of 10 mL/kg is expected to increase hemoglobin count by 3
    b) FFP: Diffuse microvascular bleeding and/or Prothrombin Time (PT) > 2× control; transfusion of 10 mL/kg is expected to increase clotting factors by 30% (which is typically adequate for satisfactory coagulation)
    c) Cryoprecipitate: Maintain fibrinogen > 80–100 mg/dL. Transfusion of 1 bag per 10 kg is expected to increase fibrinogen by 100 mg/dL
    d) Platelets: Maintain > 50,000 or > 100,000 depending on patient and clinical scenario; transfusion of 10 mL/kg is expected to increase platelet count by 50,000 (which is expected to result in satisfactory platelet function)
    e) Recombinant factor VIIa: Rescue measure for hemorrhage/coagulopathy refractory to surgical control and maximal component therapy. Associated with thrombotic complications; use reserved for life-threatening situations where other measures have failed
    f) Surgical: Strongly consider surgical causes and maneuvers to decrease bleeding (direct pressure, packing abdomen, tourniquet, temporarily pausing surgical procedure to allow volume resuscitation).

5. Prevention

    a) Increased vigilance and communication during procedures at risk for severe hemorrhage
    b) Acquire blood products in advance for procedures at risk for severe hemorrhage
    c) Obtain appropriate vascular access for procedures at risk for severe hemorrhage
    d) Understand and become familiar with institutional massive transfusion protocols
    e) Hemostatic resuscitation approach in which higher FFP:PRBC and platelet transfusion are aimed at preventing dilutional coagulopathy
    f) Antifibrinolytic agents may be considered where massive blood loss is anticipated in absence of contraindications. Supporting evidence varies by clinical scenario with efficacy shown in adult trauma, scoliosis surgery, and craniosynostosis surgery
    g) Hyperkalemia prevented by use of PRBCs stored < 7 days, use of washed PRBCs.

Further reading

Bhananker SM, Ramamoorthy C, Geiduschek JM et al. Anesthesia-related cardiac arrest in children: update from the Pediatric Perioperative Cardiac Arrest Registry. *Anesth Analg.* 2007; 105:344–50.

Brown KA, Bissonnette B, McIntyre B. Hyperkalaemia during rapid blood transfusion and hypovolaemic cardiac arrest in children. *Can J Anaesth.* 1990; 37:747–54.

Cote CJ, Liu LM, Szyfelbein SK et al. Changes in serial platelet counts following massive blood transfusion in pediatric patients. *Anesthesiology* 1985; 62:197–201.

Hiippala ST, Myllyla GJ, Vahtera EM. Hemostatic factors and replacement of major blood loss with plasma-poor red cell concentrates. *Anesth Analg.* 1995; 81:360–5.

Practice guidelines for perioperative blood transfusion and adjuvant therapies: an updated report by the American Society of Anesthesiologists Task Force on Perioperative Blood Transfusion and Adjuvant Therapies. *Anesthesiology* 2006; 105:198–208.

Part F Hematology

Chapter 69 Sickle cell crisis

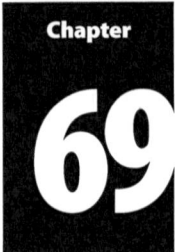

Tae W. Kim

1. Presentation
   a) Sickle cell disease – incidence 1:375 in African-Americans
   b) Moderate to severe anemia, hemoglobin typically 5–9 g/dL
   c) Vaso-occlusive crisis: sickle cells are predisposed to thrombosis of vessels resulting in ischemia, pain, necrosis, and end-organ damage
   d) Splenic sequestration: trapping of sickle cells causes acute, precipitous fall in hemoglobin levels resulting in possible hypovolemic shock
   e) Aplastic anemia: worsening of baseline anemia triggered by parvovirus B19 infection
   f) Hemolytic anemia: accelerated hemolysis associated with G6PD deficiency
   g) Acute chest syndrome: respiratory symptoms such as hypoxemia, cough, dyspnea, fever, chest pain.

2. Risk factors
   a) Blood type: SS, Sβthal, SC
   b) African, Mediterranean, Indian, and Middle Eastern descents
   c) Infection, dehydration, acidosis, hypothermia, stress.

3. Differential diagnosis
   a) Leukemia
   b) Aplastic anemia
   c) Autoimmune disorder
   d) Osteomyelitis/avascular necrosis of femoral head
   e) Primary pulmonary or cardiac etiologies for chest pain/respiratory distress
   f) Acute abdomen.

4. Pathophysiology
   a) Single nucleotide mutation of the β-globin gene on chromosome 11
   b) Substitution of valine for glutamic acid at position 6 – hemoglobin S
   c) Substitution of lysine for glutamic acid at position 6 – hemoglobin C
   d) Sickle hemoglobin susceptible to forming tactoids (spindle shaped red blood cells) when exposed to risk factors (e.g., hypoxia, dehydration, acidosis)
   e) Sickled red blood cells interact with vascular endothelium resulting in activation of inflammatory pathways and coagulation cascade resulting in tissue ischemia and infarction. Cell membrane fragility occurs from repeated transformation from normal state to sickle state as RBC traverses the circulatory system

Handbook of Critical Incidents and Essential Topics in Pediatric Anesthesiology, ed. David A. Young and Olutoyin A. Olutoye. Published by Cambridge University Press. © Cambridge University Press 2015.

f) Cell lysis results in release of hemoglobin (a nitric oxide scavenger) and iron (an irritant) to vascular endothelium
g) Life span of sickle cell much less (5–15 days) than a regular RBC (120 days)
h) Autosplenectomy from recurrent infarction of spleen occurs typically by age 7
i) Cerebral vasculopathy resulting in Moyamoya syndrome and risk for cerebrovascular accident occurs at increased frequency
j) Cardiopulmonary disease – possible development of pulmonary hypertension and pneumonia
k) Renal insufficiency/end-stage renal disease
l) Liver disease/failure – cholelithiasis/cholecystitis.

5. Management
   a) No evidence exists for superiority of any anesthesia technique
   b) Blood transfusion recommended prior to moderate to high-risk surgery or procedures: (intraabdominal, intrathoracic, intracranial)
   c) No transfusion required for minimal-risk surgery or procedures (e.g., examination under anesthesia, ear tubes, diagnostic studies)
   d) Transfusion targets: exchange: Hgb 10 g/dL, HgbS ≤ 30%, simple transfusion: Hgb 10 g/dL
   e) No superiority of exchange transfusion vs. simple transfusion
   f) Maintain normovolemia and normothermia
   g) Pain management – priority to have effective perioperative pain control; increased tolerance to opioids may be present
   h) Supplemental oxygen and intravenous fluids have been recommended in the preoperative and postoperative periods.

6. Prevention
   a) No technique is superior in prevention
   b) Preoperative identification of patients with SCD; no additional therapies required for patients only with sickle cell trait (8% of African-American population)
   c) Supplemental oxygen
   d) Adequate fluid hydration
   e) Normothermia
   f) Effective pain control including regional anesthesia when appropriate
   g) Blood transfusions as indicated.

Further reading

Coté CJ, Lerman J, Anderson BJ. *Coté and Lerman's A Practice of Anesthesia for Infants and Children,* 5th edition. Philadelphia, PA: Elsevier, 2013; 183–7.

Davis PJ, Cladis FP, Motoyama EK. *Smith's Anesthesia for Infants and Children,* 8th edition. Philadelphia: Elsevier Mosby, 2011; 1130–7.

Dobson SR, Holden KR, Nietert PJ, et al. Moyamoya syndrome in childhood sickle cell disease: a predictive factor for recurrent cerebrovascular events. *Blood.* 2002; 99(9):3144–50.

Firth PG, Head CA. Sickle cell disease and anesthesia. *Anesthesiology.* 2004; 101(3):766–85.

Howard J, Malfroy M, Llewelyn C, et al. The Transfusion Alternatives Preoperatively in Sickle Cell Disease (TAPS) study: a randomized, controlled, multicentre clinical trial. *Lancet* 2013; 381:930–8.

Part F — Hematology

Chapter 70

Transfusion reaction

Tae W. Kim

1. Presentation/epidemiology
   a) Transfusion-related fatalities estimated at 12.5 deaths per year
   b) Life-threatening transfusion reaction estimated at 1:139,908 units
   c) Febrile non-hemolytic transfusion reactions estimated at 2%
   d) Transfusion-related acute lung injury (TRALI) estimated at 0.81 per 10,000 transfused blood components and is more common after plasma-rich components such as fresh frozen plasma (FFP); presents as respiratory compromise and can have a similar presentation and management as acute respiratory distress syndrome (ARDS)
   e) Transfusion-associated circulatory overload (TACO) – development of cardiogenic pulmonary edema; may require cardiopulmonary support
   f) Transfusion reactions can be categorized by timeframe of presentation: acute (< 24 h) vs. delayed (> 24 h), the presence of an immune-mediated response and if a hemolytic reaction has occurred
      i) Types of immune-mediated responses include: hemolytic (ABO incompatibility), febrile non-hemolytic, anaphylactic, transfusion-related acute lung injury, graft vs. host, post transfusion purpura.
   g) Patients may exhibit: tachycardia, hypotension, hemoglobinuria, oozing, fever, chills, urticaria, bronchospasm; many signs/symptoms may be difficult to identify under general anesthesia.

2. Risk factors
   a) Prior blood transfusions or pregnancy leading to alloimmunization
   b) Storage temperature above 20–24°C
      i) Platelet transfusion – leading cause of death due to bacterial contamination.
   c) Estimated risk for acquiring the following infectious diseases:
      i) HIV – 1:2,300,000
      ii) HCV – 1:1,800,000
      iii) HBV – 1:350,000
      iv) Undetectable: Malaria, Chagas disease, variant Creutzfeldt-Jakob disease.
   d) Clerical errors, administration errors (hemolytic ABO incompatibility)
   e) Preexisting immunosuppression.

Handbook of Critical Incidents and Essential Topics in Pediatric Anesthesiology, ed. David A. Young and Olutoyin A. Olutoye. Published by Cambridge University Press. © Cambridge University Press 2015.

3. Differential diagnosis
   a) Hypersensitivity reactions, medications
   b) Anaphylaxis – medications, contrast, latex
   c) Hemolytic anemia
   d) Pulmonary edema, cardiogenic
   e) Septic shock
   f) Sudden cardiac death.
4. Pathophysiology
   a) Hemolytic reactions
      i) IgM and/or IgG antibody with complement activation
      ii) Release of bradykinin – fever, hypotension
      iii) Release of histamine and serotonin – bronchospasm
      iv) Coagulopathy development in 30–50%.
   b) Non-hemolytic reactions
      i) Release of cytokines from leukocytes (white blood cells)
      ii) Most common with platelet transfusions.
5. Management
   a) Immediately stop administration of product if transfusion reaction is present or suspected
   b) Alert surgeon, halt surgery if indicated
   c) Check labels, forms, and identification for possible clerical errors
   d) Send remaining blood product and new blood specimen from patient to the blood bank for analysis
   e) Consider blood cultures if bacterial contamination suspected
   f) Consider O negative blood if emergency transfusion is required
   g) Contact blood bank/transfusion medicine physician for consultation
   h) Maintain brisk diuresis if hemoglobinuria is present or suspected
   i) Administer intravenous acetaminophen, steroids, and/or diphenhydramine for supportive care
   j) Administer vasopressors (e.g., epinephrine) as indicated for circulatory support
   k) Consider diuretics for volume overload
   l) Consider admission to the intensive care unit for continued perioperative management.
6. Prevention
   a) Check often for signs/symptoms of possible reaction during and after transfusion of all blood products
   b) Check ABO compatibility prior to administration of blood products
   c) Check for history of previous transfusion reactions
   d) Consider blood conservation strategies: autologous blood donation, erythropoietin, cell saver, meticulous surgical hemostasis, induced hypotension, hypervolemic hemodilution

e) Consider pretreatment for febrile or allergic non-hemolytic transfusion reactions: acetaminophen, diphenhydramine, and steroids.

Further reading

American Society of Anesthesiologists Task Force on Perioperative Blood Transfusion and Adjuvant Therapies. Practice guidelines for perioperative blood transfusion and adjuvant therapies: an updated report by the American Society of Anesthesiologists Task Force on Perioperative Blood Transfusion and Adjuvant Therapies. *Anesthesiology.* 2006; 105(1):198–208.

Barash PG. *Clinical Anesthesia*, 7th edition. Philadelphia: Wolters Kluwer/Lippincott Williams & Wilkins, 2013; 408–44.

Carson JL, Grossman BJ, Kleinman S, et al. Red blood cell transfusion: a clinical practice guideline from the AABB. *Ann Intern Med.* 2012; 157(1):49–58.

Gregory GA, Andropoulos DB. *Gregory's Pediatric Anesthesia*, 5th edition. Hoboken: Wiley-Blackwell, 2012; 224–54.

Part G Renal

Chapter 71 Oliguria

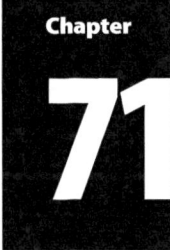

Amy Graham-Carlson

1. Presentation
   a) Urine output < 0.5 mL/kg/hr
   b) Variable volume status depending on underlying cause
   c) Signs and symptoms include tachycardia, dizziness, polydipsia, weight loss or gain, hypertension or hypotension, edema, pelvic pain.
2. Risk factors
   Prerenal, renal or post-renal etiologies
   a) Prerenal (most common cause of oliguria)
      i) Relative hypovolemia (prolonged fasting, hemorrhage)
      ii) Diarrhea and vomiting
      iii) Renal losses: salt wasting, osmotic diuresis, syndrome of inappropriate antidiuretic hormone (SIADH)
      iv) Third space losses: sepsis, liver failure, capillary leak
      v) Shock: anaphylaxis, septic, hypovolemic or cardiogenic
      vi) Congenital or acquired heart disease with reduced cardiac output.
   b) Renal
      i) Glomerulonephritis
      ii) Acute tubular necrosis
      iii) Nephritis: vascular or interstitial
      iv) Post-renal transplant rejection
      v) Toxins: drugs (e.g., amphotericin, cyclosporine, contrast), hemoglobin, myoglobin.
   c) Post-renal
      i) Vesicoureteral reflux or posterior urethral valves
      ii) Occluded urinary catheter
      iii) Ureteral obstruction (nephrolithiasis, strictures, tumors)
      iv) Rupture or trauma to urinary excretory pathway.
3. Differential diagnosis
   See Risk factors.

Handbook of Critical Incidents and Essential Topics in Pediatric Anesthesiology, ed. David A. Young and Olutoyin A. Olutoye. Published by Cambridge University Press. © Cambridge University Press 2015.

4. Pathophysiology
   a) Prerenal
      i) During hypovolemia and hypoperfusion, kidneys limit water loss to preserve total body fluid and attempt to maintain normovolemia
      ii) Hypovolemia and increased plasma osmolality induce antidiuretic hormone (ADH) formation and release which induces water absorption but reduces urine output.
   b) Renal: direct renal parenchymal impairment results in reduced glomerular permeability, leakage of filtrate from damaged renal tubules, intratubular obstruction, extensive loss of nephrons, and high resistance in afferent vessels
   c) Post-renal: obstruction to outflow of urine output.
5. Management
   a) Prerenal
      i) Correct hypovolemia with crystalloid bolus 20 mL/kg or packed red blood cells if indicated by significant anemia
      ii) Consider administration of diuretics to stimulate urine production after correction of hypovolemia/hypoperfusion
      iii) Consider blood pressure support with vasopressors during fluid resuscitation if indicated.
   b) Renal
      i) Supportive; remove offending agent(s) if toxic agent/medication is identified
      ii) Correct electrolyte disturbances (e.g., hypercalcemia).
   c) Post-renal
      i) Consider flushing, repositioning or reinsertion of urinary catheter
      ii) Surgery to repair outflow tract if traumatic injury is precipitating factor.
6. Prevention
   a) Maintain increased vigilance of urine output, especially during complex cases and in patients with impaired renal function
   b) Prerenal: maintain adequate renal perfusion with volume and blood pressure support
   c) Renal: monitor for signs of impaired renal function in patients receiving medications known to cause renal toxicity or with a history of renal impairment
   d) Post-renal: monitor urinary output and catheter patency; rapid diagnosis and surgical intervention for amenable issues may reduce oliguria from post-renal causes.

Further reading

Albright RC. Acute renal failure: a practical update. *Mayo Clini Proc.* 2001; 76(1):67–74.

Bissonnette B. *Pediatric Anesthesia: Basic Principles – State of the Art – Future.* Shelton, CT: People's Medical Publishing House, 2011; 157–60.

Coté CJ, Lerman J, Anderson BJ. *Coté and Lerman's A Practice of Anesthesia for Infants and Children*, 5th edition. Philadelphia, PA: Elsevier, 2013; 577.

Gregory GA. *Gregory's Pediatric Anesthesia*, 5th edition. Hoboken: Wiley-Blackwell, 2012; 977–80.

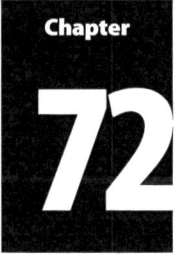

Part G Renal

Chapter 72 Polyuria

Amy Graham-Carlson

1. Presentation
    a) Urine production of > 4 mL/kg/hr
    b) Hypo-, hyper- or normovolemia depending on etiology
    c) May occur along with polydipsia
    d) Hypotension and tachycardia may be present if patient is hypovolemic.
2. Risk factors
    a) Excessive volume resuscitation
    b) Hyperglycemia
    c) Intracranial tumors or craniotomy
    d) Traumatic brain injury
    e) Renal pathology of the distal tubules and collecting ducts
    f) Medications (diuretics, antipsychotics, lithium, caffeine).
3. Differential diagnosis
    a) Excessive hydration: fluid administration that exceeds maintenance, surgical and insensible losses
    b) Diabetes mellitus: hyperglycemia resulting in an osmotic diuresis
    c) Diabetes insipidus (DI): vasopressin challenge test (administration of vasopressin) can distinguish between central or nephrogenic causes:
        i) Central DI: occurs secondary to defect in antidiuretic hormone (ADH) production or transport (responds to vasopressin test)
        ii) Nephrogenic DI: occurs secondary to decreased renal responsiveness to ADH (Decreased urine production is not observed following the vasopressin test).
    d) Cerebral salt wasting syndrome (CSW): urine sodium loss causes osmotic diuresis, hyponatremia (< 130 mEq/L) and dehydration
    e) Drug induced: elicited through medical history (history of diuretic, caffeine, alcohol or antipsychotic use)
    f) Psychogenic polydipsia: history reveals increased fluid intake due to sensation of dry mouth (associated with phenothiazines)
    g) Medullary cystic diseases: decreased ability to concentrate urine.

Handbook of Critical Incidents and Essential Topics in Pediatric Anesthesiology, ed. David A. Young and Olutoyin A. Olutoye. Published by Cambridge University Press. © Cambridge University Press 2015.

4. Pathophysiology
   a) Polyuria may result in dehydration, increased serum osmolality, and features of conditions mentioned above
   b) Specific gravity (SG) of urine may either be normal, decreased or increased depending on etiology:
      i) Central or nephrogenic DI, psychogenic polydipsia: decreased SG (1.001–1.005 g/mL)
      ii) CSW: increased SG (> 1.035) and increased serum osmolality
      iii) Overhydration: normal (1.003–1.035) or decreased SG, decreased serum osmolality.
5. Management
   a) Diabetes insipidus
      i) Central: desmopressin (ADH analog) administration
      ii) Nephrogenic: maintain fluid intake; hydrochlorothiazide administration.
   b) Central salt wasting syndrome: volume repletion with normal or hypertonic saline, correction of hyponatremia; possible mineralocorticoid therapy
   c) Diabetes mellitus: manage hyperglycemia with insulin therapy
   d) Excessive hydration: fluid restriction
   e) Drug induced: avoid offending drug (if possible) & replace losses as deemed appropriate
   f) Psychogenic polydipsia: fluid restriction, behavioral therapy, possible therapy with diuretics and/or angiotensin receptor blockade agents; adjustment of antipsychotic therapy
   g) Medullary cystic diseases: depending on type: provide adequate maintenance, control hypertension, prevent infection, and provide salt replacement for wasting varieties.
6. Prevention
   a) Maintain increased vigilance of urine output and consider evaluation of electrolytes in patients at increased risk (e.g., brain surgery)
   b) Avoid excessive hydration by calculating fluid requirements and having increased awareness for changes to intraoperative fluid demands.

Further reading

Bissonnette B. *Pediatric Anesthesia: Basic Principles – State of the Art – Future.* Shelton, CT: People's Medical Publishing House, 2011; 159–62.

Caletti MG. Pre- and post-treatment urinary tract findings in children with nephrogenic Diabetes Insipidus. *Pediatr Nephrol.* 2013 Dec 14. Epub ahead of print.

Coté CJ, Lerman J, Anderson BJ. *Coté and Lerman's A Practice of Anesthesia for Infants and Children*, 5th edition. Philadelphia, PA: Elsevier, 2013; 533–47.

Kasper D, et al. *Harrison's Principles of Internal Medicine*, 16th edition. New York: McGraw-Hill, 2005; 251–5, 2098.

Section 2
Essential topics

Part A Basic concepts in pediatric anesthesiology

Chapter 73

Development
General concepts
Shakeel Siddiqui

Introduction
- An understanding of the normal pattern of development and physical growth is important for identifying expected milestones or conversely, developmental delay.
- Awareness of milestones:
    - Allows the anesthesiologist to know what to expect during the preoperative evaluation.
    - Tailors perioperative management accordingly.
    - Builds appropriate expectations for the postoperative period.

Development of the newborn to 5 years
See Table 73.1.

Table 73.1 Normal ages for major developmental milestones.

Age	Motor	Language	Adaptive	Social
Neonatal period	Moro reflex Grasp reflex			Visual preference to human faces Fixes on light
1 month	Turns head Momentary head lifts			Smiles Body movements to sound Follows objects with eyes
2 months	Lifts head when prone Tonic neck posture	Gurgles and coos		Notices hand Follows objects to 180 degrees
3 months	Lifts head and chest when prone Loss of Moro reflex Selective withdrawal Early head control	Says aah and ngah		Waves at objects Sustained social contact
4 months	Hands to midline Grasps objects to mouth No head lag in sitting stance	Laughs	Sees object but makes no move to it	Laughs Signs of displeasure Excited at sight of food

Handbook of Critical Incidents and Essential Topics in Pediatric Anesthesiology, ed. David A. Young and Olutoyin A. Olutoye. Published by Cambridge University Press. © Cambridge University Press 2015.

Table 73.1 (cont.)

Age	Motor	Language	Adaptive	Social
5 months	Plays with hands and feet			Recognizes sounds and turns
6 months	Sits with support Rolls over in both directions	Imitates sounds		
7 months	Facial expressions Sits without support Crawls	Nonverbal communication Polysyllabic vowel sounds	Reaches and grasps objects	Displays parental preference Enjoys mirror
8 months	Begins standing with support	Says mama and dada	Transfers objects within hands Searches for hidden objects	Responds to vocal tones
9 months	Stands with support		Grasps objects Object constancy	Uncovers hidden toys
10 months	Stands and walks with support		Grasps objects with thumb and fingers Retrieves dropped objects	Responds to name Waves "bye-bye" Plays "peek a boo"
11 months	Walks with one hand held		Understands "No"	Autonomy emerges
12 months	Rises independently Plays simple ball games	More words than mama and dada	Releases objects to others on request Postural changes to dressing	Understand names of objects Shows interest in pictures
15 months	Walks alone Crawls upstairs	Follows simple commands Names simple objects	Draws a line with crayon	Hugs parents Points to object of need
18 months	Runs rigidly Sits in small chair Explores drawers	10 words average Identifies parts of the body Names pictures	Creates tower of 4 cubes Imitates vertical strokes	Feeds self Protests when soiled Seeks help
24 months	Runs well Walks upstairs Climbs on furniture	Puts 3 words together Half of speech comprehensible	Creates tower of 7 cubes Circular and imitated scribbling	Listens to stories with pictures
30 months	Climbs stairs with alternating feet	Knows full name Identifies self by "I"	Tower of 9 cubes Makes vertical and horizontal lines	Helps put things away Pretend plays
36 months	Stands on one foot momentarily	Knows age and sex Counts 3 objects Repeats sentences of 6 syllables	Tower of 10 cubes Imitates a cross Copies a circle	Plays simple games Washes hands

Table 73.1 (cont.)

Age	Motor	Language	Adaptive	Social
48 months	Hops on one foot Throws ball over head Climbs well Uses scissors	Tells a story Counts up to 4	Bridge of 5 cubes Draws a man of 2–4 parts	Plays with several children Goes to toilet alone
60 months	Skips	Names 4 colors Repeats a sentence of 10 syllables Counts up to 10	Draws a triangle	Dresses and undresses Role playing Asks question and meanings

Adapted from *Nelson Textbook of Pediatrics*, 17th edition, 2004

Early school years

Physical development
- Irregular spurts of physical growth: head growth is only 2–3 cm throughout this period.
- Lymphoid hypertrophy occurs leading to enlarged tonsils and adenoids.
- Muscular growth, coordination, and stamina increases progressively to perform complex movements.

Cognitive and language development
- School-age children increasingly apply the rule of concrete logical thinking.
- Children effortlessly voice their needs, likes, and dislikes.

Social and emotional growth
- Decreased emotional lability with parents and increasing involvement outside of home.
- Despite the move towards independence, school-age children are often nervous during the preoperative period.

Adolescence
- Between the ages of 10 and 19, children undergo rapid changes in body size, shape, physiology, psychology, and social function.
- Hormones and social agendas with transition from childhood to adulthood have effects on developmental course.
- Have greater emotional lability and are more likely to be involved in risk taking behavior (e.g illicit drug use, tobacco use). History should therefore be sought during the preoperative evaluation.
- Increasing sexual activity also occurs during this time, emphasizing the need to consider preoperative pregnancy tests prior to elective surgery.

Development characteristics of adolescence
See Table 73.2.

Table 73.2 Key development characteristics of adolescence.

	Early adolescence	Middle adolescence	Late adolescence
Age (years)	10–13	14–16	17–20
Sexual maturity rating	1–2	3–5	5
Somatic	Secondary sexual characteristics Rapid growth	Height growth, body shape Acne and odor Menarche and spermarche	Slower overall growth
Cognitive and moral	Concrete operation	Emergence of abstract thought Questioning more	Idealism
Self-concept	Preoccupation with changing body Self-consciousness	Concern with attractiveness	Relatively stable body image
Peers	Same sex group conformity	Dating, peer groups less important	Intimacy, possible commitment

Adapted from *Nelson Textbook of Pediatrics,* 17th edition, 2004

Further reading

Gregory GA, Andropoulos DB. *Gregory's Pediatric Anesthesia*, 5th edition. Hoboken: Wiley-Blackwell, 2012.

Part A Basic concepts in pediatric anesthesiology

Chapter 74

Anatomy
General concepts
Shakeel Siddiqui

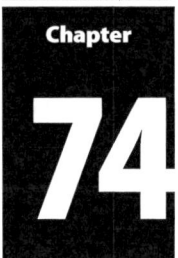

- There are several significant anatomical differences between the infant/child and an adult.
- The anatomical differences in the neonate or child which may impact anesthetic management are discussed below.

Head, neck, chest, and respiratory system
- Neonates and infants have a relatively large head, short neck and a prominent occiput.
- Neonates preferentially breathe through their nose. The narrow nasal passages are easily blocked by secretions and may be traumatized by a nasogastric tube or nasal intubation.
- The tongue is relatively large and occupies a large portion of the mouth; this can contribute to airway obstruction when oropharyngeal muscles relax.
- The larynx is more cephalad and anterior, located at the level of C3–C4. The epiglottis is long and U-shaped.
- The airway is funnel shaped and is narrowest at the level of the cricoid cartilage. Trauma to the airway results in edema; 1 mm of edema can narrow a neonate's airway up to 60% (resistance $\propto 1/radius^4$).
- Adequate placement of the endotracheal tube is approximately 1 cm above the carina in order to prevent endobronchial intubation.
- The neonate and infant have limited respiratory reserve.
- Horizontal ribs limit the ability to increase tidal volume.
- Ventilation is primarily diaphragmatic. Bulky abdominal organs or a stomach filled with air from poor bag mask ventilation can impair respiration.
- The chest wall is significantly more compliant than that of an adult, resulting in lower functional residual capacity (FRC).
- The closing volume is greater than the FRC until 6–8 years of age. This results in an increased tendency for airway closure at end expiration.
- Respiratory muscles develop fatigue more rapidly due to a low percentage of type I muscle fibers in the diaphragm. The number of these fibers increases to the adult level over the first year of life.
- At birth, alveoli are thick walled and account for only 10% of the total number found in adults. Alveoli clusters develop gradually over the first 8 years of life.

Handbook of Critical Incidents and Essential Topics in Pediatric Anesthesiology, ed. David A. Young and Olutoyin A. Olutoye. Published by Cambridge University Press. © Cambridge University Press 2015.

Cardiovascular system

- Decreased contractility of the myocardium causes the ventricles to be less compliant and unable to generate adequate tension during contraction. This limits the amount of stroke volume; cardiac output is therefore rate dependent.
- Vagal parasympathetic tone is predominant, making neonates and infants more prone to bradycardia.
- The ductus arteriosus functionally contracts in the first few days of life and anatomically closes within 2–4 weeks.
- Closure of the foramen ovale is pressure dependent and occurs in the first day of life.
- Transitional or fetal circulation may recur with alterations in atrial pressure, hypoxia, and/or acidosis.

Thermoregulation

- Infants are unable to shiver; metabolism of brown fat is required for non-shivering thermogenesis.
- Brown fat comprises 2–6% of neonatal body weight and is located in small amounts around the scapula, mediastinum, kidneys, and adrenal glands.

Central nervous system

- Head circumference increases markedly during the first postnatal year due to the progressive and rapid growth of the brain. The important relationship of brain and cranium size can be demonstrated on a percentage basis.
- 70% of the adult brain weight is achieved at 18 months, 80% at 3 years, 90% at 5–8 years; and approximately 95% by the 10th year.
- The cerebral vessels in the preterm infant are thin-walled, fragile, and are therefore prone to intraventricular hemorrhage. Risk of hemorrhage is increased with hypoxia, hypercarbia, hypernatremia, low hematocrit, awake airway manipulation, rapid bicarbonate administration, as well as fluctuations in blood pressure and cerebral blood flow.
- The cranium of the infant and child is pliable due to the segmental development and arrangement of the skull bones. The individual bones are flexible and extremely thin. The skull develops as a loosely joined system of bones formed in the soft tissue matrix surrounding the brain. Junctions between bones (fontanelles) are broad and large.
  - The fontanelles are most obvious in the anterior and posterior skull regions.
  - The posterior fontanelle, between the occipital and parietal bones, closes about 1–3 months after birth but the larger anterior fontanelle, between the frontal and parietal bones, does not close until 12–18 months old.

Further reading

Coté CJ, Lerman J, Anderson BJ. *Coté and Lerman's A Practice of Anesthesia for Infants and Children*, 5th edition. Philadelphia, PA: Elsevier, 2013; 12.

Gregory GA, Andropoulos DB. *Gregory's Pediatric Anesthesia*, 5th edition. Hoboken: Wiley-Blackwell, 2012; 304.

Part A Basic concepts in pediatric anesthesiology

Chapter 75

Anatomy
Airway
Rachel A. Koll and Jacquelyn Morillo-Delerme

Developmental anatomy of the larynx
- Laryngotracheal tube (LTT) develops at 3 weeks gestation from the ventral wall of the foregut.
- LTT grows caudally into the splanchnic mesoderm, dividing into bilateral lung buds.
- Aryepiglottic folds develop from the 4th branchial arch between epiglottis and arytenoid eminence around the 5th week of gestation.
- Incomplete development of these structures results in laryngeal cleft.
- Cricoid and thyroid cartilage develop around 7 weeks of gestation.
- Glottis deepens and true vocal cords align within thyroid laminae.
- Rapid growth of the subglottic airway occurs during the first 2 years of life.
- Cricoid and thyroid cartilages reach adult proportion by 10–12 years, eliminating the angulation of the vocal cords and the narrow subglottic area.

Innervation of airway
- Sensory innervation to the supraglottic region is via the internal branch of the superior laryngeal nerve.
- External branch of the superior laryngeal nerve (SLN) innervates the cricothyroid muscle.
- Sensory innervation to the infraglottic region is via the inferior laryngeal nerve (a branch of the recurrent laryngeal nerve).
- The recurrent laryngeal nerve provides most of the motor innervation of the airway (only the cricothyroid muscle is innervated by the SLN).

Blood supply
Arterial supply to the larynx is via the superior and inferior thyroid arteries.

Major anatomic differences between the pediatric and adult airway
- Tongue: Large in proportion to oral cavity in infants, resulting in development of airway obstruction.

Handbook of Critical Incidents and Essential Topics in Pediatric Anesthesiology, ed. David A. Young and Olutoyin A. Olutoye. Published by Cambridge University Press. © Cambridge University Press 2015.

- Larynx position
    - More cephalad in the neck in younger patients.
        - Preterm: C3 vertebra.
        - Term: C3–4 interspace.
        - Adult: C4–5 interspace.
    - Increased angle between the plane of the tongue and the glottic opening in infants.

Epiglottis
- Narrow, floppy, omega-shaped, and angled away from the axis of the trachea in neonates – may be more challenging to displace with laryngoscope blade.
- Adults: epiglottis is broad, flat, and parallel to axis of trachea.

Vocal cords
- Neonates: anterior attachment is more caudal than the posterior attachment; endotracheal tube may get stuck on the anterior commissure of the vocal cords during endotracheal intubation.
- Adults: vocal cords are perpendicular to the trachea.

Subglottic region
- Traditional teaching is that the cricoid cartilage is the narrowest portion of the airway in infants vs. the glottis in adults.
- Cricoid ring is the only complete ring of cartilage in the trachea and cannot expand.
- Both magnetic resonance imaging (MRI) and pediatric bronchoscopy studies in children reveal a cylindrical, not funnel-shaped, pediatric airway with the narrowest point located at the vocal cords.

Further reading

Coté CJ, Lerman J, Anderson BJ *Coté and Lerman's A Practice of Anesthesia for Infants and Children*, 5th edition. Philadelphia, PA: Elsevier, 2013; 237–43.

Davis PJ. *Smith's Anesthesia for Infants and Children*, 8th edition. Philadelphia: Mosby, Inc., 2011; 350.

Part A Basic concepts in pediatric anesthesiology

Chapter 76

Anatomy
Central
Nitin Wadhwa

Intracranial compartment
Three components make up the intracranial compartment:
- Brain and interstitial fluid (80%).
- Cerebrospinal fluid-CSF (10%).
- Blood (10%).

Vertebral column
- Vertebral bones and fibrocartilaginous vertebral disks make up the spinal column.
- There are 7 cervical, 12 thoracic, 5 lumbar, and 5 fused sacral vertebrae (sacrum).
- Paired spinal nerves exit at each vertebral level.
- The first cervical vertebra (atlas) has unique attachments to the base of the skull and also to the 2nd cervical vertebra (axis).
- All thoracic vertebrae attach to their corresponding rib.
- Each vertebra consists of an anterior vertebral body. A hollow ring is encompassed between each vertebral body and the posterior spinous processes. This ring is bound laterally by the pedicles and transverse processes.
- The pedicles exist between the transverse process and the vertebral body. The pedicles have notches superiorly and inferiorly forming the intervertebral foramina through which paired spinal nerves exit at each level.
- The laminae exist between the transverse processes and the spinous processes.
- Compared to adults, pediatric vertebral laminae are incompletely ossified.
- The vertebrae are interconnected by synovial joints (facet joints) and intervertebral disks.
- The spinal cord sits in the spinal column formed by the hollow rings stacked vertically.
- The order of ligaments which provide structural support to the vertebrae from ventral to dorsal include: anterior longitudinal ligament, posterior longitudinal ligament, ligamentum flavum, interspinous ligament, and supraspinous ligament.

Spinal cord
- In neonates and infants, the conus medullaris is at L3 and the dural sac ends at S3.
- After age 1 and in adults, the conus medullaris is at L1 and the dural sac ends at S1.

Handbook of Critical Incidents and Essential Topics in Pediatric Anesthesiology, ed. David A. Young and Olutoyin A. Olutoye. Published by Cambridge University Press. © Cambridge University Press 2015.

- The spinal cord is covered by three meningeal layers (pia mater, arachnoid mater, dura mater).
- The layers that are traversed in order to reach the spinal cord from dorsal to ventral are: skin → subcutaneous fat → supraspinous ligament → interspinous ligament → ligamentum flavum → epidural space → dura mater → subdural space (a potential space) → arachnoid mater → subarachnoid space (contains CSF) → pia mater → spinal cord.

Caudal space anatomy

- Caudal space exists due to nonfusion of the fifth sacral vertebral arch.
- This nonfusion creates the sacral hiatus which provides the landmark for performing a caudal block.
- The sacral cornua, posterior superior iliac spines, and the coccyx form the other landmarks around the sacral hiatus.
- The caudal space exists beneath the sacrococcygeal ligament.
- This space may become more difficult to access in children older than 6 years.
- Compared to adults, neonates have a narrower and flatter sacrum which allows for a more direct approach to the dural sac from the caudal space.

Epidural space anatomy

- The epidural space is encompassed between the ligamentum flavum and the dura mater.
- Compared to adults, the ligamentum flavum is thinner and less dense in neonates and children.
- The intercristal line (Tuffier's line) – the line drawn between the highest points of the iliac crest, is the preferred landmark to perform a lumbar epidural block. Its location varies:
    - L5–S1 in neonates.
    - L4–5 in infants below one year of age.
    - L3–4 in children and adults.
- Thoracic spine vs. lumbar spine
    - Thoracic spine has longer spinous process and narrower interspinous processes.
    - The ligaments are more relaxed in the thoracic region.
    - Smaller distances exists between the spinal cord and the epidural space in the thoracic region.

Congenital anomalies of the central nervous system

Encephalocele – dysraphism of the head

- Can occur anywhere from the frontal area to the occiput.
- May present as "nasal polyps" if they invade through the cribiform plate.
- May contain CSF.

Myelodysplasia – dysraphism of the spine
- Failure of the neural tube to close: spina bifida.
- Failure of the vertebrae to close: spina bifida occulta – the spinal column does not close, but the meninges and spinal cord do not protrude through the defect. May be associated with a sacral dimple.
- Meningocele (meningeal cyst) – part of the meninges protrudes through the defect, but the spinal cord is not involved.
- Myelomeningocele: protrusion of the meninges and the spinal cord.
- Rachischisis: open neural tissue without any overlying membrane.

Chiari malformations
- Type I: herniation of the cerebellar tonsils below the plane of the foramen magnum.
- Type II (Arnold Chiari malformation): 4th ventricle, cerebellar vermis, and lower brainstem are caudally displaced below the plane of the foramen magnum.
  - May be associated with myelodysplasia.
  - May be associated with a dysplastic brainstem.
- Type III: the brainstem and cerebellum herniate caudally into a cervical meningocele.
- Type IV: cerebellar hypoplasia.

Further reading
Coté CJ, Lerman J, Anderson BJ. *Coté and Lerman's A Practice of Anesthesia for Infants and Children*, 5th edition. Philadelphia, PA: Elsevier, 2013; 528–32.

Davis PJ. *Smith's Anesthesia for Infants and Children*, 8th edition. Philadelphia: Mosby, Inc., 2011; 7.

Gregory GA, Andropoulos DB. *Gregory's Pediatric Anesthesia*, 5th edition. Hoboken: Wiley-Blackwell, 2012; 119–20.

Part A **Basic concepts in pediatric anesthesiology**

Chapter
Anatomy
77 Peripheral

Nitin Wadhwa

Head and neck

- Supraorbital nerve and supratrochlear nerve
    - End branches of the ophthalmic division (V1) of the trigeminal nerve (CN 5).
    - Located above the eyelid.
    - Supraorbital nerve is sensory to the scalp anterior to the coronal suture.
    - Supratrochlear nerve is sensory to the lower forehead.
- Infraorbital nerve
    - End branch of the maxillary division (V2) of the trigeminal nerve.
    - Its path runs from the skull through the foramen rotundum to the pterygopalatine fossa to the infraorbital foramen where it splits into four branches: external nasal, internal nasal, superior labial, and inferior palpebral nerves.
    - Sensory to the vermilion, upper lip and mucosa, lateral inferior portion of the nose, and lower eyelid.
- Greater occipital nerve
    - Originates from the dorsal rami of C2.
    - Sensory to majority of the posterior scalp.
- Greater auricular nerve
    - Originates from branches of C3 which itself is part of the superficial cervical plexus (C2–4).
    - Sensory to the mastoid and external ear.
    - At the level of the cricoid, it follows the belly of the sternocleidomastoid muscle.

Brachial plexus

- Formed from anterior branches of spinal **roots** C5–T1.
- Contained in a sheath that runs between the anterior and middle scalene muscles in the neck.
- These roots then form three **trunks** (superior, middle, inferior) that exit the interscalene groove and run posterior to the subclavian artery.

Handbook of Critical Incidents and Essential Topics in Pediatric Anesthesiology, ed. David A. Young and Olutoyin A. Olutoye. Published by Cambridge University Press. © Cambridge University Press 2015.

- The trunks give rise to anterior and posterior **divisions** which then combine to form the lateral, posterior, and medial **cords**.
- The cords give rise to the major nerves (**branches**) of the upper extremities.
- Musculocutaneous nerve
    - Arises from the lateral cord.
    - Innervates the coracobrachialis, biceps, and brachialis muscles.
    - Provides cutaneous innervation to lateral forearm.
    - Injury leads to loss of biceps reflex.
- Axillary nerve
    - Terminal branch of posterior cord.
    - Innervates the deltoid and provides sensory innervation to lateral upper arm.
    - Injury from a surgical neck fracture of humerus or anterior dislocation of shoulder leads to inability to abduct the arm to 90°.
- Radial nerve
    - Arises from the posterior cord and is posterior to the axillary artery.
    - Innervates the triceps, brachioradialis, and extensors of the wrist and fingers.
    - Provides sensory innervation to the dorsal aspect of the upper extremity including the thumb, index, middle, and half of ring finger.
    - Injury from a midshaft fracture of humerus leads to compromised wrist extension (wrist drop) and impaired supination.
- Median nerve
    - Arises from the lateral and medial cord.
    - Innervates the flexors of the wrist and fingers.
    - Sensory innervation to palmar aspect of thumb along with palmar and dorsal aspect of index, middle, and half of ring finger.
    - Supracondylar humerus fracture leads to compromise of pronation and wrist flexion. Thumb abduction, opposition, and flexion are also lost.
- Ulnar nerve
    - Termination of the medial cord.
    - Sensory innervation to palmar and dorsal aspects of little finger and half of ring finger.
    - Fracture of medial epicondyle results in loss of adduction and abduction of fingers. Adduction of the thumb, flexion and extension of 4th and 5th digits is also compromised.

Lumbar plexus

- Formed from anterior rami of lumbar nerves L1–4. As the plexus exits the paravertebral space, it gives rise to three major nerves as described below.
- Femoral nerve
    - Located lateral to the femoral artery which is lateral to the femoral vein.

- Provides motor innervation to the quadriceps and sensory innervation to the anterior thigh.
- Saphenous nerve is a branch of the femoral nerve that provides sensory innervation to the medial lower leg and foot.
- Injury from a pelvic fracture causes compromise of thigh flexion and leg extension.
- Lateral femoral cutaneous nerve
  - Sensory innervation to the lateral thigh.
- Obturator nerve
  - Primary motor nerve to the thigh adductors and sensory innervation to the medial thigh.
  - Anterior hip dislocation may injure nerve.
  - The fascia iliaca block can anesthetize all three nerves (femoral, lateral femoral cutaneous, and obturator) as they run along the fascia.

Sacral plexus

- Originates from anterior rami of L4–5 and S1–3 and forms the sciatic nerve and posterior cutaneous nerve.
- Sciatic nerve
  - Provides motor innervation to the posterior thigh (semimembranosus, semitendinosus, biceps femoris muscles) and sensory innervation to the posterior thigh, gluteal area, and posterior lower leg.
  - Separates into the common peroneal nerve and tibial nerve in the mid-thigh.
- Common peroneal nerve
  - Provides sensory innervation to the dorsum of the foot and the anterolateral leg.
  - Responsible for eversion and dorsiflexion of the foot, along with extension of the toes.
  - Can be injured from fracture of neck of the fibula.
- Tibial nerve
  - Sensory innervation to sole of the foot.
  - Responsible for plantar flexion and inversion of the foot, along with flexion of the toes.
  - Can be injured at the popliteal fossa.

Further reading

Coté CJ, Lerman J, Anderson BJ. *Coté and Lerman's A Practice of Anesthesia for Infants and Children*, 5th edition. Philadelphia, PA: Elsevier, 2013; 854–77.

Gregory GA, Andropoulos DB. *Gregory's Pediatric Anesthesia*, 5th edition. Hoboken: Wiley-Blackwell, 2012; 431–6.

Part A   Basic concepts in pediatric anesthesiology

Chapter 78

Pharmacology
General concepts
Carlos Rodriguez

Pharmacokinetics
- Refers to the relationship of drug dose and the concentration within the body in the plasma or at the site of action.
- The processes of absorption, distribution, and elimination (clearance, metabolism, transport, and excretion) all have an impact on this relationship.

Absorption
- Absorption is not relevant to intravenous medications.
- Gastric absorption is variable among neonates, infants, and children. This is largely due to differences in gastric pH, gastric emptying times (slower in neonates), and intestinal maturity.
- Absorption via skin (e.g., ointments) is increased in younger patients in part due to thinner layers (neonates), increased perfusion, and larger surface area ratios.
- Neonates and infants have increased capillary density in skeletal muscle and therefore increased intramuscular bioavailability.

Distribution
- Volume of distribution is the ratio of amount of drug administered to the measured concentration of the drug.
- Volumes of distribution differ among neonates, infants, and children. The volume of distribution of hydrophilic drugs is higher in neonates and infants when compared to older children. This is largely due to the total body water (TBW) in these age groups. TBW = 80% in premature neonates, 75% in full term neonates, 60% in adolescents.
- Binding proteins (mainly albumin and α1-acid glycoprotein) contribute to the amount of unbound drug available. Neonates have decreased amounts of these proteins and therefore have a relatively increased proportion of unbound (pharmacologically active) drugs present.

Clearance/Metabolism
- Clearance refers to the removal of a drug from the body. The three main modes of clearance include hepatic, renal and tissue (e.g., pulmonary, blood hydrolysis).

Handbook of Critical Incidents and Essential Topics in Pediatric Anesthesiology, ed. David A. Young and Olutoyin A. Olutoye. Published by Cambridge University Press. © Cambridge University Press 2015.

- The liver uses oxidation, reduction, hydrolysis, or conjugation to metabolize drugs. Oxidation and reduction occur in the cytochrome P450 system. The cytochrome P450 system is not fully established in younger patients (neonates).
- Hepatic clearance is mostly dependent on hepatic blood flow and the hepatic extraction ratio for a particular drug. Hepatic extraction ratios can be high (e.g., lidocaine, fentanyl) or low (e.g., methadone). Clearance of drugs with high hepatic extraction ratios is primarily dependent on hepatic blood flow; clearance of low hepatic extraction ratio drugs is mostly dependent on metabolism and is essentially independent of hepatic blood flow.
- As a rule, hepatic drug metabolism and clearance is low during the first month of life; it is similar to that of adults by the age of one year. The prepubescent age group has the most efficient hepatic function; which declines in adulthood.
- Clearance in the kidneys occurs by filtration in the glomerulus. Renal blood flow can impact the degree of drug clearance. Renal blood flow and creatinine clearance are both inversely proportional to age. The function of the kidney is immature at birth and renal excretion reaches full function by the age of 2–3 years. Clearance via the kidney is perhaps the most important process for the elimination of water-soluble drugs.
- Tissue esterases contribute to the clearance of certain anesthetic drugs such as remifentanil. Tissue clearance is dependent on blood flow to the specific tissue and the overall tissue capacity.

Pharmacodynamics

Refers to the physiologic effects of a drug on the body. This is best characterized by the terms potency and efficacy.

- Potency is characterized by the effective dose of a drug that will lead to a clinical effect. Minimum alveolar concentration (MAC) is the term used to compare potency among general anesthetic inhalational agents.
- Efficacy refers to the maximum possible response of a drug at its maximum possible concentration.

Further reading

Davis PJ, Cladis FP, Motoyama EK. *Smith's Anesthesia for Infants and Children*, 8th edition. Philadelphia: Elsevier Mosby, 2011; 179–96.

Gregory GA, Andropoulos DB. *Gregory's Pediatric Anesthesia*, 5th edition. Hoboken: Wiley-Blackwell, 2012; 168–73.

Miller RD. *Miller's Anesthesia*, 7th edition. Philadelphia: Churchill Livingstone, 2010; 1140–79.

Part A Basic concepts in pediatric anesthesiology

Chapter 79
Pharmacology
Inhaled anesthetic agents
Carlos Rodriguez

General concepts
- The uptake and elimination of inhaled anesthetic agents occurs in the lungs.
- Factors that influence the uptake of an inhaled agent include the inspired concentration, total fresh gas flow, alveolar ventilation, cardiac output, and the solubility of the agent.
- Slower uptake is due to increased solubility of the agent, increased cardiac output, and lower alveolar ventilation.
- Uptake is dependent on age. Uptake is faster in infants when compared to adults.
  - Infants have increased ventilation relative to functional residual capacity.
  - Agents tend to be less soluble in infants which leads to less peripheral tissue uptake.
- Insoluble agents (e.g., sevoflurane) are not affected as much by the influence of age when compared with soluble agents (e.g., isoflurane).
- Elimination of inhaled anesthetic agents is influenced by solubility (blood and tissue) and alveolar ventilation.
- Potency of inhaled agents is age dependent and is commonly described using minimum alveolar concentration (MAC), i.e. amount/concentration of volatile anesthetic at which 50% of individuals will not respond to noxious stimuli.
  - MAC increases from the neonatal period and peaks during infancy.
  - After infancy, MAC decreases throughout life.
  - Many factors also impact MAC such as acid–base status, temperature, and the co-administration of other medications.
- Neonates are more sensitive to the myocardial effects of inhaled agents; a more pronounced decrease in blood pressure occurs in infants than in older children.
- Inhalational agents depress ventilatory drive and the response to carbon dioxide (CO_2) in a dose-dependent manner.
- Sevoflurane is minimally irritating to the airway; conversely, desflurane has significant degrees of airway irritability.
- All volatile inhalational agents cause dose-dependent cerebral vasodilation (desflurane > sevoflurane); sevoflurane and isoflurane decrease the cerebral metabolic oxygen consumption rate of oxygen ($CMRO_2$).

Handbook of Critical Incidents and Essential Topics in Pediatric Anesthesiology, ed. David A. Young and Olutoyin A. Olutoye. Published by Cambridge University Press. © Cambridge University Press 2015.

- Cerebral blood flow increases with all agents in a dose-dependent manner (halothane > desflurane > isoflurane > sevoflurane).
- Sevoflurane, isoflurane, and desflurane can all trigger malignant hyperthermia.

Nitrous oxide

- Commonly used in pediatric anesthesia especially during inhalation induction. Using a 70% concentration of nitrous oxide (N_2O), rapid equilibrium of the agent occurs. N_2O may increase the rate of uptake for other inhaled agents (second gas effect).
- N_2O is rapidly diffusible and may lead to diffusion hypoxia and hypoxemia especially during emergence if high concentrations of N_2O are present.
- The use of N_2O results in a lower overall requirement for inhaled volatile agents.
- N_2O is rapidly diffusible which can result in expansion of air-filled cavities (e.g., pneumothorax, bowel, middle ear).
- N_2O increases cerebral blood flow and $CMRO_2$.
- N_2O is not a trigger for malignant hyperthermia.
- Controversial if it is associated with an increased risk of postoperative nausea and vomiting.
- Controversial if it results in toxicity to several sites of the hematologic system.

Sevoflurane

- Most common inhalational agent used in pediatric anesthesia.
- Nitrous oxide has a limited effect on the MAC of sevoflurane (decreases by only 25%). The reason is unclear. Nitrous oxide decreases the MAC of other inhalational agents in proportion to its concentration.
- Well-tolerated for inhalational inductions due to minimal airway pungency.
- EEG stimulation and seizure activity has been reported with induction of sevoflurane.
- May lead to emergence agitation primarily in preschool-aged children.
- Approximately 5% of sevoflurane is metabolized.
- Compound A is a byproduct of degraded sevoflurane and has been associated with pathologic changes only in animal studies.

Desflurane

- Desflurane is the most insoluble inhalational volatile agent currently available.
- MAC of desflurane increases during infancy and then decreases after the age of one year.
- Nitrous oxide also has a blunted effect on the MAC of desflurane (decreases by only 25%).
- It is not recommended for inhalational induction due to increased airway irritability and pungency.
- Rapid increases in dose is associated with sympathetic stimulation.
- Desflurane has minimal metabolism (0.02%).

Isoflurane

- Isoflurane is not recommended for inhalation induction due to increased airway irritability and pungency.
- Isoflurane overall maintains blood pressure and often increases heart rate.
- Isoflurane is the most soluble of the commonly utilized inhalational agents.
- Isoflurane has minimal metabolism (0.2%).

Further reading

Cote CJ. *A Practice of Anesthesia for Infants and Children*, 4th edition. Philadelphia, PA: Elsevier, 2013; 107–13.

Davis PJ, Cladis FP, Motoyama EK. *Smith's Anesthesia for Infants and Children*, 8th edition. Philadelphia: Elsevier Mosby, 2011; 223–32.

Gregory GA. *Gregory's Pediatric Anesthesia*, 5th edition. Hoboken, NY: Wiley-Blackwell, 2012; 174–80.

Part A Basic concepts in pediatric anesthesiology

Chapter 80

Pharmacology
Hypnotics and anxiolytics
Kha M. Tran

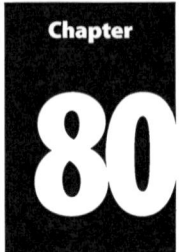

Barbiturates
- May be used as a sole sedative; do not offer any analgesia.
- Mode of action is as a gamma amino butyric acid (GABA) agonist.

Methohexital
- Quick acting but associated with side effects such as involuntary movements, hiccups, respiratory irregularity and seizure exacerbation in patients with history of epilepsy.
- Rapid recovery time (greater than thiopental).
- Routes of administration: intravenous (IV), intramuscular (IM) and rectal.
- Dose:
  - IV: 1–3 mg/kg: dose for infants (2.5–3 mg/kg) is twice that required for older children (1–1.5 mg/kg).
  - Rectal (< 5 years of age): 25–30 mg/kg. Rectal dosing induces sleep in 6 minutes; may cause mucosal damage if high concentrations are used and should be avoided in the presence of injured or inflamed mucosa, as this may cause unpredictably fast absorption.

Thiopental
- No longer available in the United States.
- Ultra-shortacting barbiturate.
- Decreases intraocular pressure and cerebrospinal fluid pressure (of benefit in patients with increased intracranial pressure).
- Dose for induction of anesthesia higher in infants (6–7 mg/kg) and children (5 mg/kg) than adults (4 mg/kg).
- Termination of clinical effect after single dose is via redistribution.
- Contraindicated in patients prone to develop porphyria.

Benzodiazepines
Also acts as a GABA receptor agonist.

Handbook of Critical Incidents and Essential Topics in Pediatric Anesthesiology, ed. David A. Young and Olutoyin A. Olutoye. Published by Cambridge University Press. © Cambridge University Press 2015.

Midazolam

- Most commonly used sedative premedication in pediatrics.
- Reduces separation anxiety, facilitates induction, enhances amnesia.
- Administered via oral, IM, IV, rectal, intranasal, sublingual routes.
  - Oral: 0.25–1 mg/kg.
  - Rectal 0.3–1 mg/kg.
  - Nasal and sublingual 0.2–0.3 mg/kg.
  - IV and IM 0.05–0.1 mg/kg.
- Onset of action:
  - 0.5 mg/kg orally provides anterograde amnesia at 10–20 minutes and anxiolysis after 15 minutes with minimal effects on respiration and oxygen saturations.
  - Peak concentrations after IM, rectal, and oral administrations occur at 15, 30, and 53 minutes respectively.
- Postoperative changes in behavior such as fearfulness, nightmares, food rejection, dysphoria, and paradoxical agitation may occur.
- Has bitter taste therefore many administer in a syrup or other carrier that is more palatable such as acetaminophen or ibuprofen.
- Physiologic effects:
  - Mild decreases in blood pressure (BP) and systemic vascular resistance (SVR).
  - Mild increase in heart rate (HR).
  - Respiratory depression is minimal.
  - Highly protein bound in serum and is metabolized in the liver.

Diazepam

- Indications: anxiolysis and muscle spasms.
- May be administered via oral or intravenous (IV) routes:
  - Oral 0.2–0.3 mg/kg.
  - IV 0.1–0.3 mg/kg (pain on injection may occur).
- Excreted predominantly via the kidneys.

Flumazenil

- Reversal agent for benzodiazepine induced sedation/respiratory depression.
- Dose: Initial dose of 0.01 mg/kg, may repeat every minute up to 1 mg total dose.
- Half life is short (0.7–1.3 hours); therefore resedation may occur requiring redosing.
- Adverse effects include: nausea, vomiting, blurred vision, anxiety, emotional lability, seizures and dysrhythmias.

Other drugs

Dexmedetomidine

- Central acting alpha-2 agonist.

- Has sedative, anxiolytic, and analgesic properties.
- Provides sedation without respiratory depression.
- Routes of administration: IV, IM, and nasal.
- Doses:
  - IV: 0.5–2 µg/kg loading dose over 10 minutes followed by 0.3–2 µg/kg/hr infusion if indicated.
  - IM and nasal: 1–2 µg/kg.
- Side effects:
  - Hypertension may be observed initially, followed by hypotension and bradycardia.
  - Slow recovery which may prolong time to discharge from recovery room.

Propofol

- Agonist at GABA receptor.
- Administered only via IV route: 1–3 mg/kg; associated with pain on injection and involuntary excitatory movements.
- Physiologic effects:
  - Decreases blood pressure and systemic vascular resistance.
  - Decreases cerebral blood flow.
  - Has antiemetic properties.
  - Decreases hepatic blood flow, limits its own conjugation.
  - Rapid redistribution and metabolism result in short duration of action.
  - Metabolism occurs in the liver via glucuronidation; extrahepatic metabolism also occurs and plays a role in clearance of propofol as well.
- Tolerance has been reported.
- Drug has lipid base and may support bacterial growth if aseptic precautions are not observed or if drug vial has been opened for more than 6 hours.
- Propofol infusion syndrome (PRIS):
  - PRIS involves a block in mitochondrial fatty acid oxidation.
  - More likely to occur in patients receiving high dose infusions or in sick patients also receiving catecholamine infusions or steroids.
  - Characterized by arrhythmias during infusion and one or more of the following: lipemic plasma, hepatomegaly, metabolic acidosis with or without an increase in serum lactate, or rhabdomyolysis with myoglobinuria.

Ketamine

- Cyclohexamine derivative which acts as a sedative, analgesic and causes dissociative anesthesia.
- May be administered via IV, IM or oral routes.
- Doses:
  - 1–2 mg/kg IV.
  - 3–6 mg/kg oral premedication, faster onset with larger dose.

- 4–6 mg/kg IM, may be administered with atropine 20 μg/kg and succinylcholine 2 mg/kg for IM induction in uncooperative or combative patients.
- Physiologic effects:
  - In patients with intact sympathetic autonomic nervous system: an increase in blood pressure, heart rate and cardiac output is observed.
  - Direct negative inotropy may occur in a patient with a denervated heart.
  - High doses may cause apnea in infants.
  - Pulmonary vascular resistance may increase but if airway and ventilation are maintained no marked changes should occur.
  - Increases cerebrospinal fluid pressure.
  - Increases intraocular pressure.
- Preserves gag reflexes; nystagmus may occur.
- Increased saliva production merits the co-administration of an antisialogue such as glycopyrrolate.
- Good adjunct to other anesthetic agents, has opioid sparing effect, and minimizes need for propofol or fentanyl rescue.
- Side effects: Emergence agitation may occur.

Etomidate

- Potent, short-acting, non-barbiturate, sedative-hypnotic.
- Central depression due to GABA mimetic effect.
- Administered via IV route: 0.2–0.3 mg/kg for induction, associated with pain on injection and myoclonic movements.
- Onset of action: 5–15 seconds onset, peak effect in 60 seconds, duration of action: 3–5 minutes.
- Physiologic effects:
  - Offers hemodynamic stability with little change in cardiovascular function.
  - Adrenal suppression with both single bolus and infusion.
  - Rapid redistribution and is metabolized in the liver.
- Contraindicated in patients with suspected septic shock.

Further reading

Coté CJ, Lerman J, Anderson BJ. *Coté and Lerman's A Practice of Anesthesia for Infants and Children*, 5th edition. Philadelphia, PA: Elsevier, 2013; 113–19.

Davis PJ. *Smith's Anesthesia for Infants and Children*, 8th edition. Philadelphia: Elsevier, 2011; 197–208.

Part A Basic concepts in pediatric anesthesiology

Pharmacology
Opioids, antagonists, and non-opioids
Luigi Viola and Senthilkumar Sadhasivam

Opioids
- Indication: treatment of moderate to severe nociceptive pain.
- Mechanism of action: binding to specific pre- and post-synaptic receptors causing inhibition of neurotransmitter release and hyperpolarization of post-synaptic neurons.
- Receptors and effects:
  - μ: analgesia and dependence (μ_1), respiratory depression, intestinal dysmotility, sedation, and bradycardia (μ_2).
  - κ: spinal analgesia, sedation, miosis, mild respiratory depression.
  - δ: analgesia, euphoria.
  - σ: dysphoria, hallucinations.
- Agonists: receptor-binding triggers intracellular functional change.
- Partial agonists: receptor-binding produces reduced response compared to pure agonists (e.g., buprenorphine).
- Mixed agonist-antagonists: agonists at certain receptors and antagonists at others.
- Adverse reactions from opioids include: nausea, vomiting, sedation, pruritus, urinary retention, respiratory depression, constipation, myoclonus, dysphoria, hallucinations, seizures. There is a great variability in the incidence and severity of these side effects between individuals and among specific agents.

Common opioid agonists
Morphine
- Primary metabolism is hepatic glucuronidation to inactive (morphine-3-glucuronide, M3G) and active (morphine-6-glucuronide, M6G) metabolites, both excreted by the kidneys. M6G is more potent than morphine; it may accumulate if renal insufficiency is present.
- Histamine release is possible.
- Elimination half-life: 1–3 hours; duration of action: 4–5 hours.
- Newborns have a prolonged elimination half-life due to kidney immaturity and decreased protein-binding.

Handbook of Critical Incidents and Essential Topics in Pediatric Anesthesiology, ed. David A. Young and Olutoyin A. Olutoye. Published by Cambridge University Press. © Cambridge University Press 2015.

- Recommended doses:
  - Oral: 0.1–0.2 mg/kg every 3–4 hours.
  - Intravenous: bolus 10–25 µg/kg (neonate) to 50–100 µg/kg (infants to adults) every 10 minutes (i.e., acute postoperative pain in post-anesthesia care unit) to 3–4 hours (i.e., postoperative pain on ward); infusion: 2–20 µg/kg/hr (neonate), 15–30 µg/kg/hr (children to adults).

Fentanyl

- Synthetic opioid, phenylpiperidine-related, very lipophilic, and 50–100 times more potent than morphine.
- It has a rapid redistribution to inactive sites, with rapid onset and short offset. Total body half-life is 80–370 minutes (age dependent); it can accumulate in the plasma with high or repeated doses such as an infusion.
- Patients may experience persistent sedation after fentanyl infusion discontinuation.
- Hepatic metabolism leads to inactive products, excreted by the kidneys.
- Transmucosal route is more efficient than the oral administration (onset within 20 minutes, 2 hour duration). Histamine release is not possible.

Methadone

- Synthetic opioid, equipotent to morphine, but with longer half-life (15–40 hours) and unpredictable elimination. It is also an NMDA receptor antagonist (used in hyperalgesia and opioid tolerance). Used mostly for chronic pain management.
- Possible QT interval prolongation, pre-use EKG recommended.
- Oral bioavailability: 80%.
- Recommended doses:
  - Oral: 0.1 mg/kg every 6–12 hours.
  - Intravenous: 0.05–0.1 mg/kg every 6–12 hours.

Meperidine

- Synthetic opioid phenylpiperidine-related, about one tenth as potent as morphine.
- Normeperidine is an active hepatic metabolite, with 50% of potency, and high risk for producing seizures. Minimal use in current clinical practice.
- Other use: postoperative shivering (0.5–1 mg/kg).

Oxycodone

- Semisynthetic opioid related to morphine, about 1.5 times more potent than oral morphine.
- Features: onset after 20–30 minutes (peak effect at 1–2 hours), offset after 4–5 hours, and elimination half-life 3–4 hours.
- Oxymorphone is an active metabolite (14-fold stronger than parent drug) that can accumulate in renal insufficiency. Oral solutions combined with non-opioids (i.e., acetaminophen) are commonly used for postoperative pain management.

Hydromorphone
- Semisynthetic derivative of morphine that is more lipophilic and five times more potent than morphine and has a similar half-life and duration of action.
- Clinical evidence for less nausea and pruritus when compared to morphine.
- Oral solutions combined with non-opioids (e.g., acetaminophen) are commonly used for postoperative pain management.

Tramadol
- Opioid and non-opioid activity: mainly norepinephrine and serotonin reuptake inhibitor as well as being a weak μ-agonist.
- 10–15 times less potent than morphine, but with better side effects profile (no respiratory depression, sedation or constipation).
- Recommended dose: 1–2 mg/kg oral, 2–2.5 mg/kg intravenous; every 6 hours.

Opioid antagonists
Naloxone
- Potent μ, κ, and δ antagonist, used to treat opioid-related respiratory depression and sedation (10 μg/kg) and nausea, urinary retention or pruritus secondary to opioids (0.25–2 μg/kg/hr).
- High doses in opioid-dependent patients may cause hypertension, tachycardia, seizures, pulmonary edema, and vomiting; titration to effect is safer: 0.5–1 μg/kg every minute.
- Elimination half-life is 1 hour, which is shorter than some of the opioids; therefore repeat doses and infusions may be needed.

Opioid agonist-antagonists
Nalbuphine
- Mixed agonist (κ) – antagonist (μ), often used to antagonize pruritus, nausea, and urinary retention. It also provides analgesia through κ receptors.
- "Ceiling effect": dose increase beyond 200 μg/kg may cause sedation or dysphoria but no additional analgesia.
- Intravenous administration: 10–50 μg/kg (neonate), 50–100 μg/kg (child), every 2–4 hours.

Non-opioids
- Mild to moderate pain is managed with nonsteroidal anti-inflammatory drugs (NSAIDs): they inhibit the enzyme cyclooxygenase (COX) which transforms arachidonic acid into prostaglandins and thromboxanes (pain mediators at peripheral nerve endings).

- Among all COX isoenzymes, type 1 is essential for many body functions. Unfortunately most NSAIDS are nonselective COX inhibitors, and complications from their use include gastric bleeding and renal insufficiency.
    - Acetaminophen: effective central COX inhibitor and weak peripheral inhibitor, therefore it has poor anti-inflammatory effects but is a potent antipyretic. Overdose leads to an oxidation process in the liver, which produces a highly hepatotoxic metabolite. Dose 10–15 mg/kg every 4 hours. Maximum daily dose: 75 mg/kg/day. Can be given by oral or intravenous routes.
    - Ketorolac: short-term intravenous use (less than 48–96 hours) of 0.5 mg/kg every 6 hours (maximum dose 30 mg) is recommended to avoid acute renal failure or gastrointestinal bleeding. Can be given by oral or intravenous routes.

Further reading

Coté CJ, Lerman J, Anderson BJ. *Coté and Lerman's A Practice of Anesthesia for Infants and Children*, 5th edition. Philadelphia, PA: Elsevier, 2013; 129–48.

Davis PJ, Cladis FP, Motoyama EK. *Smith's Anesthesia for Infants and Children*, 8th edition. Philadelphia: Elsevier Mosby, 2011; 208–32.

Walco GA, Goldschneider KR. *Pain in Children*. Totowa, NJ: Humana Press, 2008; 8 (73–85).

Part A Basic concepts in pediatric anesthesiology

Chapter 82
Pharmacology
Neuromuscular blocking and reversal agents
Julia Chen

Depolarizing muscle relaxants

Succinylcholine

- Pharmacology: Structure consists of two acetylcholine molecules linked by an ester bond; hydrolyzed by plasma cholinesterase.
- Dosing
  - Infants: 3 mg/kg.
  - Children: 1.5–2 mg/kg.
  - Intramuscular dose: 3–5 mg/kg.
- Rapid onset (30–60 seconds) and short duration of action (less than 10 minutes)
- Clinical use
  - Limited use in pediatrics by many providers; concerns related to the rare risk of hyperkalemic cardiac arrest in male children due to an undiagnosed muscular dystrophy.
  - Common clinical uses include emergency airway management, rapid sequence tracheal intubation, and treatment of laryngospasm.

Cholinesterase deficiency

- Genetic variations in plasma cholinesterase will affect enzyme activity resulting in varying degrees of prolongation to the duration of action of succinylcholine.
- Heterozygous atypical enzymes may prolong neuromuscular blockade by only a few minutes and be clinically undetected, while homozygous atypical enzymes may prolong neuromuscular blockade by several hours.
- The local anesthetic dibucaine normally inhibits plasma cholinesterase activity by 80%; the dibucaine number is proportional to the plasma cholinesterase function with 80 being a normal response and 20 corresponding to a homozygous atypical allele.

Side effects

- Cardiovascular: Increased incidence of bradycardia and arrhythmias in children; a vagolytic agent is often given prior to administration of succinylcholine and is effective in reducing vagal responses.

Handbook of Critical Incidents and Essential Topics in Pediatric Anesthesiology, ed. David A. Young and Olutoyin A. Olutoye. Published by Cambridge University Press. © Cambridge University Press 2015.

- Hyperkalemia
  - Transient increase in serum potassium of 0.5–1 mEq/L is expected after a standard dose.
  - Life-threatening hyperkalemia can occur in children with preexisting hyperkalemia, burns, trauma, neuromuscular diseases, prolonged immobilization, and other conditions which lead to increased proliferation of extrajunctional and immature acetylcholine receptors.
- Fasciculations
  - Gross muscle contractions usually observed in older children and adolescents and can be associated with postoperative discomfort.
  - Fasciculations after succinylcholine are rare in infants.
- Intraocular pressure elevations
  - Transient increase in intraocular pressure up to 10 mmHg; the clinical significance of this increase is unclear.
  - Caution should be taken in patients with preexisting or suspected ocular injuries.
- Temporomandibular joint stiffness
  - Increase in masseter muscle tone (trismus) that is typically mild and transient.
  - Severe trismus after succinylcholine may increase clinical suspicion for development of malignant hyperthermia.
  - Controversy exists regarding cancellation of elective procedures after the development of succinylcholine associated trismus.

Long-acting nondepolarizing muscle relaxants

Pancuronium

- Bisquaternary ammonium steroid compound.
- Pharmacology: Primarily renal excretion (80%).
- Dosing: 0.08–0.1 mg/kg, intubating dose.
- Onset of action 3–5 minutes; duration of action > 60 minutes.
- Side effects
  - Vagolytic effect including increases in heart rate.
  - No histamine release.
  - Clearance decreased if renal function is impaired.

Intermediate-acting nondepolarizing muscle relaxants

Atracurium

- Imidazoline bisquaternary compound.
- Pharmacology
  - Degradation via Hofmann elimination and nonspecific ester hydrolysis.
  - Duration of action is not dependent on renal or hepatic function.

- Dosing: 0.3–0.6 mg/kg, intubating dose.
- Onset of action 2–3 minutes; recovery after 40–60 minutes.
- Side effects
    - Patients with impaired hepatic function may accumulate increased plasma concentrations of laudanosine and have an increased risk for the development of seizures.
    - Dose-dependent histamine release may cause flushing, bronchospasm, hypotension, and tachycardia.

Cisatracurium

- Stereoisomer of atracurium.
- Pharmacology
    - Degradation via Hofmann elimination and nonspecific ester hydrolysis.
    - Duration of action not dependent on renal or hepatic function.
- Dosing: 0.1–0.2 mg/kg, intubating dose.
- Onset of action 2–3 minutes; recovery after 40–60 minutes.
- Side effects
    - Minimal histamine release.
    - Significantly decreased potential for increased plasma concentrations of laudanosine when compared with atracurium.

Vecuronium

- Monoquaternary aminosteroid compound.
- Pharmacology
    - Primarily metabolized by the liver and excreted in bile and urine.
    - Duration of action dependent mostly on redistribution.
- Dosing: 0.1–0.2 mg/kg, intubating dose.
- Onset of action 1–3 minutes and duration of action 30–40 minutes.
- Side effects
    - No histamine release.
    - Devoid of cardiovascular effects.
    - Prolonged infusions of vecuronium in the intensive care unit setting have been associated with prolonged neuromuscular blockade.

Rocuronium

- Monoquaternary aminosteroid compound.
- Pharmacology
    - Predominant hepatic metabolism (80–90%).
    - Duration of action dependent mostly on redistribution.
    - Minimal block prolongation in renal failure.

- Dosing
    - 0.6 mg/kg (elective procedure) to 1.2 mg/kg (rapid sequence induction).
    - Potency of rocuronium greater in infants compared with older children.
- Onset of action 1–3 minutes (dose dependent); duration of action 30–40 minutes for 0.6 mg/kg dose, 60 minutes for > 1 mg/kg dose; (latter dose is alternative to succinylcholine for rapid sequence induction.
- Side effects
    - Minimal histamine release.
    - A moderate increase in heart rate is common (10–15 BPM).
    - More anaphylactic type events described with rocuronium than with other nondepolarizing muscle relaxants.

Reversal agents

Anticholinesterase agents
- Clinical observation, evaluation, and monitoring should guide the need for antagonism of neuromuscular blockade.
- The administration of anticholinesterase agents inhibits acetylcholinesterase; this results in an increase of acetylcholine to competitively inhibit the nondepolarizing neuromuscular blocking agents located at the motor end plate.
- Anticholinesterase agents include edrophonium, neostigmine, and pyridostigmine.
    - Edrophonium has a more rapid onset than neostigmine.
    - Neostigmine is more potent than edrophonium.
    - Muscarinic effects of anticholinesterase agents (i.e., bradycardia, bronchospasm) are expected but can be reduced by the co-administration of anticholinergic agents such as atropine or glycopyrrolate.

Further reading

Barash PG. *Clinical Anesthesia*, 7th edition. Philadelphia: Lippincott Williams & Wilkins, 2013; 530–40, 550–4.

Coté CJ, Lerman J, Anderson BJ. *Coté and Lerman's A Practice of Anesthesia for Infants and Children*, 5th edition. Philadelphia, PA: Elsevier, 2013; 119–29.

Gregory GA, Andropoulos DB. *Gregory's Pediatric Anesthesia*, 5th edition. Hoboken: Wiley-Blackwell, 2012; 191–7.

Part A Basic concepts in pediatric anesthesiology

Chapter 83

Pharmacology
Cardiovascular agents
Premal M. Trivedi and Pablo Motta

Receptor pharmacology

α-adrenergic receptors

- $α_1$
  - Heart: increases contractility and decreases heart rate (HR).
  - Post-synaptic vascular smooth muscle: vasoconstriction.

- $α_2$
  - Pre-synaptic: decreases norepinephrine release.
  - Post-synaptic: vasoconstriction.
  - Brain: decreases sympathetic outflow and causes sedation.

β-adrenergic receptors

- $β_1$
  - Heart: increases HR, contractility, and automaticity.
- $β_2$
  - Post-synaptic: vasodilation.
  - Lungs: bronchodilation.

Inotropes

Epinephrine

- Secreted endogenously by the adrenal medulla.
- Direct, dose-dependent effects on $α_1$, $β_1$, and $β_2$ receptors.
- Dose range: 0.02–0.4 µg/kg/min
  - At lower doses: $β_1, β_2 > α_1$.
  - At higher doses: $α_1 > β_1, β_2$.

Handbook of Critical Incidents and Essential Topics in Pediatric Anesthesiology, ed. David A. Young and Olutoyin A. Olutoye. Published by Cambridge University Press. © Cambridge University Press 2015.

- Heart rate and contractility increase with all doses, but systemic vascular resistance (SVR) and peripheral vascular resistance (PVR) may initially decrease, remain unchanged, or increase markedly as the dose increases.
- Undergoes rapid metabolism by monoamine oxidase (MAO) and catechol-O-methyl transferase (COMT).

Dopamine

- Precursor to norepinephrine.
- Dose-dependent effect on dopaminergic (DA_1), $α_1$, $β_1$, and $β_2$ receptors, and also causes release of norepinephrine from nerve endings.
- Dose range: 2–20 μg/kg/min.
  - 2–5 μg/kg/min: DA1, increases renal/mesenteric blood flow.
  - 5–10 μg/kg/min: $β_1$, $β_2$ > $α_1$.
  - > 10 μg/kg/min: $α_1$ > $β_1$, $β_2$.
- High inter-patient response variability.
- Metabolized by MAO and COMT.

Dobutamine

- Synthetic catecholamine.
- Direct $β_1$ agonist with limited $β_2$ and $α_1$ effects.
- HR and contractility increase while SVR remains unchanged or decreases.
- Dose range: 2–20 μg/kg/min.
- Rapidly metabolized by COMT and by conjugation in the liver.

Milrinone

- Inhibits phosphodiesterase III, increasing cyclic adenosine monophosphate (cAMP) levels independent of adrenergic stimulation.
- Acts as an inotrope and vasodilator.
- Dose range: loading dose 25–100 μg/kg; infusion: 0.25–0.75 μg/kg/min.
- Primarily excreted via the kidneys: use cautiously in patients with renal dysfunction.

Calcium

- Acts as an inotrope when ionized serum calcium levels are low, and as a vasoconstrictor when levels are normal.
- Particularly useful in the setting of citrated blood product administration to neonates and infants.
- Two formulations:
  - Calcium chloride: higher levels of elemental Ca.
  - Calcium gluconate.
- Dose range
  - Calcium chloride: 10–20 mg/kg bolus, 10 mg/kg/hr infusion.
  - Calcium gluconate: 30–100 mg/kg bolus.

Chronotropes

Isoproterenol
- Non-selective β-agonist with minimal α-effects.
- Increases HR, and to a lesser extent, contractility, and decreases SVR.
- An infusion of isoproterenol has greater chronotropic effects than inotropic when compared to dopamine and dobutamine.
- Indications
    - Increase HR in the denervated heart following transplant.
    - Treatment of complete atrioventricular (AV) block.
    - Assess for supraventricular tachycardia (SVT) in the electrophysiology laboratory.
- Dose range: 0.05–2 µg/kg/min.

Vasoconstrictors

Phenylephrine
- Direct α-1 agonist.
- Increases SVR and causes reflex bradycardia.
- Useful in the management of "Tet spells" in patients with tetralogy of Fallot, hypertrophic cardiomyopathy, and aortic stenosis.
- Dose range: 0.5–5 µg/kg bolus dose, 0.02–0.3 µg/kg/min infusion.
- Undergoes rapid MAO metabolism.

Vasopressin
- Present endogenously in the pituitary.
- Produces intense vasoconstriction and has an antidiuretic effect via vasopressin receptors (V1 and V2).
- Can be useful in the setting of adrenergic receptor downregulation or blockade.
- Visceral perfusion may be compromised at high doses.
- Dose range: 0.01–0.05 units/kg/hr.

Norepinephrine
- Direct $α_1$, $α_2$, and $β_1$-agonist (minimal $β_2$ effect).
- Secreted by the adrenal medulla and central nervous system neurons; also acts as the primary postganglionic sympathetic neurotransmitter.
- Equipotent to epinephrine at $β_1$ receptors.
- May be useful for vasoconstriction if phenylephrine has been ineffective.
- Dose range: 0.02–0.2 µg/kg/min.

Vasodilators

Nitroprusside
- Increases cyclic guanine monophosphate (cGMP) through nitric oxide (NO) release.
- Dilates both arteries and veins, but primarily decreases SVR, thereby lowering blood pressure (BP) and increasing cardiac output (CO).
- Can cause cyanide toxicity, particularly in patients with liver failure, and also when high doses are used for extended periods of time.
- Dose range: 0.5–5 µg/kg/min.

Nitroglycerin
- Increases cGMP through nitric oxide (NO) release.
- Indicated in the management of myocardial ischemia, pulmonary or systemic hypertension, volume overload, or congestive heart failure.
- Dose-dependent effects on systemic/pulmonary arterial versus capacitance vessel dilation.
  - Higher doses can decrease SVR/PVR.
- Dose range: 0.5–5 µg/kg/min.

Phentolamine
- Competitive α-antagonist: decreases SVR.
- Indicated during cardiopulmonary bypass (CPB), in the management of α-adrenergic agonist drug extravasation, and management of hypertension in pheochromocytoma.
- Dose for CPB: 0.1–0.2 mg/kg.
- Offset occurs after 10–30 minutes.

Prostaglandin E_1
- Increases cAMP through activation of adenylate cyclase.
- Used in neonates to maintain patency of the ductus arteriosus in ductal dependent lesions (e.g., hypoplastic left heart syndrome).
- Side effects observed at higher doses: hypotension, apnea, fever.

Inhaled nitric oxide
- Increases cGMP with subsequent vasodilation.
- Results in pulmonary vasodilation and decrease in PVR.
- Oxygenation also improves through ventilation/perfusion (V/Q) matching.
- Biologic half-life ~ 6 seconds.
- Dose: 2–20 parts per million (ppm).

Rhythm agents

Amiodarone
- Used for rhythm control of ventricular tachycardia, atrial fibrillation, and SVT.
- Noncompetitive antagonist of α and β receptors.
  - Administration of loading dose may be associated with vasodilation, sinus bradycardia or heart block, and negative inotropy.
- Side effects associated with chronic use: hypo- or hyperthyroidism, pulmonary fibrosis, hepatitis, and cirrhosis.
- Long elimination half-life.

Further reading

Andropoulos DB. *Anesthesia for Congenital Heart Disease*, 2nd edition. Hoboken: Wiley-Blackwell, 2010; 292–9.

Coté CJ, Lerman J, Anderson BJ. *Coté and Lerman's A Practice of Anesthesia for Infants and Children*, 5th edition. Philadelphia, PA: Elsevier, 2013; 369–78.

Gregory GA, Andropoulos DB. *Gregory's Pediatric Anesthesia*, 5th edition. Hoboken: Wiley-Blackwell, 2012; 950–3.

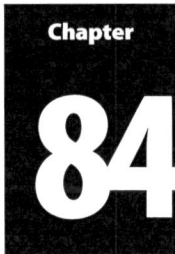

Part A Basic concepts in pediatric anesthesiology

Chapter 84

Pharmacology
Local anesthetics

Smokey Clay and Jacquelyn Morillo-Delerme

Overview

- Local anesthetics are weak bases that are composed of an aromatic ring, intermediate chain, and a hydrophilic residue.
- The pKa of these molecules ranges from 7.6 to 8.9.
- At physiologic pH, 60–85% of amide molecules are ionized and > 90% of ester molecules are ionized.
- Local anesthetics cross phospholipid membranes in their unionized form.
- Onset of action is determined by the amount of free base and pKa (lower pKa, faster onset).
- The major determinant of drug potency is lipid solubility.
- Latency of action and rate of dissociation from the receptor depend on molecular weight.
- Duration of action depends on the degree of protein binding.
- A time-dependent decrease in the effect of both esters and amides may occur (tachyphylaxis).
- Ropivacaine, which is being increasingly used, has the advantage of decreased risks of cardiac and central nervous system toxicity compared to bupivacaine.

Major classification

- Categorization of the local anesthetic depends on the link between the aromatic ring and the intermediate chain.
- Amino esters (2-chloroprocaine, procaine, and tetracaine) are metabolized in the plasma by pseudocholinesterases.
- Amino amides (lidocaine, bupivacaine, ropivacaine, prilocaine, and others) undergo hepatic metabolism.

Mechanism of action

- Nerve impulses are conducted when their sodium channels are in the resting-closed or activated open state.
- Local anesthetics enter the voltage-gated sodium channels in the open or active state and render them inactive or closed.

Handbook of Critical Incidents and Essential Topics in Pediatric Anesthesiology, ed. David A. Young and Olutoyin A. Olutoye. Published by Cambridge University Press. © Cambridge University Press 2015.

- The resulting inhibition of sodium influx blocks propagation of impulses along nerve fibers (nerve depolarization) from occurring.

Binding
- Binding of local anesthetics protects against adverse effects.
- Local anesthetics bind to blood components including red cells, alpha-1-acid glycoprotein (AAG) and albumin.
- Amide local anesthetics have a high degree of binding; binding occurs with serum proteins at a higher rate than red blood cells.
- Alpha-1-acid glycoprotein (high affinity – low capacity) and human serum albumin (low affinity – high capacity) are the main binding proteins of amide local anesthetics.
- Albumin and alpha-1-acid glycoprotein (AAG) concentrations are low at birth and increase slowly over the first year of life.
- Neonates have a lower serum AAG and albumin concentration.
- Lower binding capacity should be expected in the first 6–9 months of life.
- Acidosis decreases the affinity of AAG for local anesthetics.
    - Red blood cells may be considered a significant buffering system when local anesthetic toxicity occurs.
    - Anemia allows for higher free drug concentrations.
    - Infants < 6 months of age with lower, physiologic hematocrit are at higher risk for toxicity.
- Ester local anesthetics are mostly unbound but binding plays a role when toxic concentrations are reached.

Elimination
- Esters are metabolized by nonspecific esterases or pseudocholinesterases to inactive metabolites.
- Cocaine is unique in that it is an ester local anesthetic that undergoes significant hepatic metabolism.
- Allergic reactions may occur secondary to para-aminobenzoic acid, a metabolite of ester metabolism.
- Amides are metabolized by the cytochrome P450 (CYP450) system into active metabolites excreted by the kidneys.
- CYP3A4 enzyme which is important in the metabolism of bupivacaine, is not fully active before one year of age.
- The bupivacaine extraction ratio is lower in infants than in children and adults.
- Rate of clearance of ropivicaine and bupivacaine are lower at birth and gradually increase over the first year of life.
- The volume of distribution is high in infants and offsets low clearance after a single injection. However, this is not the case for repeat injections, in which clearance may be lower than expected.
- Tachyphylaxis occurs more slowly in infants and children.

Further reading

Bosenberg AT, Thomas J, Cronje L, et al. Pharmacokinetics and efficacy of ropivacaine for continuous epidural infusion in neonates and infants. *Paediatr Anaesth.* 2005; 15:739–49.

Coté CJ, Lerman J, Anderson BJ. *Coté and Lerman's A Practice of Anesthesia for Infants and Children*, 5th edition. Philadelphia, PA: Elsevier, 2013; 236.

Gregory GA, Andropoulos DB. *Gregory's Pediatric Anesthesia*, 5th edition. Hoboken: Wiley-Blackwell, 2012; 198.

Part A Basic concepts in pediatric anesthesiology

Chapter 85

Pharmacology
Other

Shakeel Siddiqui

Anticholinergic agents

- Atropine and glycopyrrolate are most common examples.
- Indications: bradycardia, sialorrhea, co-administration with neostigmine for reversal of neuromuscular blockade, and bronchospasm (atropine).
- Mechanism of action: non-selective competitors for acetylcholine (ACH) at the muscarinic receptors with little or no action on nicotinic receptors.
- Atropine is a tertiary amine, a natural alkaloid of *Atropa belladonna*, and glycopyrrolate is a synthetic quaternary ammonium salt.
- Supratherapeutic doses of atropine result in tachycardia, restlessness, excitement, hallucinations, delirium, and coma (CNS effects due to ability of atropine to cross the blood–brain barrier). Atropine also induces mydriasis.
- Glycopyrrolate induces tachycardia (its heart rate effects are delayed compared to that of atropine (2–3 min versus 1 min), but it does not cross the blood–brain barrier and therefore does not cause CNS effects.
- The terminal half-life of atropine is 3–4 times longer than glycopyrrolate.
- Atropine is metabolized in the liver. Glycopyrrolate is not extensively metabolized and is rapidly excreted unchanged in urine.
- Dosing:
    - Atropine: intravenous dose is 0.02 mg/kg.
    - Glycopyrrolate: intravenous dose is 0.01 mg/kg.

Nitric oxide

- Nitric oxide (NO) is an endogenous gas produced by the vascular endothelium. It is ultra-short-acting (< 5 seconds) with relatively localized action.
- Indication: pulmonary hypertension.
- Mechanism of action: following inhalation, it is released into the pulmonary blood vessels where it causes selective localized vasodilation by releasing cyclic guanine monophosphate (cGMP).
- Adverse effects include: rebound hypoxemia/pulmonary hypertension, methemoglobinemia, hyperglycemia, and hypotension.
- Dosing: 10–20 parts per million (ppm).

Handbook of Critical Incidents and Essential Topics in Pediatric Anesthesiology, ed. David A. Young and Olutoyin A. Olutoye. Published by Cambridge University Press. © Cambridge University Press 2015.

Sodium nitroprusside
- Indication: treatment of hypertension.
- Mechanism of action: direct acting, nonselective peripheral venous and arterial vasodilator through generation of nitric oxide. Onset of action is almost immediate with a short duration of action. The decrease in peripheral vascular resistance activates baroreceptor-mediated reflex tachycardia. It increases cerebral blood flow, attenuates hypoxic pulmonary vasoconstriction, causes coronary steal, inhibits platelet aggregation, and may decrease renal function.
- Adverse effects: cyanide/thiocyanate toxicity, methemoglobinemia. Occurrence of metabolic acidosis with use, mandates treatment with thiosulfate, sodium nitrate or vitamin B12.
- Dosing: Infusion of 0.25–2 µg/kg/min to a maximum of 10 µg/kg/min.

Nitroglycerin
- Indications: Relief of coronary vasospasm during periods of angina, to induce controlled hypotension and for management of cardiac failure. Relaxation of pulmonary vasculature in pulmonary hypertension as well as the smooth muscle in the gastrointestinal tract including the biliary tract and sphincter of Oddi.
- Mechanism of action: acts principally on venous capacitance. High doses also relax arterial vasculature.
- Adverse/side effects: tachycardia, hypotension, flushing, and methemoglobinemia.
- Dosing: Slow intravenous (IV) bolus of 0.5–2 µg/kg and continuous IV infusion of 0.1–4 µg/kg/min. Other routes of administration include sublingual, PO and transdermal ointment/patch.

Nicardipine
- Calcium channel blocker.
- Indications: hypertension and to induce hypotension.
- Mechanism of action: peripheral arteriolar dilatation.
- Metabolism: extensively metabolized by the liver and excreted by the kidney. Half-life is prolonged in liver disease.
- Adverse effects are minimal; the most common reported adverse effect is headache.
- Dosing: starting dose of 0.5 µg/kg/min and titrate to effect.

Labetalol
- Combined α and β adrenergic blocker.
- Indication: hypertension.
- Can be used in combination with sodium nitropusside or nicardipine to prevent reflex tachycardia.
- Adverse effects: nausea, bronchospasm, elevated liver transaminases.
- Dosing: 0.5–1 mg/kg IV, may repeat as needed.

Sildenafil
- Indication: pulmonary hypertension.
- Mechanism of action: selectively decreases phosphodiesterase type 5 which inhibits cyclic guanine monophosphate (cGMP). Increased cGMP causes smooth muscle relaxation.
- Adverse effects include headache, epistaxis, and visual defects (photophobia, blurry vision). Contraindicated in patients on nitrites.
- Dosing: Loading dose of 0.35–0.44 mg/kg over 1–3 hours and continuous infusion of 0.067 mg/kg/hr.

Dexamethasone
- Fluorinated derivative of prednisolone and isomer of betamethasone with little mineralocorticoid activity.
- Indications include: treatment of cerebral edema, bronchial asthma, allergic reactions, rejection of transplanted organs, replacement or stress dose administration in adrenocortical insufficiency, airway edema and prevention of postoperative nausea and vomiting.
- Adverse effects: may suppress adrenocortical production; impair wound healing; cause fluid retention, hyperglycemia, and myopathy. Cautious use recommended in patients with diabetes, hypertension, and gastritis.
- Dosing: Cerebral edema 0.1 mg/kg up to 10 mg. Airway edema or vomiting 0.5–1 mg/kg.

Ondansetron
- Indication: prevention and treatment of nausea/vomiting.
- Mechanism of action: 5-HT3 receptor antagonist.
- Onset of action is < 30 minutes, duration of action 12–24 hours, and half-life 3–4 hours.
- Adverse effects: headaches, prolonged QT interval. Cautious use recommended in patients with heart block and elevated liver enzymes.
- Dosing: 0.1–0.15 mg/kg for postoperative nausea and vomiting.

Albuterol
- Indication: treatment of asthma or bronchospasm.
- Mechanism of action: selective β-2 adrenergic agonist that acts on β-2 receptors in lung to cause smooth muscle relaxation.
- Onset of action: acts immediately on inhalation, peak effect in 30–60 minutes and duration of 4 hours. Response diminishes with long-term therapy.
- Adverse effects: tremor, tachycardia, hyperglycemia, hypokalemia, and hypermagnesemia.
- Dosing: Metered dose inhaler 90 µg/puff; 2–4 puffs as needed. Nebulized: 1.5–2.5 mg in normal saline.

Further reading

Coté CJ, Lerman J, Anderson BJ. *Coté and Lerman's A Practice of Anesthesia for Infants and Children*, 5th edition. Philadelphia, PA: Elsevier, 2013; 457–9.

Gregory GA, Andropoulos DB. *Gregory's Pediatric Anesthesia*, 5th edition. Hoboken: Wiley-Blackwell, 2012; 1295–6.

Part A Basic concepts in pediatric anesthesiology

Chapter 86
Fluid management
General concepts
Mary A. Felberg

Overall goals
Selection and administration of fluids to maintain or restore intravascular volume, tissue perfusion, and ensure optimal oxygen delivery to tissues.

Total body water and fluid compartments
- Total body water (TBW), as a percentage of body weight in kg, changes with age due to the reduction in surface area to volume ratio as the infant grows.
- TBW in the newborn is 80% of total body weight; this decreases and stabilizes at approximately 60% by 6 months of age.
- TBW is divided into two main compartments, intracellular and extracellular, which achieve adult distribution (67% intracellular, 33% extracellular) by age of 12 months.
- The extracellular compartment is further divided into two components:
    ○ Plasma (25%) is found within blood vessels.
    ○ Interstitial fluid (75%) is the remainder of the extracellular fluid; this includes the lymphatic fluid.

Estimated blood volume
- Fluid management involves monitoring and maintaining intravascular blood volume which contains both intracellular fluid (blood cells, platelets) and extracellular fluid (plasma).
- The estimated blood volume changes with age as indicated in Table 86.1.

Table 86.1 Estimated blood volume at different ages.

Age	Estimated blood volume (mL/kg)
Premature or low birth weight infant	100
Term infant	90
2 years old	80
> 2 years old	75–80

Handbook of Critical Incidents and Essential Topics in Pediatric Anesthesiology, ed. David A. Young and Olutoyin A. Olutoye. Published by Cambridge University Press. © Cambridge University Press 2015.

Water and sodium considerations

- The extracellular fluid compartment is regulated by the balance of water and sodium; the kidneys are the primary organs of regulation.
- Water is freely permeable and moves between fluid compartments in response to solute concentrations.
- Sodium is the primary extracellular electrolyte and is crucial to the maintenance of intravascular volume.
- Antidiuretic hormone (ADH) also has a critical role in water homeostasis by regulating the uptake of free water due to increased plasma osmolality.
- Neonates have immature renal function, as shown by their inability to concentrate urine and effectively regulate solutes such as sodium.
- Mild metabolic acidosis is common in the neonate due to immature renal function.

Preoperative assessment

- Assessment of the preoperative fluid status should consider the underlying medical conditions, current medications (including IV fluids), fasting status, pertinent laboratory values (e.g., hematocrit, electrolytes, platelets), vital signs, and physical examination.
- Clinical indicators suggestive of depleted intravascular volume may include tachycardia, orthostatic hypotension, delayed skin turgor, decreased urine output, and depressed fontanelles (in infants).
- Evaluate current intravenous access. Central line placement or ultrasound-guided placement of additional peripheral intravenous access may be indicated.
- Confirm the availability of blood components when indicated.
- Consider administering glucose-containing intravenous fluids to patients at increased risk for hypoglycemia (e.g., neonates, patients on total parenteral nutrition).

Perioperative fluid requirements

- Perioperative fluid requirements can be divided into five categories: fasting deficit, preoperative losses, maintenance fluids, ongoing operative fluid losses, and fluid derangements.
- Fasting deficit is defined as the number of hours without enteral intake (oral or enteral tube) or intravenous fluids. Permitting clear liquids up to 2 hours preoperatively can significantly decrease the fasting deficit.
- Preoperative losses contribute to volume depletion and can cause metabolic derangements. Losses can be due to excessive output (e.g., vomiting, diarrhea), lack of input (e.g., anorexia, neglect), blood loss (e.g., trauma, bleeding), or fluid shifts (e.g., ascites, edema).
- Maintenance fluids include insensible losses (e.g., respiratory tract) and urinary output.
- Ongoing operative fluid losses include blood loss, evaporative losses from the surgical field (e.g., open exploratory laparotomy), and third space losses.
- Fluid derangements due to other causes (e.g., renal dysfunction, sepsis, acid base disturbances, electrolyte abnormalities).

Calculating the fasting deficit
- Defined as the number of hours without enteral intake (oral, enteral tube) or intravenous fluids.
- The fasting deficit can be calculated using the "4–2–1" rule, the patient's weight in kilograms multiplied by the fasting time in hours to obtain the total amount of fluid deficit:
    - Use 4 mL/h for 0–10 kg, then use 2 mL/h for 11–20 kg, and finally 1 mL/h for weights > 20 kg.
- Example: weight 25 kg
    - 40 + 20 + 5 = 65 mL/h × # hours fasting = mL of total amount of fluid deficit.

Fluid replacement
- Replace the fasting deficit with non-glucose-containing isotonic crystalloid solutions (e.g., 0.9% normal saline or lactated Ringer).
- The calculated deficit should be replaced over 3 hours; ½ of the deficit replaced over the first hour, ¼ replaced over the second hour and ¼ over the third hour.
- Ongoing assessment of fluid replacement needs may include clinical signs (heart rate and blood pressure, dose of volatile agent delivered), estimated blood loss (suction canisters, weighing of sponges, visual inspection of the field, serial hematocrit levels), and estimation of surgical insensible losses due to third spacing.
- Assessment caveats for the pediatric patient:
    - Blood pressure may be preserved by increasing heart rate until significant volume loss has occurred (i.e., 30% of estimated blood volume).
    - A narrowed pulse pressure can be a warning for significant hypovolemia.
    - Due to renal immaturity, urine output may not be a reliable indicator of organ perfusion in the premature infant and neonate.
- Three categories are commonly used for the estimation of surgical insensible loss:
    - Major insensible loss is estimated at 8–10 mL/kg/hr.
    - Moderate insensible loss is estimated at 5–7 mL/kg/hr.
    - Minor insensible loss is estimated at 3–4 mL/kg/hr.
- Administer non-glucose-containing solutions to replace ongoing intraoperative losses.
- Isotonic crystalloid replacement for blood loss is estimated at 3 mL of fluid for every 1 mL of blood loss.
- Colloid replacement for blood loss is estimated at 1 mL:1 mL blood loss ratio but total dosing limits exist (i.e., hyperosmolality).
- Blood products are administered to modify oxygen-carrying capacity and normalize coagulation function.

Maintenance fluid
- The "4–2–1" rule may also be used to calculate the hourly maintenance fluid rate. (4 mL/h for 0–10 kg) + (2 mL/h for 11–20 kg) + (1 mL/h for > 20 kg) = mL/h.

- Isotonic crystalloid fluids are typically chosen for maintenance fluid replacement. Consider glucose-containing intravenous solutions for patients at risk for hypoglycemia.

Further reading

Coté CJ, Lerman J, Anderson BJ. *Coté and Lerman's A Practice of Anesthesia for Infants and Children*, 5th edition. Philadelphia, PA: Elsevier, 2013; 159–75.

Gregory GA, Andropoulos DB. *Gregory's Pediatric Anesthesia*, 5th edition. Hoboken: Wiley-Blackwell, 2012; 205–20.

Part A Basic concepts in pediatric anesthesiology

Chapter 87

Fluid management
Crystalloid/colloid
Rebecca Laurich and Jacquelyn Morillo-Delerme

Crystalloids
- Holliday and Segar's "4–2–1" rule is used to determine maintenance fluid requirements.
    - Patients < 10 kg: 4 mL/kg/hr.
    - Patients 11–20 kg: 40 mL/hr + 2 mL/kg/hr for each kilogram between 11 and 20 kg.
    - Patients > 20 kg: 60 mL/hr + 1 mL/kg/h for each kilogram > 20 kg.
- Perioperative fluid requirements
    - Current fasting requirement guidelines by the American Society of Anesthesiologists allow clear liquids up to 2 hours before procedures requiring anesthesia.
    - Furman et al. method (commonly used)
        - Multiply hourly rate of fluid requirement (calculated by Holliday and Segar method) by the number of hours the patient was NPO (*nil per os*).
        - Replace half of this calculated amount in first hour of surgery and the second half over the next 2 hours.
    - Berry's simplified method
        - Deliver a bolus of a basic salt solution to otherwise healthy children over first hour of surgery.
        - Children 3 years and younger should receive 25 mL/kg.
        - Children 4 years and older should receive 15 mL/kg.
    - Lactated Ringer's solution is an acceptable solution for fluid replacement.
    - Isotonic normal saline is also a balanced salt solution that can be used for fluid replacement; however, when administered in large amounts, hyperchloremic metabolic acidosis may develop.
- Perioperative dextrose
    - Selectively administer intraoperative dextrose (D_5LR) only to patients at greatest risk for hypoglycemia:
        - Neonates.
        - Patients receiving hyperalimentation.
        - Patients with endocrinopathies.

Handbook of Critical Incidents and Essential Topics in Pediatric Anesthesiology, ed. David A. Young and Olutoyin A. Olutoye. Published by Cambridge University Press. © Cambridge University Press 2015.

- ○ Monitor blood glucose levels and adjust the rate of dextrose infusion accordingly.
- ○ Routine dextrose administration is no longer recommended for otherwise healthy children receiving anesthesia.

Colloids

Natural protein colloids

- Albumin
    - ○ Derived from pooled human plasma by a process that heats human plasma to 60°C for 10 hours and then undergoes ultrafiltration for sterilization.
    - ○ Two concentrations of albumin are produced in the US: 5% and 25%.
        - . 5% Albumin: osmotically equivalent to an equal volume of plasma.
        - . 25% Albumin: osmotically equivalent to 5 times the volume in plasma
    - ○ Side effects
        - . Rare.
        - . Weak anticoagulation effects through inhibition of platelet aggregation or heparin like effects on antithrombin III.
        - . This effect is thought to be insignificant if volume of albumin administration is kept below 25% of the patient's blood volume.

Synthetic colloids

Not commonly utilized in pediatrics.

- Hydroxyethyl starches (HES)
    - ○ Modified, natural polysaccharide.
    - ○ Available concentrations are 3%, 6%, and 10%.
    - ○ Noted to have prolonged volume effects (lasting 2–6 hours), however, also have a greater side-effect profile.
    - ○ Hypocoagulation, renal toxicity and pruritus.
    - ○ Older, higher molecular weight HES solutions have increased risk of side effects.
    - ○ The coagulation effects are more concerning in cases involving cardiopulmonary bypass in which further coagulation and platelet dysfunction occur.
- Dextrans
    - ○ Water-soluble, glucose polymer
        - . Available concentrations: dextran 40 (10%) remains in intravascular space for 3–4 hours; dextran 70 (6%) remains in intravascular space for 5–6 hours.
        - . Current literature does not recommend use of dextrans due to coagulation effects and high anaphylactic potential.
        - . Use of dextran should be limited to 20 mL/kg.
        - . Side effects:
            - – VonWillebrand-type syndrome (dose dependent).
            - – Enhanced fibrinolysis.
            - – Dextran reactive antibodies trigger release of vasoactive mediators, leading to anaphylactic and anaphylactoid reactions.

Crystalloid vs. colloid

- There is a scarcity of evidence supporting crystalloid vs. colloid use for volume expansion in the pediatric population.
- The Cochrane Database review in adult patients (2007) concludes that there is no evidence to support the use of colloids over crystalloids in resuscitation of patients with burns, trauma, or after surgery.

Further reading

Bailey AG, McNaull PP, Jooste E, Tuchman JB. Perioperative crystalloid and colloid fluid management in children: Where are we and how did we get here? *Anesth Analg.* 2010; 110(2):375–90.

Bissonnette, B. *Pediatric Anesthesia Basic Principles – State of the Art – Future.* Shelton, CT: People's Medical Publishing House, 2011; 843–9.

Part A Basic concepts in pediatric anesthesiology

Chapter 88

Fluid management
Blood products

Premal M. Trivedi and Pablo Motta

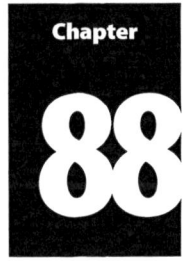

Applied immunology

- ABO system: defined by the presence or complete absence of A and/or B antigens on the red blood cell surface (Table 88.1).
- Rh blood group system: another group of surface antigens (~50) including the D antigen (most immunogenic), and Rh antigen, whose presence or absence determines Rh status (Rh+ or Rh−).
- Approximately 85% of the US population is Rh+.

Table 88.1 Red cell antigens and transfusion compatibility.

	A	B	O	AB
ABO antigen	A	B	None	AB
ABO antibodies	Anti-B	Anti-A	Anti-A, Anti-B	None
Incidence in USA	42%	10%	44%	4%
PRBC-compatible donor	A and O	B and O	O	A, B, AB, and O
Plasma-compatible donor	A and AB	B and AB	O, A, B, and AB	AB

Packed red blood cells

- Storage: Packed red blood cells (PRBCs) are stored at 1–6°C in the anticoagulant/preservative solution CPDA-1 (citrate, phosphate, dextrose, adenine–formula 1).
  ○ Hematocrit 65–80% with a shelf-life of 35 days.
- Irradiation: reduces transfusion-associated graft versus host disease.
  ○ Indicated in immunocompromised patients or transplant candidates.
  ○ Shelf-life decreases to 28 days after irradiation.
- Leukocyte reduction: can be performed pre- or post-storage using leuko-reduction filters.
  ○ Decreases the incidence of:
    . Febrile non-hemolytic transfusion reactions.
    . Alloimmunization of recipients to human leukocyte antigens.
    . Transmission of cytomegalovirus (CMV).

Handbook of Critical Incidents and Essential Topics in Pediatric Anesthesiology, ed. David A. Young and Olutoyin A. Olutoye. Published by Cambridge University Press. © Cambridge University Press 2015.

- Rationale for transfusion: to increase oxygen-carrying capacity of blood and enhance end-organ perfusion.
  - ABO and Rh factor status must be checked prior to transfusing blood products (Table 88.1).
  - Rh– individuals should receive Rh– PRBCs.
  - Initial amount: 10 mL/kg.
- Exposure to Rh+ RBCs produces anti-Rh antibodies in 30–80% of transfusion recipients.
- Transfusion triggers vary depending on patient physiology, ongoing blood loss, and adequacy of oxygenation/perfusion.
- Generally indicated in patients with hemoglobin < 7 g/dL; however, trigger may be much higher in premature infants, or patients with cyanosis, or chronic conditions.
- Physiologic nadir for hemoglobin occurs at approximately 2–3 months of age.
- Neonates and premature infants have higher fractions of fetal hemoglobin, thus influencing oxygen delivery.
- Use of somatic and cerebral oximetry can guide transfusion in critical patients.
- **Massive blood transfusion**: replacement of one or more circulating blood volumes

Estimated blood volume

- Estimated blood volume (EBV) varies with age (see Table 88.2).
- Calculation of maximal allowable blood loss (MABL):
  MABL = EBV × (starting Hct – lowest acceptable Hct)/starting Hct.

Fresh frozen plasma

- Fresh frozen plasma (FFP) is prepared from the platelet-rich plasma component of whole blood or by apheresis and contains anti-ABO antibodies.
- It is stored at –18°C or cooler.
- After 24 hours the activity of factor V and VIII is significantly diminished.
- Leukocytes are killed or nonfunctional by the freezing process so irradiation is not needed.
- Each mL of FFP contains one international unit of each coagulation factor.
- Before administration, FFP is thawed in a water bath at 30–37°C for approximately 20–30 min.
- Patients can only receive plasma with anti-ABO antibodies that will not react with the patient's ABO surface antigens (Table 88.1).

Table 88.2 Estimated blood volume and age.

Age	Estimated blood volume (mL/kg)
Premature infant	90–100
Term infant – 3 months	80–90
Children older than 3 months	70
Very obese children	65

- Indication: coagulopathy and reversal of anticoagulation.
- Dose: 10 mL/kg.

Cryoprecipitate

- Cold-insoluble white precipitate that forms when a unit of FFP is thawed at 1–6°C.
- Needs to be refrozen at −18°C or colder and has a shelf-life of 1 year.
- Components:
    - Fibrinogen (150–250 mg).
    - Factor VIII (80–150 IU).
    - Von Willebrand factor (40–70% of original plasma concentration).
    - Factor XIII (30% of original plasma concentration).
    - Fibronectin (30–60 mg).
    - Plasma 5–15 mL.
- Indication: hypofibrinogenemia.
- Dose: 1 unit per 5 kg body weight.

Platelets

- Prepared from the platelet-rich plasma component of whole blood or by apheresis.
- Single or random donor platelets.
- Stored at 20–24°C with continuous gentle agitation to prevent aggregation.
- Shelf-life is only 5 days because of the increased risk of infection.
- Irradiation is necessary to kill viable lymphocytes.
- Compatibility between recipients and donors of platelet units is recommended in infants and children.
- Indications: thrombocytopenia in symptomatic patients or patients requiring invasive procedures.
- Dose: 1 unit per 5 kg body weight.

Transfusion complications

- Metabolic
    - Hypocalcemia and hypomagnesemia can occur due to citrate toxicity.
    - Hyperkalemia secondary to PRBC leakage: more pronounced in older (> 7 days) and irradiated blood.
    - Hypothermia.
    - Acidosis due to PRBC shift to anaerobic metabolism which increases lactic acid.
- Infectious
    - Decreased by screening tests but may occur due to false-negative screen.
    - Hepatitis A, B, and C.
    - Human immunodeficiency virus (HIV).
    - Human T lymphotrophic virus I and II.
- Immune mediated

- - Incompatibility: clerical error.
  - Graft versus host disease is caused by lymphocytes contained in a transfused blood component, that proliferate and cause host tissue destruction.
- Hemolytic transfusion reactions.
- Febrile non-hemolytic transfusion reactions.
- Allergic reactions.
- Transfusion-related acute lung injury.
- Post-transfusion purpura.
- Transfusion-related immunomodulation.
- Alloimmunization.

Further reading

Coté CJ, Lerman J, Anderson BJ. *Coté and Lerman's A Practice of Anesthesia for Infants and Children*, 5th edition. Philadelphia, PA: Elsevier, 2013; 213.

Gregory GA, Andropoulos DB. *Gregory's Pediatric Anesthesia*, 5th edition. Hoboken: Wiley-Blackwell, 2012; 239–50.

Part A: Basic concepts in pediatric anesthesiology

Chapter 89

Regional anesthesia
General concepts

Nitin Wadhwa

Safety

- Unlike adults, children typically receive regional anesthesia while they are under general anesthesia.
- According to data from the Pediatric Regional Anesthesia Network (PRAN), performing regional anesthesia under general anesthesia does not lead to an increased incidence of complications.

Advantages

- Effective postoperative analgesia.
- Adverse side effects of intravenous opioids such as respiratory depression, nausea, and vomiting are reduced.
  - Avoiding opioid use is especially useful for ex-premature infants who are at increased risk for postoperative apnea.
- Decreased volatile agent requirement.
- Rapid emergence following surgery due to decreased opioid use.
- Decreased postoperative recovery time.
- Improvement of pulmonary function in patients undergoing thoracic or upper abdominal surgery.

Ultrasonography

- The use of ultrasonography has led to:
  - An increased number of blocks being performed in pediatric patients due to increased visibility of both needle location and surrounding structures.
- Lower dose of local anesthetics are required for a given block due to deposition of local anesthetic at the site of the nerve. Compared to nerve stimulator or anatomic landmark techniques, the use of ultrasound has several advantages including:
  - Shorter block performance time.
  - Higher success rate.
  - Shorter onset time.

Handbook of Critical Incidents and Essential Topics in Pediatric Anesthesiology, ed. David A. Young and Olutoyin A. Olutoye. Published by Cambridge University Press. © Cambridge University Press 2015.

- Longer block duration.
- Visibility of neuraxial structures.

Central vs. peripheral blocks

- Contraindications to central neuraxial (caudal, epidural, spinal) blockade include:
  - Coagulopathy.
  - Spinal malformations (spina bifida, myelomeningocele).
  - Post spinal surgery (spinal fusion, laminectomy).
  - Vertebral anomalies.
- Compared to central neuraxial blocks, peripheral nerve blocks:
  - Are performed at a target area.
  - Can be performed in any anatomic location (e.g., face, neck).
  - Require a smaller dose of local anesthetic and, as a result, there is decreased systemic absorption and less risk of systemic toxicity.
  - Are not associated with the risk of unintended spinal anesthesia, hypotension, or urinary retention.

Use of a test dose

- Negative blood aspiration prior to local anesthetic injection may still be associated with a needle location within the intravascular space (False negatives may occur).
- A small "test dose" of local anesthetic and epinephrine may be useful to detect intravascular injection. It identifies intravascular injection of local anesthetic and reduces the potential adverse consequences from local anesthetic toxicity.
- The recommended test dose under sevoflurane anesthesia is 0.1 mL/kg of the local anesthetic plus 5 µg/mL of epinephrine. The total volume should not exceed 3 mL.
- Indications suggestive of a positive test dose include a heart rate increase of 10 bpm or greater, a systolic blood pressure increase of 15 mmHg or greater, or a T-wave amplitude increase of 25% or greater. These symptoms usually occur for about 60–90 seconds after injection. In addition to being a marker for intravascular injection, epinephrine also decreases systemic absorption of local anesthetic due to its vasoconstrictive properties.

Anatomic and physiologic differences vs. adults

- In neonates and infants, the dural sac ends at S3, while the conus medullaris is at L3.
- After age 1 and in adults, the dural sac ends at S1 and conus medullaris at L1.
- Due to the lower position of the spinal cord in neonates, it is important to perform a spinal anesthetic at L4–5 or L5–S1.
- Due to the more caudal position of the dural sac in neonates and infants, there is a higher risk of inadvertent dural puncture while performing a caudal block, compared to children and adults.
- Compared to adults, higher doses of local anesthetic are required for effective spinal anesthesia in neonates and young children. This is attributed to increased cerebrospinal fluid volume as a percentage of body weight.

- Despite higher doses of local anesthetics used for spinal blocks, the duration of spinal block is shorter in neonates and young children due to the higher rate of cerebrospinal fluid (CSF) turnover.
- Neonates are at highest risk for local anesthetic toxicity compared to older children and adults:
    - Lower levels of albumin and alpha-1-acid glycoproteins lead to less plasma protein binding of amide local anesthetics, which results in an increase of free plasma concentrations of local anesthetic.
    - As a result, bolus and infusion doses of local anesthetics should be decreased by 30% for infants less than 6 months of age.

Central blockade and hypotension

- Unlike adults, children less than 5 years of age may not exhibit hypotension or bradycardia secondary to administration of local anesthetic into the caudal or neuraxial space.
- This is attributed to:
    - Decreased vagal tone that allows the heart rate to compensate for changes in peripheral vascular resistance.
    - Immature sympathetic nervous system.
    - Insignificant volume for venous pooling in the lower extremities.
- As a result, no volume loading is necessary prior to performance of central blockade.

Further reading

Coté CJ, Lerman J, Anderson BJ. *Coté and Lerman's A Practice of Anesthesia for Infants and Children*, 5th edition. Philadelphia, PA: Elsevier, 2013; 843–50.

Davis PJ. *Smith's Anesthesia for Infants and Children*, 8th edition. Philadelphia: Mosby, Inc., 2011; 458.

Marhofer P, et al. Everyday regional anesthesia in children. *Paediatr Anaesth*. 2012; 22(10):995–1001.

Part A Basic concepts in pediatric anesthesiology

Chapter 90

Regional anesthesia techniques
Central

Amanda K. Brown and Rhonda A. Alexis

Central blockade

- Includes spinal, caudal and epidural anesthesia.
- May be used as a primary anesthetic or combined with general anesthesia; combination with general anesthesia is common practice in children.
- Represents at least half of most pediatric regional practices and is applicable to surgical procedures of the thorax, abdomen or lower extremity.
- Contraindications:
  - Coagulopathy.
  - Congenital abnormalities, previous spinal instrumentation.
  - Infection.
- All regional anesthetic techniques should incorporate sterile preparation and draping.

Spinal blockade

- Local anesthetics administered into the subarachnoid space result in rapid central neuraxial anesthesia.
- As a primary anesthetic, spinal anesthesia may reduce the risk of postoperative apnea in preterm infants < 60 weeks post-conceptual age. Avoiding mechanical ventilation in this scenario may also be beneficial in the setting of preexisting respiratory dysfunction.
- Equipment selection is guided by age.
  - A spinal block may be placed in infants utilizing a 1½ inch 22g spinal needle as the reduced integrity of the ligamentum flavum in infancy hinders detection with smaller needles.
  - Higher gauge needles can be selected for older children to reduce the risk of post-dural puncture headache.
- A supported sitting position for this block in the infant may optimize flow of cerebrospinal fluid (CSF). Baseline reductions in the opening CSF pressure in infancy may preclude brisk flow in the lateral decubitus position.
- Anatomical differences must be considered. Placement at L4–5 is recommended to avoid the conus medullaris, which is located at L3 prior to 1 year of age.

Handbook of Critical Incidents and Essential Topics in Pediatric Anesthesiology, ed. David A. Young and Olutoyin A. Olutoye. Published by Cambridge University Press. © Cambridge University Press 2015.

- Neonates and infants require higher dosing of local anesthetic per weight compared to adults. Neonates have a relatively larger CSF volume (4 mL/kg) with half of the volume being present in the spinal subarachnoid space, causing a more rapid decline in sensory blockade.
- Dose: hyperbaric 1% tetracaine 0.4–0.5 mg/kg with a minimum of 1.5 mg tetracaine, is recommended; the addition of epinephrine will achieve 90–120 min of surgical anesthesia blockade.
- Post-dural puncture headache may occur in approximately 10% of children older than 10 years of age.
- Inadvertent high spinal blockade in infants may present as apnea without hypotension or bradycardia.

Caudal block

- Indications: commonly utilized during inguinal hernia repair, circumcision, and orchiopexy. Commonly performed as a single injection technique but catheter placement can be incorporated with this technique.
- The reliability and ease of performance of the caudal block are responsible for the increased frequency of its use.
- The caudal space (also the epidural space) can be approached easily through the sacral hiatus. Lateral positioning of the child with hip flexion aids in landmark palpation.
    - The sacral cornu, bony prominences of the non-fused fifth sacral vertebral, are palpable cephalad to the coccyx and form the lateral boundary of the sacral hiatus.
    - The sacrococcygeal ligament (continuation of the ligamentum flavum) is located within the sacral hiatus.
- A 22g short beveled needle or angiocatheter is inserted into the caudal space at a 45° angle. A distinctive loss of resistance is observed once the sacrococcygeal ligament has been penetrated. The angle of the needle is then lowered, needle is slightly advanced, and local anesthetic is injected into the caudal space.
- Lack of subcutaneous swelling cephalad to site of injection and ease of injection supports an effective technique.
- Needle aspiration to confirm absence of blood and CSF is mandatory prior to medication administration.
- Initial injection of a small volume is recommended to rule out intravascular injection.
- The use of epinephrine (1:200,000) to detect intravascular administration remains controversial and unreliable.
- Dose: 0.5–1 mL/kg of local anesthetic (0.2% ropivacaine or 0.25% bupivacaine) is commonly utilized.
- Preservative-free morphine, a hydrophilic opioid, is an additive occasionally administered with local anesthetics. It is characterized by cephalad spread and is therefore useful for thoracic procedures. It is associated with adverse effects such as itching and late onset respiratory depression.

Epidural

- Placement of epidural catheters is typically performed under general anesthesia.
- Epidural catheters may also be inserted via the caudal space and threaded up to the desired vertebral level.
- Epidural catheters inserted through caudal space:
  - Required catheter length for appropriate dermatomal coverage should be measured externally prior to placement.
  - Radiographic confirmation of placement by infusion of nonionic contrast or insertion under fluoroscopy is strongly suggested.
  - Catheter placement via this route may prove difficult after 24 months of age due to changes in the epidural patency at this site.
  - Catheter aspiration is important to assess for blood or CSF.
  - Tunneling of catheter reduces the risk of catheter contamination.
- An approximation of the distance from the skin to the epidural space can be made utilizing the formula of 1.0 mm catheter per kg ideal body weight.
- Continuous epidural infusions typically do not exceed 0.2 mg/kg/hr for use in neonates or with thoracic catheters.
- Dose of 0.4 mg/kg/hr is appropriate for children more than 1 year of age for lumbar or caudal catheters.
- Epidural and caudal additives include fentanyl (1–3 µg/mL) to increase the effects of analgesia.
  - While opioids may improve the analgesic efficacy of blocks, their use introduces risks of respiratory depression, nausea, urinary retention and pruritus.

Further reading

Davis PJ. *Smith's Anesthesia for Infants and Children*, 8th edition. Philadelphia: Mosby,Inc., 2011; 474–6.

Gregory GA, Andropoulos DB. *Gregory's Pediatric Anesthesia*, 5th edition. Hoboken: Wiley-Blackwell, 2012; 427–30.

Part A **Basic concepts in pediatric anesthesiology**

Regional anesthesia techniques
Peripheral
Diane Gordon and Jacquelyn Morillo-Delerme

- Use of regional anesthesia, especially peripheral nerve blocks in children, has increased over the past two decades, partly due to increasing use of ultrasound.
- Ultrasound has gained popularity for a number of reasons:
    - It allows for clear visibility of the needle or catheter being placed.
    - It also allows for the use of a smaller amount of local anesthetic since the drug is deposited close to the nerve bundles.
- There is also an increasing trend in the placement of peripheral nerve catheters for intra- and postoperative analgesia.
- Any peripheral nerve block performed in an adult can also be performed in a child, although nerve blocks are usually placed under general anesthesia for pediatric patients.
- Techniques for placement of pediatric peripheral nerve blocks is similar to adults – both nerve stimulation and ultrasound-guided techniques are utilized.
- Ropivacaine 0.2% and bupivacaine 0.25% are commonly used concentrations of local anesthetics employed in peripheral nerve blocks.
- Dose of local anesthetic depends on the block. Additives such as clonidine 1 μg/kg (up to 100 μg) have been shown to increase duration of sensory analgesia when included in peripheral nerve blocks.
- Readers are referred to textbooks on regional anesthesia for in-depth descriptions of peripheral nerve block techniques.

Types of peripheral nerve block

Facial blocks

- Supraorbital nerve blocks: The supraorbital nerve and supratrochlear nerves are terminal branches of the ophthalmic division of the trigeminal nerve. Blockade provides pain relief for procedures on the anterior scalp and forehead.
- Infraorbital nerve block: The infraorbital nerve is derived from the second maxillary division of the trigeminal nerve. This block provides effective analgesia for cleft lip repair, endoscopic sinus surgery, nasal septal reconstruction and rhinoplasty.

Handbook of Critical Incidents and Essential Topics in Pediatric Anesthesiology, ed. David A. Young and Olutoyin A. Olutoye. Published by Cambridge University Press. © Cambridge University Press 2015.

- Great auricular nerve block: This is a sensory nerve branch of the superficial cervical plexus. This nerve innervates the mastoid and external ear. Sensory blockade provides anesthesia for tympanoplasty. This nerve is close to the carotid artery and jugular veins therefore this block may be complicated by intravascular injection as well as inadvertent phrenic nerve block, cervical plexus block, and Horner syndrome.

Upper extremity blocks

- Axillary nerve block: Indication is for surgery on the arm or hand. This block is frequently used due to its low complication rate. Anatomical landmarks include: axillary artery, pectoralis major muscle, and the coracobrachialis muscle. Recommended dose of local anesthetic is 0.3–0.5 mL/kg, not to exceed a total volume of 20 mL. Supplemental blockade of the musculocutaneous nerve may be required.
- Interscalene block: Provides anesthesia for surgery of the shoulder and upper extremity. It reliably blocks the musculocutaneous nerve as well; however, the ulnar nerve may occasionally be missed. This block is associated with significant side effects such as pneumothorax, epidural spread of medication, subarachnoid block and phrenic nerve block with ipsilateral hemidiaphragm paralysis and as a result, this block is not commonly performed in children.
- Supraclavicular block: Commonly employed as it provides anesthesia to all sections of the arm and is useful for almost all upper extremity procedures. Despite the ubiquitous application of this nerve block for most upper extremity procedures, the risk of pneumothorax is high. Needle-tip visualization under ultrasound allows this block to be performed with a low incidence of pneumothorax.
- Infraclavicular block: Offers anesthesia and analgesia to the distal upper extremity and covers most of the areas the axillary block covers. It is associated with a risk of pneumothorax therefore the ultrasound-guided approach is recommended. The median nerve may be missed with a single injection and therefore may require a separate, targeted injection. This site is commonly used for insertion of continuous catheters as it offers stability and secure positioning of catheters.

Truncal blocks

- Tranversus abdominis plane (TAP) block: Provides sensory blockade to the entire anterolateral abdominal wall from a single injection of 0.5 mL/kg local anesthetic. It is more commonly performed via ultrasound with insertion of the needle between the internal oblique muscle and the tendinous insertion of the tranversus abdominis. Complications include solid organ injury, bowel perforation and intravascular injection.
- Rectus sheath blocks: Best performed under ultrasound guidance, provides sensory blockade to the anterior abdominal wall lateral to the linea semi lunaris. Can be performed for umbilical and epigastric hernia repairs, pyloromyotomy and laparascopic procedures. Once appropriate needle location is confirmed, injection of 0.1–0.2 mL/kg of local anesthetic on each side provides satisfactory anesthesia.

Lower extremity blocks

- Ilioinguinal/Iliohypogastric block: This provides sensory blockade for surgery such as inguinal hernia repair, orchiopexy and hydrocelectomy. Both nerves originate from the

lumbar plexus and pierce the tranversus abdominis muscle. They are blocked as they pass superficial to the tranversus abdominis muscle near the anterior superior iliac spine. These nerves may also be blocked by the surgeon under direct vision.
- Sciatic nerve block: Indications include surgical procedures of the lower extremity below the knee. The entire lower extremity can be blocked if this nerve block is combined with a lumbar plexus block. The sciatic nerve, the largest nerve in the body, originates from the anterior rami of L4-S3 and consists of the tibial and common peroneal nerves which travel in a common sheath in the upper part of the lower extremity. It divides at the superior portion of the popliteal fossa and innervates the leg below the knee. It innervates the posterior thigh above the knee and the hamstring muscles. The posterior, lateral and anterior approaches to sciatic nerve blockade have all been employed in children. However, a higher success rate with the posterior approach has been described in children.
- Popliteal fossa block: also blocks the sciatic nerve proximal to the knee. The advantage of this block is patients can remain supine for the block. The block is performed with the patient supine, leg raised with the knee and thigh flexed.
- Femoral nerve block: Provides analgesia of the anterior thigh. Indications include surgery above the knee. The femoral nerve is derived from L1–L3 and it enters the thigh in the femoral triangle below the inguinal ligament. The 3-in-1 block is a modification of this block which incorporates blockade of the lateral femoral cutaneous nerve and the obturator nerve. Landmarks for this modified block are the same as for femoral block but a larger amount of local anesthetic is injected and distal pressure is applied in order to facilitate proximal spread of the local anesthetic.
- Fascia iliaca block: believed to be more effective than the 3-in-1 block as all three nerves (femoral, lateral femoral cutaneous and obturator nerves) are more effectively blocked with this technique, providing anesthesia to the entire lower extremity above the knee. It also anesthetizes the femoral branch of the genitofemoral nerve. The effectiveness of this block allows its use for muscle biopsy with intravenous sedation.
- Ankle block: simple block that provides anesthesia to the foot. The five nerves of the foot are blocked:
  - Saphenous nerve located on the medial side of the foot; is blocked anterior to the medial malleolus.
  - Sural nerve innervates lateral aspect of foot; is blocked posterior to the lateral malleolus.
  - Tibial nerve: located immediately posterior to the posterior tibial artery and the medial malleolus; is blocked posterior to the medial malleolus.
  - Superficial peroneal nerve which innervates the medial and lateral aspects of the dorsum of the foot.
  - Deep peroneal nerve which innervates the web space between the first and second toes.
    - Superficial and deep peroneal nerves are blocked with a ring of local anesthetic infiltrated across the dorsum of the foot between the medial and lateral malleolus.

Further reading

Coté CJ, Lerman J, Anderson BJ. *Coté and Lerman's A Practice of Anesthesia for Infants and Children*, 5th edition. Philadelphia, PA: Elsevier, 2013; 854–78.

Davis PJ. *Smith's Anesthesia for Infants and Children*, 8th edition. Philadelphia: Mosby, Inc., 2011; 476–508.

Polaner D, Dresher J. Pediatric regional anesthesia: what is the current safety record? *Pediatr Anesth*. 2011;21: 737–42.

Polaner DM, Tenser AH, Walker BJ et al. Pediatric regional anesthesia network (PRAN): A multi-institutional study of the use and incidence of complications of pediatric regional anesthesia. *Anesth Analg*. 2012; 115:1353–64.

Rossetti V, Ivana G. Controversial issues in pediatric regional anesthesia. *Pediatr Anesth*. 2012; 22(1):109–14.

Part A Basic concepts in pediatric anesthesiology

Chapter 92

Airway management
General concepts

Graciela Argote-Romero and Jacquelyn Morillo-Delerme

Physiology
The upper airway
- Infants are obligate nasal breathers.
- The epiglottis is located relatively more cephalad than in adults.
- The oropharynx is relatively smaller when compared with adults.

The lower airway
- Noisy breathing (stridor)
    - Causes include congenital, inflammatory, traumatic and foreign bodies.
    - Increased inspiratory efforts and noisy breathing are signs of stridor.
    - Inspiratory stridor usually indicates upper airway lesions and expiratory stridor is almost always associated with lesions below the vocal cords.
    - Biphasic stridor is most characteristic of obstruction in the subglottic region.
    - Severe obstruction may result in respiratory distress or even death.
    - Surfactant
        - Mixture of lipids secreted by the type 2 respiratory epithelial cells.
        - Decreases wall tension and reduces alveolar collapse during normal breathing cycles.
        - Deficiency results in reduced compliance, decreased alveolar ventilation, respiratory distress syndrome and bronchopulmonary dysplasia.

Basic airway management
Mask ventilation
- Loss of pharyngeal tone leading to airway obstruction occurs commonly during inhalation induction.
- The upper and lower esophageal sphincters (LES) maintain a resting tone of 10–30 mmHg.
- Premature infants and neurologically impaired children have reduced LES tone and are more susceptible to gastro-esophageal reflux and pulmonary aspiration.

Handbook of Critical Incidents and Essential Topics in Pediatric Anesthesiology, ed. David A. Young and Olutoyin A. Olutoye. Published by Cambridge University Press. © Cambridge University Press 2015.

Face masks
Proper technique is more important that the type of mask used. Compression of the submental soft tissue must be avoided to prevent airway obstruction.

Oral airways
- Correct size can be determined by approximating the distance from the teeth to the base of the tongue.
- Inappropriately sized oral airways may obstruct the airway by pushing the base of tongue towards the pharynx.
- Oral necrosis may also occur if an oral airway is left in place for long periods of time especially if the space is tight.

Nasopharyngeal airways
- Proper length can be determined by measuring the distance between the auditory meatus and the tip of the nose.
- Lubrication and gentle insertion is recommended as trauma to the turbinates or adenoids may occur during insertion.
- Avoid use in patients with coagulation defects and bleeding diathesis.

Supraglottic airway devices
- Commonly utilized for routine pediatric cases.
- Also useful as a temporizing measure in management of a difficult airway.
- Only 50% of insertions are adequately seated at the laryngeal inlet, nevertheless, the incidence of major respiratory complications or aspiration with supraglottic airway devices is low.

Endotracheal tubes
- In general, the size of the endotracheal tube (ETT) is more related to the child's age rather than size of the child. Uncuffed ETTs have been used previously in children but the development of low-pressure micro-cuffed endotracheal tubes has allowed for an airway seal at pressures of 20 cmH$_2$O (below the trigger for mucosal ischemia) which may be less than that from a tight-fitting uncuffed ETT.
- Therefore cuffed endotracheal tubes are now used more commonly in the pediatric population.
- A deflated cuff adds 0.5 mm to the external diameter of the ETT. Avoid cuff pressures > 25 mmHg to prevent mucosal injury. Use of a cuffed ETT has decreased the number of laryngoscopy attempts, reintubations, and incidence of post-intubation croup.

Laryngoscope blades
- A straight blade is better suited for infants and young children by providing full exposure of the vocal cords.
- Curved blades are satisfactory for older children and children with large tongues (e.g., Down syndrome).

Further reading

Coté CJ, Lerman J, Anderson BJ. *Coté and Lerman's A Practice of Anesthesia for Infants and Children*, 5th edition. Philadelphia, PA: Elsevier, 2013; 237–58.

Davis PJ, Cladis FP, Motoyama EK. *Smith's Anesthesia for Infants and Children*, 8th edition. Philadelphia: Elsevier, 2011; 351–7.

Part A   Basic concepts in pediatric anesthesiology

Chapter 93

Airway management techniques
Direct
Paul A. Stricker

General considerations
- Direct airway management techniques involve achieving direct exposure and line-of-sight visualization of the larynx.
- This technique remains the predominant airway management modality in children.
- A variety of conditions such as micrognathia, cervical immobility, limited mouth opening, and temporomandibular joint (TMJ) dysfunction may make direct airway management techniques difficult.
- Unfortunately, risk factors for predicting difficult direct laryngoscopy in children have not been adequately validated.
- Advantages
    - Simple and effective in the vast majority of patients once the technique has been mastered.
    - Rapid securement of the airway when performed by a proficient operator, associated with a low incidence of complications.
    - Can be used for performing both orotracheal and nasotracheal intubation.
    - Laryngoscopes and blades are relatively inexpensive and simple to maintain.
    - Battery-powered laryngoscopes are portable and can be used in a wide range of settings including most off-site environments.
- Disadvantages
    - May require significant forces delivered to tongue, pharynx, and hypopharynx which can result in soft tissue injury and inflammation.
    - Dental injury is also possible.
    - Not intuitive to learn; requires at least 50 attempts to become moderately competent.

Specific devices
- Macintosh blade: A curved blade with which the blade tip is advanced along the base of the tongue into the vallecula; the epiglottis is lifted indirectly. Many prefer to use this blade in older pediatric patients (adolescents).
- Miller blade: A straight blade that can be used to directly lift the epiglottis to expose the laryngeal inlet or can be used in the same manner as the Macintosh blade. This is the

---

Handbook of Critical Incidents and Essential Topics in Pediatric Anesthesiology, ed. David A. Young and Olutoyin A. Olutoye. Published by Cambridge University Press. © Cambridge University Press 2015.

predominant blade for neonates and infants. Sweeping the tongue to expose the larynx can be more difficult to achieve with this blade.
- Wis-Hipple blade: A straight blade similar to a Miller but with a slightly broader blade and less curvature at the tip. Technique for airway management is similar to the Miller blade.
- Anterior commissure scope: Can be useful for patients with difficult direct laryngoscopy, especially in infants with micrognathia. This device has a tubular blade through which the tracheal tube is passed once the larynx is visualized.

Further reading

Davis PJ, Cladis FP, Motoyama EK. *Smith's Anesthesia for Infants and Children*, 8th edition. Philadelphia: Elsevier Mosby, 2011; 317.

Mulcaster JT, Mills J, Hung OR et al. Laryngoscopic intubation: learning and performance. *Anesthesiology* 2003; 98:23–7.

Part A Basic concepts in pediatric anesthesiology

Chapter 94
Airway management techniques
Indirect
Paul A. Stricker

General considerations
- Indirect airway management techniques involve tracheal intubation without direct line-of-sight to visualize the larynx.
- Many patients with difficult airways are challenging due to lack of laryngeal exposure with conventional direct laryngoscopy; indirect techniques are commonly selected for use in these patients.
- Many indirect devices deliver an image for visualization using fiberoptics, prisms, or mirrors, alone or in combination.
- Several indirect tracheal intubation modalities do not involve actual visualization of the larynx (e.g., lighted stylet, ultrasound-guided intubation).

Specific tools, devices, and techniques
Flexible fiberoptic bronchoscope
- The "gold standard" modality for difficult airway management.
- Mandatory skill set for all anesthesiologists.
- Advantages
    - The most versatile airway management device.
    - Suitable for both orotracheal and nasotracheal intubation.
    - Minimal mouth opening required.
    - Can be combined with other devices (i.e., fiberoptic-assisted tracheal tube placement via a supraglottic airway).
    - Many bronchoscopes have the ability to connect to operating room video screens for group viewing.
    - Many bronchoscopes have the ability via a side-port to delivery oxygen, suction, and local anesthetics.
- Disadvantages
    - Not intuitive, can be difficult to learn and maintain proficient skills.
    - Secretions, blood, and fogging can make visualization difficult to impossible.
    - Expensive and fragile equipment; multiple sizes with differing capabilities (lack of suction port in neonatal versions).

Handbook of Critical Incidents and Essential Topics in Pediatric Anesthesiology, ed. David A. Young and Olutoyin A. Olutoye. Published by Cambridge University Press. © Cambridge University Press 2015.

- ○ Tracheal tube passage over scope into trachea can be difficult and time consuming.
- ○ Typically increased time to secure airway when compared with other techniques.
- ○ Additional steps and time required for setup when compared with other techniques.

Fiberoptic-guided intubation through a supraglottic airway

- Technique with a high success rate when mastered.
- Can transition from emergent supraglottic airway placement for unexpected difficult airway.
- Advantages
  - ○ Ventilation can be delivered via supraglottic airway throughout intubation attempts.
  - ○ Ventilation is rapidly reestablished between intubation attempts if an apnea technique is used.
  - ○ Navigation of fiberoptic scope to glottis is greatly simplified by using the supraglottic airway as a conduit; typically the glottis can be identified just inferior to the distal aperture of the supraglottic airway.
- Disadvantages
  - ○ Useful only for orotracheal intubations.
  - ○ Requires adequate mouth opening for supraglottic airway insertion.
  - ○ Removal of supraglottic airway following intubation is recommended and allows for proper securing of tracheal tube. If improperly executed, inadvertent tracheal tube dislodgment can occur.
  - ○ The pilot balloon of a cuffed tracheal tube may not fit through some brands of supraglottic airway devices. This can be addressed by using an uncuffed tube and performing a tube exchange if undersized.

Video/indirect laryngoscope

- Provides ability to "see around the corner."
- Mechanical skill set similar to that for direct laryngoscopy. Despite similarities, the required skill set to insert the tracheal tube is distinct.
- Advantages
  - ○ Intuitive for operators facile with direct laryngoscopy.
  - ○ Most devices are relatively portable and require minimal preparation when compared to a fiberoptic bronchoscope.
- Disadvantages
  - ○ Not useful in patients with severely limited mouth opening.
  - ○ Operator's attention is directed to a video screen or eyepiece; careful attention must be paid during insertion of the laryngoscope and tracheal tube.
  - ○ Secretions, blood, and fogging can interfere with visualization/optics.

Optical stylet

- A rigid or malleable stylet with optics that deliver an image from the stylet tip to the eyepiece or video screen. The tracheal tube is loaded directly onto the stylet.

- Advantages
    - Intuitive, shorter learning curve for the operator.
    - Portable, minimal setup required.
    - Relatively inexpensive and reusable.
    - The operator can visualize the tube as it passes into the larynx.
- Disadvantages
    - Secretions, fogging, and blood can make visualization difficult.
    - Poorly suited for nasotracheal intubations.

Lighted stylet

- A malleable stylet with a light source at the tip. It is configured as a J-shaped stylet and a tracheal tube is loaded onto it. Correct position for intubation is identified by a bright light seen in the center of the neck when the tip enters the larynx.
- Advantages
    - Direct visualization not required.
    - Simple, rapidly learned technique.
    - Inexpensive, portable, minimal setup required.
    - Visualization is not reduced when airway secretions are present.
- Disadvantages
    - Room lights must be dimmed for optimal use.
    - Potential for causing traumatic injuries during placement.
    - Poorly suited for nasotracheal intubations.

Ultrasound-guided intubation

- Technique uses surface ultrasound of the neck to guide intubation using a styletted tracheal tube configured in a shape similar to a lighted stylet.
- Advantages
    - Direct visualization not required.
    - Not hindered by fogging, blood, or secretions.
    - Tracheal intubation can be confirmed with ultrasound.
- Disadvantages
    - New technique; also requires proficiency with ultrasound.
    - Large learning curve; success rates and complications remain unexplored.
    - Additional time requirements when compared with traditional techniques.

Further reading

Choo MK, Yeo VS, See JJ. Another complication associated with videolaryngoscopy. *Can J Anaesth*. 2007; 54:322–4.

Coté CJ, Lerman J, Anderson BJ. *Coté and Lerman's A Practice of Anesthesia for Infants and Children*, 5th edition. Philadelphia, PA: Elsevier, 2013; 267–75.

Fiadjoe JE, Stricker P, Gurnaney H et al. Ultrasound-guided tracheal intubation: a novel intubation technique. *Anesthesiology.* 2012; 117:1389–91.

Kovatsis PG, Fiadjoe JE, Stricker PA. Simple, reliable replacement of pilot balloons for a variety of clinical situations. *Paediatr Anaesth.* 2010; 20:490–4.

Nestler C, Reske AP, Reske AW et al. Pharyngeal wall injury during videolaryngoscopy-assisted intubation. *Anesthesiology.* 2013; 118:709.

Part A **Basic concepts in pediatric anesthesiology**

Malignant hyperthermia
General concepts
Tae W. Kim

Introduction
Malignant hyperthermia (MH) is a rare and potentially fatal pharmacogenetic disorder. Individuals possessing the gene defect are at risk for developing a hypermetabolic state when exposed to triggering anesthetic agents. These "triggering agents" are halogenated volatile anesthetic gases and succinylcholine. The incidence of malignant hyperthermia is variable and has been reported to be 1:15,000 for children and 1:50,000 for adults. Treatment requires intensive care and the emergent administration of dantrolene sodium. Dantrolene administration stops the progression of the hypermetabolic process.

Genetics
The *RYR1* gene defect is located on chromosome 19q13.1, which codes for the ryanodine receptor. The pattern of inheritance is autosomal dominant. However, the gene expression has been characterized as reduced penetrance with variable expressivity. Offspring of a MH-susceptible parent have a 50% chance of inheritance. Another gene defect predisposing to MH involves the *CACNA1S*, calcium channel, voltage-dependent, L type, alpha 1S subunit, gene on chromosome 1q32. The CACNA1S protein interacts with the ryanodine receptor protein to stimulate release of calcium from the sarcoplasmic reticulum into the myoplasm. However, this genetic defect accounts for only 1% of MH-related events.

Pathophysiology
The exposure to anesthetic triggering agents results in the unregulated release of calcium from the sarcoplasmic reticulum via the ryanodine receptor protein. This uninhibited release of calcium causes a generalized contraction of skeletal muscles as actin and myosin fibrils interact. Free myoplasmic calcium is pumped back into the sarcoplasmic reticulum; these processes require a great deal of energy (ATP), oxygen, and substrate (glucose). The exhaustion of energy, oxygen, and substrate forces the muscle cells to convert to anaerobic metabolism, causing a combined respiratory and metabolic acidosis. As the metabolic process overwhelms the muscle cell's ability to maintain homeostasis, there is breakdown of cellular integrity resulting in the release of potassium, creatine kinase, and myoglobin.

Handbook of Critical Incidents and Essential Topics in Pediatric Anesthesiology, ed. David A. Young and Olutoyin A. Olutoye. Published by Cambridge University Press. © Cambridge University Press 2015.

Clinical presentation
Many individuals are unaware that they harbor the genetic predisposition for malignant hyperthermia. The realization occurs when they undergo general anesthesia for surgery and suddenly develop MH. The earliest sign of malignant hyperthermia is nonspecific tachycardia, followed by a rapid increase in end-tidal CO_2 (most sensitive), truncal rigidity (regardless of whether neuromuscular blocking agents have been administered), a rapidly rising temperature (1°C every 5 minutes), and brown colored urine due to myoglobinuria.

Treatment
See Chapter 51, Malignant hyperthermia, for detailed management guidelines.

Associated conditions
- Central core disease
  - Autosomal dominant inheritance pattern predominates.
  - Caused by mutations in the *RYR1* gene.
  - Spectrum of skeletal muscle weakness.
  - Result of disorganized areas, lacking mitochondria and oxidative enzyme activity in the center of muscle fibers.
- Multiminicore disease
  - Autosomal recessive inheritance pattern.
  - Caused by mutations in the *RYR1* or *SEPN1* gene.
  - Only *RYR1* gene defect causing MH susceptibility.
  - Four subtypes with the most common presenting in infancy or early childhood.
  - Spectrum of skeletal muscle weakness.
- King–Denborough syndrome
  - Autosomal dominant with variable expression.
  - Congenital myopathy associated with susceptibility to malignant hyperthermia, skeletal abnormalities, and dysmorphic features.
- Conditions currently controversial regarding MH susceptibility and requirement for non-triggering anesthetic techniques
  - Muscular dystrophy.
  - Masseter muscle spasm.

Testing
- Caffeine–halothane contracture test (CHCT, gold standard)
  - Non-triggering anesthetic to harvest 2 g of quadriceps femoris muscle.
  - Three sets of muscle are examined for force generated when exposed to 3% halothane and separately to 2 mmol/L of caffeine in a physiologic bath.
  - If muscle specimen has abnormal response to halothane and caffeine, then the patient is MH positive.

- ○ If muscle specimen has normal response to both halothane and caffeine, then the patient is MH negative.
- ○ If muscle specimen has abnormal response to one agent, then the patient is MH positive.
- ○ The test is 97% sensitive, 78% specific.
- Genetic test
  - ○ Recommended for those individuals related to a person known to have MH, who have already been tested positive for MH susceptibility or in whom specific gene defect has been identified.
  - ○ Requires only DNA-containing tissue (e.g., blood).
  - ○ Convenient, less time consuming and costly.
  - ○ Sensitivity only 30%.
  - ○ Test predominantly used to confirm diagnosis of MH susceptibility; negative test result does not confirm lack of MH susceptibility.

Further reading

Allen GC, Larach MG, Kunselman AR. The sensitivity and specificity of the caffeine-halothane contracture test: a report from the North American Malignant Hyperthermia Registry. *North American Malignant Hyperthermia Registry of MHAUS. Anesthesiology*. 1998; 88:579–88.

Coté CJ, Lerman J, Anderson BJ. *Coté and Lerman's A Practice of Anesthesia for Infants and Children*, 5th edition. Philadelphia, PA: Elsevier, 2013; 817–34.

Larach MG, Brandom BW, Allen GC, Gronert GA, Lehman EB. Cardiac arrests and deaths associated with malignant hyperthermia in North America from 1987 to 2006: a report from the North American Malignant Hyperthermia Registry of the Malignant Hyperthermia Association of the United States. *Anesthesiology*. 2008; 108:603–11.

Rosero EB, Adesanya AL, Timarra CH, Joshi GP. Trends and outcomes of malignant hyperthermia in the United States 2000–2005. *Anesthesiology*. 2009; 110:89–94.

Stewart SL, Hogan K, Rosenberg H, Fletcher JE. Identification of the Arg1086His mutation in the alpha subunit of the voltage-dependent calcium channel (CACNA1S) in a North American family with malignant hyperthermia. *Clin Genet*. 2001; 59:178–84.

Part A   Basic concepts in pediatric anesthesiology

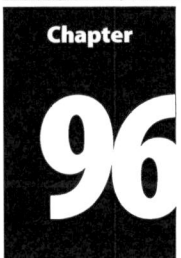

Chapter 96

Resuscitation
General concepts
Matthew D. Sjoblom and Jacquelyn Morillo-Delerme

Epidemiology
- Incidence of childhood cardiopulmonary arrest is estimated to be 16,000 per year in the United States.
- Survival to discharge after in-hospital cardiopulmonary arrest has improved from < 10% in the 1980s to about 27%.
  - ~75% of survivors have favorable neurologic outcome.
  - Survival in children is higher than in adult patients: 27% vs. 17%.
- This difference is driven primarily by better survival among infants and pre-school-aged children.
- Factors that influence outcome:
  - The nature of the preexisting condition.
  - Location where the cardiac arrest occurs.
    - Only 30% of children receive bystander cardiopulmonary resuscitation (CPR).
  - Initial rhythm.
  - Duration of pulselessness.
  - Quality of post-resuscitation care.

Phases of resuscitation
Pre-arrest phase
- Preexisting conditions and precipitating events
  - Interventions are focused on prevention:
    - Early recognition and treatment of impending respiratory failure and shock.
  - In-hospital medical emergency teams or rapid response teams (RRT):
    - Available to evaluate patients and transfer to intensive care unit (ICU), as necessary.
    - Decrease the number of patients that progress to full arrest.
    - Limits pulselessness time in patients that do arrest.

Handbook of Critical Incidents and Essential Topics in Pediatric Anesthesiology, ed. David A. Young and Olutoyin A. Olutoye. Published by Cambridge University Press. © Cambridge University Press 2015.

No flow/low flow phase

- Effective CPR improves coronary perfusion pressure and cardiac output to vital organs.
  - Push hard, push fast, allow full chest recoil, and minimize interruptions to compressions.
- Rapid detection and defibrillation of shockable rhythms is essential.

Interventions

Airway and ventilation

- Establishing an airway with effective gas exchange is critical to successful resuscitation.
- Initial bag-valve-mask ventilation is followed by endotracheal intubation as soon as possible with minimal interruption to chest compressions.
- Exhaled carbon dioxide (CO_2) detection is standard of care for pediatric resuscitation.
- Absence of CO_2 can indicate esophageal intubation or ineffective CPR resulting in very low or absent pulmonary blood flow.
  - Using an appropriately sized calorimetric CO_2 detector will avoid false-negative detection that may result from using an adult size device on a small child.
- Increased intrathoracic pressure impedes venous return, therefore caution should be employed to avoid overventilation.
- Adequate ventilation is of supreme importance in arrest due to asphyxia.

Circulation

Effective circulation is accomplished by: "push hard, push fast" motto.

- The goal of chest compressions is to maximize myocardial perfusion pressure (MPP).
- Myocardial perfusion occurs during the recoil phase of the compression. MPP = aortic diastolic pressure – right atrial pressure.
- Push hard
  - Current recommendations for appropriate depth of pediatric chest compressions ranges from 1/3 to 1/2 of the antero-posterior diameter of the chest.
- Push fast
  - > 100 compressions/minute.
  - The American Heart Association recommended ratio of compressions to ventilation is 15:2 for two rescuers and 30:2 for a single rescuer.
  - In infants, compressions are best delivered by the two-thumb encircling hands technique.

Vascular access

- Obtaining vascular access is crucial and can be challenging in hospitalized children who have undergone multiple medical interventions.
- Traditional peripheral intravenous access is the first option, with intraosseous (IO) access as the next best choice.

- Central venous access is often difficult to obtain during resuscitation and can cause undesirable interruptions to chest compressions.
- In the absence of vascular access, lidocaine, atropine, naloxone, and epinephrine (LANE) can be administered via the endotracheal tube (ETT).

Medications
See Table 96.1.

Table 96.1 Medications and dosages used in resuscitation.

Medication	Dosing
Adenosine	0.1 mg/kg IV (max 6 mg) Repeat: 0.2 mg/kg (max 12 mg)
Amiodarone	5 mg/kg IV Repeat up to 15 mg/kg (max 300 mg)
Atropine	0.02 mg/kg IV/IO/IM 0.03 mg/kg ETT (min 0.1 mg; max 0.5 mg child, 1 mg adolescent)
Calcium Chloride	20 mg/kg IV
Epinephrine	0.01 mg/kg IV/IO 0.1 mg/kg ETT
Lidocaine	Bolus: 1 mg/kg IV/IO; 2–3 mg/kg ETT (max 100 mg) Infusion 20–50 µg/kg/min
Magnesium sulfate	25–50 mg/kg IV over 10–20 min (max 2 g)
Naloxone	< 5 y or ≤ 20 kg IV: 0.1 mg/kg ≥5 y or > 20 kg IV: 2 mg
Sodium bicarbonate	1 mEq/kg IV per dose

Post-resuscitation care
- Goals include: adequate tissue oxygen delivery, treatment of myocardial dysfunction, minimizing secondary organ injury, and prevention of recurrent arrest.
- Arrhythmias and reperfusion injuries are common in this phase.
- Temperature
    - Mild induced hypothermia (32–34°C) has been shown to improve neurologic outcome in adults after ventricular fibrillation and cardiac arrest. Efficacy of this strategy in children has not been established.
    - Hyperthermia has been shown to worsen outcome and should be avoided.
- Glucose control
    - Both hypo- and hyperglycemia worsen neurologic outcome.
    - Tight control of hyperglycemia often leads to hypoglycemia.
    - Strong recommendations regarding glucose control are lacking at this time.

- Blood pressure management
    - Blood pressure lability is common after resuscitation.
        - Hypotension is often due to myocardial dysfunction.
        - Hypertension may be due to administration of vasoactive drugs.
        - Autoregulation of cerebral blood flow is often impaired after resuscitation.

Further reading

Coté CJ, Lerman J, Anderson BJ. *Coté and Lerman's A Practice of Anesthesia for Infants and Children*, 5th edition. Philadelphia, PA: Elsevier, 2013; 804–16.

Davis PJ. *Smith's Anesthesia for Infants and Children*, 8th edition. Philadelphia: Elsevier, 2011; 1200–49.

Gregory GA, Andropoulos DB. *Gregory's Pediatric Anesthesia*, 5th edition. Hoboken: Wiley-Blackwell, 2012; 255–72.

Part A Basic concepts in pediatric anesthesiology

Chapter 97

Monitoring
General concepts
Olutoyin A. Olutoye

Pulse oximetry

- Most important monitor responsible for increased perioperative safety.
- Pulse oximetry is able to detect hypoxemia before clinically apparent cyanosis.
- Utilizes differences of light absorption between oxyhemoglobin (660 nm) and deoxyhemoglobin (940 nm) to estimate arterial oxygen saturation.
- Also indirectly evaluates heart rate, rhythm regularity and perfusion.
- Accuracy of pulse oximetry is ± 2% for estimating PaO_2 unless SpO_2 < 90%, when correlation is inversely related.
- False readings can be due to:
  ○ Direct ambient light, motion of the probe, and hypothermia.
  ○ Poor perfusion from hypovolemia, vasoconstriction, and cardiogenic shock.
  ○ Intravascular dyes absorbing light with similar wavelengths as hemoglobin (e.g., methylene blue, indocyanine green, and indigo carmine).
- Abnormal hemoglobin
  ○ Carboxyhemoglobin: pulse oximetry falsely overestimates PaO_2.
  ○ Methemoglobin: pulse oximetry value approaches 85%.
- Newer pulse oximetry technology uses at least seven different wavelengths, detects abnormal hemoglobin variants, and has reduced artifacts compared with the traditional technology.

Electrocardiogram

- Three-lead electrocardiogram (EKG): is mostly used to detect arrhythmias (best by observing the P wave in Lead II).
- Five-lead EKG: can also detect myocardial ischemia or injury (by observing the ST segments for depression and elevation typically in Lead V5).

Non-invasive blood pressure

- Blood pressure (BP) cuff size should cover two-thirds of the length of the upper arm or leg, with the bladder placed over the artery.

Handbook of Critical Incidents and Essential Topics in Pediatric Anesthesiology, ed. David A. Young and Olutoyin A. Olutoye. Published by Cambridge University Press. © Cambridge University Press 2015.

- Values between upper and lower extremities may correlate poorly but either site can be used to effectively follow trends.

Capnography
- Gold standard for qualitative and quantitative assessment of ventilation.
- Common uses: confirmation of endotracheal tube placement, evaluation of ventilation, and estimation of the arterial carbon dioxide tension ($PaCO_2$) with the end-tidal carbon dioxide ($EtCO_2$) value.
- Waveform shape can detect extubation, airway obstruction, and spontaneous ventilation.
- Common sampling techniques
  - Mainstream: gas analyzed near the connector of the endotracheal tube.
  - Sidestream: most common method; easier to use and less bulky, gas analyzed at elbow of breathing circuit distal to Y piece.
- False-positive $EtCO_2$ detection may occur due to: esophageal intubation, tracheal tube in oropharynx, machine malfunction, and carbon dioxide in the stomach.
- False-negative $EtCO_2$ detection may occur due to: bronchospasm, airway obstruction, or large air leak.
- Normal $PaCO_2$–$EtCO_2$ gradient is 3–5 mmHg. This gradient may be higher in conditions that increase the dead space such as:
  - Dead space within the breathing circuit, endotracheal tubes, endotracheal tube connectors, Y piece, elbows (flow of gas occurs but no gas exchange).
  - Cyanotic heart disease.
  - Pulmonary disease: embolic events, hypoperfusion, and obstructive disease (e.g., chronic lung disease).
- Increased pulmonary shunt has minimal effect on the $PaCO_2$–$EtCO_2$ gradient.

Temperature monitoring
- Two methods: peripheral or central (core).
- Core temperature: measured in mid-esophagus in the retrocardiac position, rectum, nasopharynx (correlating to inferior surface of the cribiform plate), or bladder. Core temperature should be measured during major surgery.
- Inhaled anesthetic agents cause peripheral vasodilation and heat redistribution from the core to periphery, resulting in reduction of core temperature during the first hour.

Central nervous system monitoring
- Several types of processed EEG monitors are available to estimate anesthetic depth; the bispectral index (BIS®) monitor (Covidien, Mansfield, MA) is the most common.
- These monitors have been promoted to evaluate and reduce the occurrence of intraoperative awareness.
- Incidence of intraoperative awareness in children under general anesthesia is estimated at approximately 0.5–1%. No monitor has been shown to definitively decrease intraoperative awareness in children.

- The BIS monitor measures anesthetic depth by converting the processed EEG into a single value reported on a scale of 0–100. Adequate depth of anesthesia is 40–60.
- BIS values are less reliable in younger children compared to older children (due to maturation of the EEG from birth to adulthood).
- Utility of the BIS monitor is also unclear in patients with underlying medical conditions (e.g., epilepsy, developmental delay).

Near-infrared spectroscopy

- Near-infrared spectroscopy (NIRS) is a non-invasive method of continuous tissue oxygenation monitoring by determination of oxy and deoxyhemoglobin concentrations in non-pulsatile blood flow.
- Unlike pulse oximetry, NIRS values are not affected by poor perfusion.
- Similar to pulse oximetry, NIRS values can be affected by motion and light interference.
- Measures combined arterial and venous blood oxygen saturation; NIRS measures the venous and arterial oxygen saturation and reports the average oxygen saturation within the blood vessels and tissue.
- Normal NIRS values range from 60–80%.
- Infrared light is measured at two different wavelengths: 730 nm and 810 nm.
- Reflects balance between oxygen delivery and consumption. Original use started with monitoring trends in cerebral oxygenation.
- Can also monitor regional oxygenation (rSO_2) in skin, splanchnic, and renal regions (somatic NIRS).
- Decrease in somatic oxygenation may be associated with renal dysfunction and organ failure; intervention may improve outcome.
- A change in rSO_2 baseline value of 20% or more requires intervention.
- NIRS values will increase with the following: hypercarbia (increases in cerebral blood flow), increased hemoglobin concentration, hypothermia, increased oxygen saturation, and a decrease in cerebral metabolic rate (deep anesthesia).

Further reading

Coté CJ, Lerman J, Anderson BJ. *Coté and Lerman's A Practice of Anesthesia for Infants and Children*, 5th edition. Philadelphia, PA: Elsevier, 2013; 1068–78.

Gregory GA, Andropoulos DB. *Gregory's Pediatric Anesthesia*, 5th edition. Hoboken: Wiley-Blackwell, 2012; 401–8.

Part A **Basic concepts in pediatric anesthesiology**

Monitoring
Neurophysiologic monitors

Veronica O. Busso, Senthilkumar Sadhasivam and Mohamed Mahmoud

Somatosensory evoked potentials
- Monitoring provides valuable information concerning the integrity of the sensory tract from the peripheral nerves to the primary sensory cortex.
- Signal is generated by stimulation of peripheral nerves (e.g., median, ulnar, posterior tibial nerve).
- Signal travels ipsilaterally by ascension in the dorsal columns to the medulla, crosses over to the contralateral thalamus, then to the cortex in the internal capsule.
- Intraoperative somatosensory evoked potentials (SSEPs) are intermittently captured and compared to the baseline signals to assess for acute intraoperative changes. The surgeon and anesthesia providers are immediately notified of any significant change from the initial baseline potentials.
- A significant change is a more than 50% decrease in amplitude or a 10% increase in latency.
- SSEP can also help to optimize patient positioning by monitoring median or ulnar nerve changes due to traction on the brachial plexus.

Motor evoked potentials
- Motor evoked potentials (MEPs) can provide information regarding the functional integrity of the motor tracts of the spinal cord.
- Stimulus is conducted along the primary motor cortex via the cortico-spinal tract to the alpha motor neurons and a target muscle group.
- A significant change is a decrease in MEP amplitude of > 50–75%.
- Absolute contraindication to MEP use is presence of a cochlear implant.

Electromyography
- Electromyography (EMG) may be monitored from any muscle group that does not interfere with the surgical field.
- Any area that is at risk due to surgical intervention or patient positioning may be monitored.
- Provides real-time information regarding nerve root or peripheral nerve irritation.

Handbook of Critical Incidents and Essential Topics in Pediatric Anesthesiology, ed. David A. Young and Olutoyin A. Olutoye. Published by Cambridge University Press. © Cambridge University Press 2015.

- When a nerve root or motor axons are irritated the muscle fiber is activated by depolarization.
- "Burst" of EMG indicates a brief moment of irritation, while a "train" implies sustained irritation.
- Sustained "trains" may lead to chronic nerve damage, paresthesias or muscle weakness.
- A severely injured nerve may continue to fire even after the mechanism of injury has been removed.

Electroencephalography

- Electroencephalography (EEG) activity represents cortical neuron activity and is age- as well as anesthetic-dependent.
- EEG activity can be recorded and analyzed by direct inspection of waveform patterns and density spectral array.
- A normal EEG should be symmetric across hemispheres and the pattern should be synchronized.
- This modality may be used intraoperatively to assess cerebral perfusion, presence of after-discharge patterns following cortical stimulation, and to estimate the depth of anesthesia.
- Sharp wave activity and spikes are indicative of a seizure.
- Drug-induced burst suppression may be used as a means of decreasing cerebral metabolic demands and therefore provides cerebral protection.
- Asymmetries in EEG waveforms between hemispheres may indicate a unilateral hematoma or vascular insufficiency.

Brainstem auditory evoked response

- Brainstem auditory evoked response (BAER) evaluates the ascending auditory pathway from the eighth cranial nerve to the level of the inferior colliculus.
- BAERs are often studied during select posterior fossa craniotomies, acoustic neuroma resections, meningiomas, and ponto-medullary tumor resections.
- A significant change in the BAER is defined as more than a 50% decrease in amplitude or a 1 ms increase in absolute latency of any wave.

Near-infrared spectroscopy (NIRS)

- A non-invasive monitoring method that measures the concentration of oxyhemoglobin and deoxyhemoglobin to determine the cerebral tissue oxygen saturation.
- Commercially available devices use two wavelengths (730 nm and 810 nm) that pass through brain tissue 2–5 cm beneath the probe in the frontal cortex.
- NIRS may also be applied to assess the oxygenation of other organs such as an extremity (muscle), liver, and kidney.

Bispectral index

- Bispectral index (BIS) monitoring uses a form of processed cortical EEG to quantify the hypnotic effects of anesthetic agents.
- Uses both Fourier transformation and bispectral analysis to compute a single number.

- The BIS may range from 100 (awake) to 0 (isoelectric EEG).
- Surgical anesthesia depth is obtained at values of 40–60.

Acute loss of somatosensory or motor evoked potentials during spine surgery

Differential diagnosis

- Anesthetic agents
    - Volatile anesthetic agents
        - Dose-dependent decrease in amplitude and increase in latency.
        - SSEP: cortical potentials are susceptible to anesthetic effects.
        - MEP: all commonly used volatile anesthetics depress MEP more than SSEP (including significant depression with nitrous oxide).
    - Intravenous anesthetic agents
        - Most intravenous anesthetic agents cause dose-dependent changes in amplitude and latency of SSEPs and MEPs.
        - MEP and EMG signals are eliminated by the presence of clinically significant neuromuscular blockade.
- Physiologic events
    - Decreased spinal cord perfusion.
    - Hypotension.
    - Hypovolemia.
    - Anemia.
    - Severe hypothermia.
    - Hypocapnea: CO_2 < 20 mmHg due to decreased spinal cord perfusion.
- Medication error.
- Neuromonitoring equipment malfunction.
- Trauma to spinal cord or nerves.

Management

- Inform surgical and anesthesia team immediately to determine if there is a reversible surgical or anesthetic intervention or perhaps a technical explanation.
- Simultaneously ensure adequate perfusion pressures.
- Mean arterial blood pressure (MAP) should be raised to > 90 mmHg.
    - Administer vasoactive infusion (phenylephrine or dopamine).
    - Infuse crystalloids, colloids, or blood products.
- Reduce the anesthetic agent for appropriate depth of anesthesia.
- If there is no signal improvement, prepare for a "wake-up" test (anesthesia is discontinued to allow the patient to wake up, demonstrate muscle function, and then anesthetics are restarted).

Further reading

Cheufler KM, Zentner J. Total intravenous anesthesia for intraoperative monitoring of the motor pathways: an integral view combining clinical and experimental data. *J Neurosurg.* 2002; 96:571–9.

Coté CJ, Lerman J, Anderson BJ. *Coté and Lerman's A Practice of Anesthesia for Infants and Children*, 5th edition. Philadelphia, PA: Elsevier, 2013; 636–8.

Lo YL, Dan YF, Tan YE, Nurjannah S, Tan SB, Tan CT, Raman S. Intraoperative motor-evoked potential monitoring in scoliosis surgery: comparison of desflurane/nitrous oxide with propofol total intravenous anesthetic regimens. *J Neurosurg Anesthesiol.* 2006;18:211–14.

Mahmound M, Sadhasivam S, et al. Susceptibility of transcranial electric motor-evoked potentials to varying targeted blood levels of dexmedetomidine during spine surgery. *Anesthesiology.* 2010; 112(6): 1364–73.

Nathan N, Tabaraud F, Lacroix F, et al. Influence of propofol concentrations on multipulse transcranial motor evoked potentials. *Br J Anaesth.* 2003; 91:493–7.

Zhou HH, Zhu C. Comparison of isoflurane effects on motor evoked potential and F wave. *Anesthesiology.* 2000; 93:32–8.

Part A Basic concepts in pediatric anesthesiology

Chapter 99
Preoperative care
General concepts
Mary A. Felberg

Preoperative evaluation

History
The history portion of evaluation should focus on the following:
- Birth history, including gestational age, complications
  - Current gestational age < 60 weeks increases risk of postoperative apnea, especially with a history of prematurity or apnea.
- Patient's anesthetic history and associated complications
  - Difficult airway or vascular access.
  - Emergence agitation.
  - Postoperative nausea and vomiting.
- Family anesthetic history
  - Malignant hyperthermia susceptibility.
- Chronic medical conditions
  - Cardiac system: current status of defects, exercise tolerance, the need for infective endocarditis prophylaxis, baseline oxygen saturation, etc. (e.g., single ventricle physiology).
  - Respiratory system: respiratory symptoms, recent/current upper respiratory tract infection (URI), stridor, etc. (e.g., asthma, airway foreign body).
  - Gastrointestinal system: gastroesophageal reflux, full stomach risk based on procedure (e.g., bowel obstruction, failure to thrive).
  - Nervous system: baseline deficits, acute injuries, seizures, developmental delay (e.g., epilepsy, autism).
  - Immune system: immunosuppressed state, comorbidities related to immunosuppression (e.g., leukemia, status post kidney transplantation).
  - Metabolic disorders: status and presence of comorbidities (e.g., diabetes mellitus, hypothyroidism).
  - Hematologic system: current status, up-to-date on required medications such as factor replacement, presence of comorbidities (e.g., sickle cell disease, hemophilia).
  - Chromosomal abnormalities: presence of comorbidities (e.g., Down syndrome).

Handbook of Critical Incidents and Essential Topics in Pediatric Anesthesiology, ed. David A. Young and Olutoyin A. Olutoye. Published by Cambridge University Press. © Cambridge University Press 2015.

- Allergies
  - History of previous drug allergies (e.g., antibiotics).
    - Latex allergy is one of the most common causes of intraoperative anaphylactic reactions in children.
    - At-risk children include those with need for frequent urinary catheterization (e.g., neural tube defects, urinary malformations), or atopic individuals.
    - A history of tropical foods allergies (e.g., banana, avocado, or kiwi) is a risk factor for latex allergy.
- Current medications, including over-the-counter and herbal remedies.
- Fasting status
  - The most recent (2011) American Society of Anesthesiologists fasting guidelines for healthy patients:
    - Clear liquids may be consumed up to 2 hours prior to procedure.
    - Breast milk may be consumed up to 4 hours prior to procedure.
    - Full liquids or a "light meal" (formula, plain toast) may be consumed up to 6 hours prior to procedure; this does not include meats, fried or fatty foods.
    - All other foods may be consumed up to 8 hours prior to procedure.

Physical examination

The examination may be limited by the patient's ability to cooperate and underlying medical conditions. Some pertinent findings include:

- Vital signs: temperature (particularly if > 101°F), oxygen saturation (deviation from known baseline), tachypnea (especially if associated with respiratory distress), tachycardia (especially if associated with hypotension), blood pressure.
- Airway
  - Look for evidence predicting difficult mask airway or intubation (i.e., hypoplastic mandible, large tongue, limited oral opening, restricted neck mobility).
  - Note any dental abnormalities such as damaged or loose teeth, dental appliances.
    - Deciduous teeth are typically shed between ages 6–9 years.
    - Very loose teeth may need to be empirically extracted, typically after induction.
- Cardiovascular
  - Auscultation of rate, rhythm, and the presence of murmurs should be elicited.
  - Assess peripheral pulses, the presence of cyanosis with or without clubbing, signs of heart failure (e.g., tachycardia, tachypnea, sweating).
- Respiratory
  - Assess for signs of an upper respiratory infection (URI), (e.g., rhinorrhea, coughing, wheezing).
- Medical devices
  - Implanted devices (e.g., vagal nerve stimulators, insulin pumps, pacemakers)
    - These devices may require preoperative interrogation or mode alteration.
  - Tracheostomy tubes

- Determine size and type of tracheostomy.
- Uncuffed tubes may have large leaks and need modification prior to the surgical procedure.
- Metal tubes typically require replacement with nonferrous tubes prior to diagnostic imaging procedures (e.g., MRI).
- Ensure availability of appropriate sized backup tracheostomy tubes.
- Spinal anatomy
  - The presence of a sacral dimple or spinal curvature may impact plans for regional anesthesia (e.g., caudal block).

Laboratory testing
- Routine testing for healthy children undergoing minor procedures is not required.
- Selective testing is guided by the patient's medical conditions and the planned surgical procedure.
- Pregnancy testing for menstruating females is controversial.

Age-related risk factors
- Younger patients are at greater risk for serious perioperative adverse events.
- Infants accounted for 36% of the anesthesia-related cardiac arrests reported to the Pediatric Perioperative Cardiac Arrest registry between 1998 and 2002.
- The overall risk of cardiac arrest during anesthesia for children is in the range of 0.65–1.4/10,000 anesthetics. Risk is highest for age < 1 year and if preexisting heart disease is present.
- Older children have more adverse events overall but these events are associated with less morbidity and mortality.
- The risk of an adverse event significantly increases with a current or recent URI.
- Allergic reactions and pulmonary aspiration are uncommon.
- Anesthesia-related neurotoxicity of the developing brain is being studied. There is no evidence to guide anesthetic management. Current recommendations are to avoid unnecessary anesthetic exposure in young children.
- Awareness under anesthesia has an incidence of 0.8%; this is higher than the estimated risk for adults.

Informed consent
- Required portion of the preoperative process.
- Informed permission from the parent or legal guardian is obtained.
- Verbal assent from the child should be sought after age 8 (the accepted age of reason) in developmentally capable children.

Psychological preparation
- The anesthetic plan should include the goal of decreasing stress for the child associated with:

- ○ Separation from the family.
- ○ Acceptance of the mask for induction of anesthesia.
- A smooth separation/induction may also decrease the incidence of postoperative maladaptive behaviors (e.g., nightmares, eating disturbances, regression with developmental milestones, enuresis).
- Children aged 1–6 years old are at increased risk for separation anxiety.
- Knowledge of the patient's age, developmental stage, and personality traits in conjunction with current medical conditions can guide interventions to optimize separation.
  - ○ Non-pharmacologic interventions include tours, interaction with child life specialists, distraction techniques (electronic devices such as movies on a smartphone), or parental presence at induction.
  - ○ Pharmacologic interventions usually include anxiolytic medications (e.g., midazolam).
    - · Most studies demonstrate more effective separation with pharmacologic interventions.
    - · Routes of administration can include oral, IV, intranasal, IM, or rectal.
    - · Uncooperative patients with potential harm to self or others may benefit from ketamine 2–5 mg/kg IM.

Further reading

Coté CJ, Lerman J, Anderson BJ. *Coté and Lerman's A Practice of Anesthesia for Infants and Children*, 5th edition. Philadelphia, PA: Elsevier, 2013; 1–3, 37–44, 59–69.

Gregory GA, Andropoulos DB. *Gregory's Pediatric Anesthesia*, 5th edition. Hoboken: Wiley-Blackwell, 2012; 1–8, 273–84, 290–293, 330–8.

SmartTots. Neurotoxicity of Anesthetics in the Developing Brain: Summary Points; www.smarttots.org/about.html.

Part A Basic concepts in pediatric anesthesiology

Preoperative care
Separation anxiety/upper respiratory infections

Nancy S. Hagerman and Senthilkumar Sadhasivam

Preoperative anxiety

Incidence and risk factors

- Approximately 50–75% of children experience fear and anxiety preoperatively.
- The induction of anesthesia is one of the most stressful periods for children.
- Risk factors for increased preoperative anxiety include:
    - Young age (ages 1–5 years; separation anxiety typically does not peak until age 1 year).
    - Children with increased baseline anxiety.
    - Previous history of anxiety with prior medical encounters.
    - Increased parental anxiety.

Expected outcomes associated with "stormy" inductions

- Increased postoperative pain as well as analgesic requirements.
- Increased incidence of emergence agitation.
- Increased postoperative nausea and vomiting.
- Delayed discharge from the post-anesthesia care unit.
- Undesirable postoperative behavioral changes including:
    - Separation anxiety.
    - Generalized anxiety.
    - Night time crying.
    - Enuresis.
    - Eating difficulties.
    - Apathy.
    - Withdrawal.
    - Aggression toward authority.
- Behavioral changes are observed in 40–55% of children 2 weeks postoperatively; this reduces to approximately 19% at 6 months and 6% at 1 year.

Handbook of Critical Incidents and Essential Topics in Pediatric Anesthesiology, ed. David A. Young and Olutoyin A. Olutoye. Published by Cambridge University Press. © Cambridge University Press 2015.

Behavioral interventions
- Preoperative preparation programs; most effective when performed 5–7 days versus 1 day before surgery.
- Parental presence during anesthesia induction.
    - Parental presence does not reliably decrease child's anxiety.
    - Parental presence is associated with increased parental satisfaction.

Pharmacologic interventions
- Midazolam is the most popular preoperative anxiolytic in the United States.
    - Commonly given orally but can also be administered intravenously, nasally, rectally, and intramuscularly.
    - Decreases preoperative anxiety and postoperative maladaptive behaviors.
    - Patients may experience anterograde amnesia and loss of explicit memory; implicit memory is preserved.
    - Risk of paradoxical reaction; characterized by increased agitation.
- Other commonly used medications include:
    - Ketamine
        - May be given orally or intramuscularly.
        - Associated with increased secretions and bronchodilation.
    - Alpha-2-antagonists (clonidine and dexmedetomidine)
        - No effect on memory.
        - Minimal respiratory depression.
        - Decreases anesthetic requirements and postoperative pain scores.

Upper respiratory tract infections
- Extremely common in children (average of 6–8 episodes per year, possibly more frequent in children who attend daycare).
- Associated with an increased risk of adverse perioperative respiratory events including laryngospasm, bronchospasm, oxygen desaturation, breath holding, and severe coughing.
- Highest risk extends to the first 2 weeks after the infection has resolved.
- Although perioperative risk is increased, these events are typically managed easily, promptly and with minimal morbidity.
- Predictors of adverse perioperative respiratory events in a child with an active or recent upper respiratory tract infection (URI) include:
    - History of prematurity.
    - History of reactive airway disease.
    - Exposure to passive smoking.
    - Comorbidities.
    - Presence of sputum.
    - Presence of nasal congestion.

- Airway management (ETT (endotracheal tube) > LMA > mask).
- Surgery involving the airway.

Preoperative assessment

- History – assess for presence/severity of URI, and other predictors of adverse events. If decision is made to proceed with case, this allows for appropriate modification of intraoperative management.
- Physical – auscultation of lung fields to evaluate for lower respiratory infection, wheezing, dyspnea, preoperative vital signs including respiratory rate, and room air oxygen saturation value.
- Decision to proceed to the OR requires a risk/benefit analysis. Consider:
  - Urgency of procedure.
  - Patient's age.
  - Severity of symptoms.
  - Vital signs (i.e., fever > 38°C).
  - Comorbidities (e.g., asthma or cardiac disease).
  - Use of tracheal tube.
  - Presence of copious mucopurulent secretions, nasal congestion, productive cough.
  - Exposure to passive smoking.
  - Airway surgery.
  - History of prematurity.
  - Social issues.

Intraoperative management

- Increased incidence of adverse respiratory events in children with URIs is attributed to increased airway inflammation, reactivity, and interaction with the autonomic nervous system.
- Consider suctioning the airway after confirming that a deep level of general anesthesia is present; this may decrease future airway irritation and coughing and reduce the incidence of mucous plugging.
- Adequate intravenous hydration and airway humidification may minimize drying of secretions and reduce airway reactivity.
- Patients with a URI who have a tracheal tube placed are more likely to develop adverse respiratory events. Ensure that tracheal intubation is performed after a deep plane of general anesthesia has been established.
- The optimal depth of anesthesia for extubation is not clear. Some advocate deep extubation to avoid bronchial constriction; others argue that an awake extubation is preferable to allow the patient to have intact reflexes to control airway secretions.
- Consider avoidance of airway manipulation if feasible (i.e., providing mask general anesthesia).
- Consider administration of glycopyrrolate for the anticholinergic and antisialagogue effects.

- Consider administration of beta-2 agonists if wheezing is present.
- Consider empiric administration of topical local anesthetic to the airway (e.g., tracheal lidocaine).

Further reading

Coté CJ, Lerman J, Anderson BJ. *Coté and Lerman's A Practice of Anesthesia for Infants and Children*, 5th edition. Philadelphia, PA: Elsevier, 2013; 55–7.

Kain ZN, Caldwell-Andrews AA. Preoperative psychological preparation of the child for surgery: an update. *Anesthesiol Clin N Am.* 2005; 23(4):597–614.

Rosenbaum A, Kain ZN, Larsson P, Lonnqvist PA, Wolf AR. The place of premedication in pediatric practice. *Paediatr Anaesth.* 2009; 19(9):817–28.

Tait AR, Malviya S. Anesthesia for the child with an upper respiratory tract infection: still a dilemma? *Paediatr Anaesth.* 2005 100:59–65.

Varughese AM, Nick TG, Gunter J, Wang Y, Kurth CD. Factors predictive of poor behavioral compliance during inhaled induction in children. *Anesth Analg.* 2008; 107(2):413–21.

Von Ungern-Sternberg BS, Boda K, Chambers NA, et al. Risk assessment for respiratory complications in paediatric anaesthesia: a prospective cohort study. *Lancet.* 2010; 376:773–83.

Part A Basic concepts in pediatric anesthesiology

Chapter 101
Postoperative care
General concepts
Carlos Rodriguez

- Patients arriving in the post-anesthesia care unit (PACU) should initially receive an evaluation of oxygenation, ventilation, circulation, level of consciousness, and temperature.
    - Vital signs should be taken and compared with the preoperative and intraoperative trends.
    - Continuous pulse oximetry and electrocardiographic monitoring is used routinely in most PACU settings.
    - Selective use of capnography may also be beneficial in select patients.
    - Supplemental oxygen is routinely administered upon arrival.
    - Complete evaluation of cardiopulmonary function typically occurs.
    - Emergency equipment and medications (e.g., defibrillator, succinylcholine) should be immediately available.
- Parental presence is not a universal practice in the PACU; significant variation exists among institutions.
- Airway-related problems are one of the most common issues encountered in the PACU among the pediatric population.
    - Deep extubation may lead to laryngospasm.
    - Patients may have decreased airway tone and develop airway obstruction.
    - Postoperative apnea may occur in high-risk patients (e.g., premature neonates).
    - Patients with obstructive sleep apnea (OSA) have an increased risk for postoperative airway obstruction.
    - Patients below the age of 3 years undergoing adenotonsillectomy should undergo prolonged postoperative observation.
    - Patients with reactive airway disease and upper respiratory symptoms may develop bronchospasm.
    - Inadequate reversal of neuromuscular blockade can result in weakness and respiratory distress.
    - Airway edema can lead to post-intubation croup; a common trigger is the absence of an audible leak when utilizing an endotracheal tube. Treatment includes:
        . Humidified oxygen.
        . Nebulized racemic epinephrine.

Handbook of Critical Incidents and Essential Topics in Pediatric Anesthesiology, ed. David A. Young and Olutoyin A. Olutoye. Published by Cambridge University Press. © Cambridge University Press 2015.

- Dexamethasone.
- Consider reintubation for severe respiratory distress.
• Postobstructive pulmonary edema may occur by a forced inspiration against a closed glottis leading to significantly negative intrathoracic pressures. Signs include: hypoxemia, rales, and frothy airway secretions. Treatment should be supportive and may include oxygen, diuretics, and continuous positive airway pressure (CPAP). Mechanical ventilation using positive end-expiratory pressure (PEEP) may also be required.
• Cardiovascular instability is uncommon in the postoperative period. However, hypovolemia may be present due to inadequate fluid resuscitation or substantial blood loss. Tachycardia may be in response to hypovolemia, uncontrolled pain, anxiety, or as a result of previously administered anticholinergic agents.
• Postoperative nausea and vomiting (PONV) is one of the most common situations addressed in the PACU. Risk stratification is important in the management of PONV. Multimodal therapy has been proven to be effective in the treatment of nausea and vomiting after receiving anesthesia.
• Hypothermia can occur in the perioperative period and efforts should be made to keep patients warm using methods such as blankets and forced air warming devices. Neonates are at increased risk of developing apnea and bradycardia in the presence of hypothermia. Other problems associated with hypothermia include coagulation dysfunction, cardiovascular simulation, shivering, and increased susceptibility to infection. Special attention should be given to patients who develop hyperthermia. This may be an indicator of infection, malignancy or rarely malignant hyperthermia.
• Emergence agitation (EA) has a broad presentation and can include disorientation, crying, and uncontrollable behavior. The patient may have an altered perception of their surroundings. There is a higher incidence of EA with insoluble volatile agents such as sevoflurane and desflurane. Type of surgery, age, temperament, and preoperative anxiety are risk factors for the development of EA.
• The assessment of postoperative pain in the child may be challenging, particularly in patients that are preverbal or who have developmental disorders. Physiologic signs and communication with the patient and parent should be used in order to guide management of analgesia. Non-opioid agents (e.g., acetaminophen, ketorolac) should also be considered to either replace or complement traditional opioid therapy.
• Prior to discharge from the PACU, every patient must meet specific criteria. Traditional scoring systems include the following factors for otherwise healthy patients:
  - Appropriate vital signs which are similar to preoperative values.
  - Airway stability without the requirement for supplemental oxygen.
  - Neurologic status at baseline.
  - Minimal pain.
  - Absence of vomiting.
  - Ambulation (if applicable).

Further reading

Coté CJ, Lerman J, Anderson BJ. *Coté and Lerman's A Practice of Anesthesia for Infants and Children*, 5th edition. Philadelphia, PA: Elsevier, 2013; 980–91.

Gregory GA, Andropoulos DB. *Gregory's Pediatric Anesthesia*, 5th edition. Hoboken: Wiley-Blackwell, 2012; 361–80.

Part A   Basic concepts in pediatric anesthesiology

Postoperative care
Emergence agitation/PONV

David Moore and Senthilkumar Sadhasivam

Emergence agitation

- Emergence agitation (EA) is a dissociative state of consciousness noted during recovery from general anesthesia characterized by lack of coherence, restlessness, and inconsolability. Patients with EA are often noted to have the triad of consciousness, altered mental status, and perceived noxious stimuli.
- Risk factors for EA include age < 5 years, short duration outpatient surgery, use of insoluble volatile anesthetics such as sevoflurane, prior episodes of EA, excessive preoperative anxiety, and poor perioperative coping ability.
- Diagnosis of EA is often by exclusion of other conditions such as postoperative pain, anxiety, hypoxemia/hypercarbia.

Prevention of emergence agitation

- Avoidance of volatile anesthetics such as sevoflurane in patients with a previous history of significant EA.
- Avoidance of midazolam in patients with history of paradoxical agitation to benzodiazepines.
- Judicious use of regional anesthesia, and/or opioids for postoperative pain control. Propofol, fentanyl, clonidine, and dexmedetomidine have all been associated with reducing EA.
- Reduce postoperative anxiety in children by providing a rapid reunion with parents in the recovery room.

Management of emergence agitation

- Rule out hypoxemia, hypercarbia, postoperative pain, and anxiety.
- Treatment focused on altering one or more aspects of the triad of consciousness, altered mental status, and postoperative pain. Residual postoperative pain can be treated with pain medications such as fentanyl because of rapid onset. Sedatives can also be used to reduce anxiety. If EA is severe, flumazenil may be considered to reverse a suspected paradoxical reaction due to midazolam. In refractory cases of EA, propofol may be useful while ruling out other potential causes such as hypoglycemia.

Handbook of Critical Incidents and Essential Topics in Pediatric Anesthesiology, ed. David A. Young and Olutoyin A. Olutoye. Published by Cambridge University Press. © Cambridge University Press 2015.

Postoperative nausea and vomiting

- Incidence: Postoperative nausea and vomiting (PONV) is a very common perioperative problem; it is one of the most common reasons for unexpected postoperative admission. Patients often rate severe postoperative nausea and vomiting worse than postoperative pain. The overall incidence of PONV varies between 10% and 80% depending on patient and surgical risk factors. With the use of prophylactic antiemetics, the incidence of PONV is typically reduced to 10% or less.

Clinical and economic implications

- PONV can lead to delayed discharge from the recovery room, emergency room visits due to refractory PONV and dehydration, and unanticipated hospital admission in addition to adverse clinical outcomes (e.g., rupture of sutures, surgical bleeding).
- After outpatient surgery, the overall incidence of post-discharge nausea and vomiting (PDNV) has been reported to be between 8% and 17%. Patients who experience PDNV are typically unable to quickly resume their normal daily activities.
- Risk factors
    - Previous history of PONV.
    - Parental history of PONV.
    - Motion sickness.
    - Post-pubertal girls.
    - Use of volatile anesthetics, nitrous oxide, perioperative opioids.
    - Longer duration of surgery.
    - Type of surgery: adenotonsillectomy, strabismus repair, laparoscopic procedures, orchiopexy.
    - Postoperative pain.
    - Premature ambulation.
    - Premature or excessive oral intake.

Risk prediction and scoring system

- Risk of PONV in children can be estimated based on presence of four risk factors:
    - Surgery duration > 30 minutes.
    - Age > 3 years.
    - Previous PONV history.
    - Strabismus surgery.
- When 0, 1, 2, 3, and 4 of the risk factors are present, the estimated risk of PONV in children is approximately 10%, 10%, 30%, 55%, and 70% respectively.

Strategies to reduce risk

- Use of propofol for general anesthesia and avoid/minimize use of volatile anesthetics and nitrous oxide.
- Minimization of perioperative opioids by using regional analgesia, opioid-sparing analgesics such as intravenous acetaminophen and NSAIDs (e.g., ketorolac).

- Maintaining adequate hydration.
- Avoiding neostigmine.
- Consider performing gastric decompression.
- Use of prophylactic antiemetic drugs.

Prophylactic and therapeutic antiemetics

- The American Society of Anesthesiologists Task Force on Post-anesthetic Care recommends prophylaxis and treatment of nausea and vomiting. Antiemetic agents should be used for the prevention and treatment of PONV when indicated.
    - Commonly used antiemetics include 5-HT3 receptor antagonists (e.g., ondansetron, dolasetron, granisetron, tropisetron, palonosetron, ramosetron), dexamethasone, metoclopramide, scopolamine patch. Occasionally antihistamines and neuroleptics (e.g., droperidol) are used for refractory PONV.
    - Antiemetic drug selection depends on efficacy, cost, safety, and ease of dosing. Safety concerns have arisen regarding the side effects of antiemetics, specifically the effect on the QT interval of the EKG with use of butyrophenones and the first-generation 5-HT$_3$ receptor antagonist class of antiemetics.
- Combination of two or more prophylactic antiemetics from different classes may be considered when the risk of PONV is high and its clinical and economic implications are significant (e.g., combination of ondansetron and dexamethasone for outpatient adenotonsillectomy in children).
- Non-pharmacologic means such P6 point acupressure may also be beneficial in reducing PONV.

Further reading

Apfelbaum JL, Silverstein JH, Chung FF, et al. Practice guidelines for postanesthetic care: an updated report by the American Society of Anesthesiologists Task Force on Postanesthetic Care. *Anesthesiology.* 2013; 118(2):291–307.

Cole JW, Murray DJ, McAllister JD, Hirshberg GE. Emergence behavior in children: defining the incidence of excitement and agitation following anaesthesia. *Paediatr Anaesth.* 2002; 12:442–7.

Davis PJ, Cladis FP, Motoyama EK. *Smith's Anesthesia for Infants and Children*, 8th edition. Philadelphia: Elsevier Mosby, 2011; 1074–5.

Fronapfel PJ. Prevention of emergence delirium. *Paediatr Anaesth.* 2008; 18:1113–14.

Kovac AL. *Update on the Management of Postoperative Nausea and Vomiting. Drugs.* September 2013.

Uezono S, Goto T, Terui K, Ichinose F, Ishguro Y, Nakata Y, Morita S. Emergence agitation after sevoflurane versus propofol in pediatric patients. *Anesth Analg.* 2000; 91(3):563–6.

Part A — Basic concepts in pediatric anesthesiology

Chapter 103: Pediatric critical care medicine
General concepts
Amanda K. Brown and Rhonda A. Alexis

Acute respiratory failure
- Children, particularly infants, suffer increased morbidity and mortality from respiratory insufficiency.
- There is a predisposition to develop respiratory failure due to the increased compliance of the thoracic cage, underdeveloped intercostal musculature, and immaturity of the diaphragm.
- Etiology in children is similar to adults (e.g., acute respiratory distress syndrome (ARDS) and interstitial pneumonia) but specific precipitating pathology occurs in children (e.g., congenital adenomatoid malformation and bronchopulmonary dysplasia).
- Non-invasive ventilator strategies are increasingly employed to limit lung barotrauma and hypoxemia, particularly in neonates.

Cardiopulmonary resuscitation and pediatric advanced life support
- Cardiopulmonary resuscitation (CPR) of a child achieves higher success rates than observed in the adult population.
- Resuscitation outcomes are influenced by arrest location, existing comorbidities, initial EKG rhythm, quality of basic and advanced life support, and the time duration of arrest prior to implementation of life support.
- Ventricular fibrillation is detected in 25% of in-hospital pediatric arrests.
- Return of spontaneous circulation (ROSC) is achieved through algorithmic implementation of Airway, Breathing, Circulation, and Evaluation (ABCE). The preferred order for implementation is C-A-B.
- Asphyxia precedes many pediatric cardiac arrests. Optimal airway positioning with rescue breathing, bag-mask ventilation and advanced airway support remain key components of pediatric basic and advanced life support.
- Prompt initiation of effective chest compressions with minimal interruption is imperative, with a compression rate of 100 BPM. A depth of 1/3 the antero-posterior diameter should be achieved, allowing full chest recoil between compressions.

Handbook of Critical Incidents and Essential Topics in Pediatric Anesthesiology, ed. David A. Young and Olutoyin A. Olutoye. Published by Cambridge University Press. © Cambridge University Press 2015.

- In the infant, two-thumb encircling hand technique at the mid-sternum is an alternative to two-finger compression. In the child up to age 8 years, the heel of the hand should be used.
- The chest compression to ventilation ratio should be 30:2 for all ages, except with two rescuers available; in this situation a ratio of 15:2 should be implemented.
- Following endotracheal intubation, ventilation can be asynchronous and interruption of compressions is no longer necessary.
- Early utilization of an automated electrical defibrillator (AED) is essential (if a standard defibrillator is not available). Chest compressions should resume immediately following each defibrillation attempt. Chest compressions should be continued for approximately five cycles (or about 2 minutes).
- Vascular access should be established early. If difficult to secure, intraosseous (IO) line access should be strongly considered; the antero-medial surface of the proximal tibia 2 cm below the tibial tuberosity is the most common location utilized for IO placement.
- Medication therapy in cardiopulmonary resuscitation increases coronary and cerebral perfusion, myocardial contractility and rate, and treats arrhythmias.
- While epinephrine and vasopressin may improve ROSC rates, no single medication has demonstrated improved survivability to discharge. Use of empiric calcium therapy may be deleterious. Vasopressin is not included in any of the PALS algorithms.
- Reversible conditions may be amenable to extracorporeal membrane oxygenation (ECMO) following CPR.
- Post-resuscitation reperfusion injury poses specific neurologic and cardiac challenges.
- Avoiding hyperthermia and hyperglycemia minimizes secondary neurologic injury.
- Post-arrest myocardial dysfunction and hypotension are common.

Shock

- Pathophysiologic events requiring intensive critical care management vary, but a common denominator for many of the conditions is the evolution of shock.
- Shock develops from a failure of the circulation supply to meet the metabolic demands of the body.
- Compensated shock in the pediatric patient may mask significant circulatory dysfunction.
- Uncompensated shock may evolve rapidly into cardiovascular collapse.
  - General management principles include:
    - The primary principle of management is early recognition.
    - Investigation of the etiology for tachycardia, tachypnea, narrowed or diminishing peripheral pulses, abnormal capillary refill, and hypotension is mandatory but may be challenging.
    - Supportive management includes mechanical ventilation, volume resuscitation, administration of vasoactive medications, invasive monitoring, evaluation of laboratory studies, and frequent bedside assessment.
    - The primary therapeutic goal is to improve oxygen delivery and meet the metabolic demands.

- Aggressive fluid resuscitation, inotrope support, and antibiotic therapy (if indicated) within the first hour of presentation may be required.
- Tachycardia is a sensitive but non-specific marker of shock.
- Resolution of tachycardia is a useful indicator of successful treatment.
- Specific interventions are guided by the etiology and/or pattern of shock observed.

- Shock may be hypovolemic, cardiogenic, obstructive and distributive (septic, anaphylactic or neurogenic shock).
- Hypovolemic shock may occur following hemorrhagic or non-hemorrhagic conditions.
  - Intravenous fluid therapy in incremental boluses of 20 mL/kg up to 60 mL/kg may be required.
  - Detection of significant hemorrhage mandates repletion with blood products in order to maintain oxygen-carrying capacity and minimize coagulopathy.
- Cardiogenic shock may be due to a cardiogenic abnormality or rhythm disturbance.
  - Fluid resuscitation in cardiogenic shock is more cautious, as additional preload may not improve contractility and can actually worsen the overall function.
  - Treatment strategies may rely on the diagnostic yield of chest radiography, EKG and echocardiography.
  - Administration of inotropic medications may be required (e.g., milrinone, dobutamine).
- Obstructive shock occurs following potentially reversible etiologies, including tension pneumothorax, cardiac tamponade, and pulmonary emboli.
  - Circulatory support with fluid therapy and inotropic support are mainstays of therapy until successful identification and therapeutic reversal are achieved.
- Distributive shock is due to low systemic vascular resistance and impaired circulatory flow.
  - Evaluation to identify the etiology of distributive shock must be robust, as different strategies are employed to address sepsis, anaphylaxis, and neurologic injury.
  - Loss of vasomotor tone may occur following septic, anaphylactic, or neurogenic shock.
  - Inotropic support may be required to increase circulatory volume and improve systemic vascular resistance.

Further reading

Davis PJ. *Smith's Anesthesia for Infants and Children*, 8th edition. Philadelphia: Mosby, Inc., 2011; 1258–62.

Hay WW, Levin MJ, Sondheimer JM et al. *Current Pediatric Diagnosis & Treatment*. New York: McGraw Hill, 2005.

Topjian A. Advances in recognition, resuscitation and stabilization of the critically ill child. *Pediatr Clin North Am.* 2013; 60(3):605–20.

Part A Basic concepts in pediatric anesthesiology

Chapter 104
Pediatric critical care medicine
ECMO
Kha M. Tran

Extracorporeal membrane oxygenation (ECMO) is the use of a modified heart-lung machine; blood drains via gravity from a central vein, passes through a membrane oxygenator, and is pumped back into the patient through a central artery or central vein.

Indications

- Neonatal conditions (most common):
  - Persistent pulmonary hypertension of the newborn.
  - Meconium aspiration.
  - Congenital diaphragmatic hernia.
  - Respiratory distress syndrome.
- May also be of benefit in pediatric patients.
- Disease process MUST BE REVERSIBLE.
- Respiratory or cardiac failure.
- Congenital heart disease or cardiac surgery
  - Promotes healing by reducing ventricular work and reducing wall tension.
  - Serves as a bridge to transplant.
  - Can be initiated following failure to wean from bypass.
- May be instituted as an adjunct to cardiopulmonary resuscitation (CPR):
  - Up to 35% survival to discharge, with mean of 50 minutes of CPR before ECMO.
  - Good neurologic outcomes reported in 75% of patients placed on ECMO following CPR.

Contraindications

- Severe prematurity or small size, making cannulation difficult or impossible (< 34 weeks or < 2 kg).
- Conditions precluding heparinization (i.e., intracranial bleed, coagulopathy, active hemorrhage).
- Irreversible disease processes.

Handbook of Critical Incidents and Essential Topics in Pediatric Anesthesiology, ed. David A. Young and Olutoyin A. Olutoye. Published by Cambridge University Press. © Cambridge University Press 2015.

Types of ECMO cannulation

- Veno-venous (VV)
    - Instituted solely for respiratory support.
    - Does not support cardiac function.
    - Pulsatile systemic flow is preserved.
    - No vessels need to be ligated after discontinuation.
    - Cerebral venous congestion may occur with large catheters.
        - Recirculation may occur in VV ECMO as both inflow and outflow of blood from the catheter occurs in the right atrium, in contrast to veno-arterial ECMO where inflow is from the right atrium and outflow is into the aortic arch.
- Veno-arterial (VA)
    - Typically jugular vein and carotid artery are cannulated.
    - Femoral vessels (older children) or central (mediastinal) cannulation may also be used.
    - Allows for both cardiac and respiratory support.
    - Carotid artery is typically ligated.
    - Non-pulsatile systemic flow occurs.
    - Left ventricular stunning may occur resulting in poor myocardial function.
    - Aortic valve is exposed to high back pressure and this may increase left ventricular work requiring medications to decrease afterload.
    - Decreased pulmonary blood flow.
    - Minimal oxygenation occurs in the lungs.
    - Blood flowing to the left atrium and left ventricle does not have much oxygen, resulting in decreased coronary artery perfusion.

ECMO circuit

- At least 300–400 mL volume is required for neonatal circuits.
- Blood is heparinized to an activated clotted time (ACT) of 180–200 seconds (for comparison, full cardiopulmonary bypass ACT is 300–400 seconds).
- Flow rates range from 100–150 mL/kg/min.
- Normal cardiac output for comparison:
    - Neonate at birth: 400 mL/kg/min.
    - Infant: 200 mL/kg/min.
    - Adolescent: 100 mL/kg/min.

Catheters

- Single lumen venous catheters are multiorifice, wire reinforced.
- Single lumen arterial catheters are single orifice, wire reinforced, and the tip should be at the junction of the brachiocephalic artery and the aortic arch.
- Double lumen catheters may be used for VV ECMO; they sit deeper in the right atrium, with the arterial port ejecting into the right ventricle via the tricuspid valve to minimize recirculation.

Bladder

- A venous reservoir.
- Located between venous cannula and pump.
- Gives the circuit compliance.
- Pressure is monitored. A negative pressure in the bladder means that not enough blood is being drained from venous cannulas to go to the pump.
- If venous flow is less than pump flow, the pump will slow or stop to prevent damage to the atria or entrainment of air.

Tubing

- The "raceway" is where the pump rollers are working to achieve flow in the circuit.

Pump

- Blood is propelled through the tubing by the pump.
- The pump can be a roller pump or a centrifugal pump.
- In the roller pump, a roller displaces volume and propels blood forward.
- In the centrifugal pump, the blood is propelled by centrifugal force.
- Identify the hand crank which can manually operate the pump if power failure occurs.

Membrane lung (oxygenator)

- For gas exchange. Semipermeable membrane. Gas flows on one side and blood on the other side in a countercurrent fashion.
- Surface area is important for gas exchange.
- Carbon dioxide exchange is six times faster than oxygen exchange.
- Membrane lungs have a "rated flow."
- There is a point where increased flow will not help with oxygenation as there is not enough time for the blood to pick up oxygen from the membrane oxygenator.

Sweep gas

- This is oxygen, air, and carbon dioxide flowing in a countercurrent manner to the blood in the oxygenator.
- Inspired oxygen and carbon dioxide tensions are adjustable.
- Flow of the sweep is the major determinant of carbon dioxide removal (1–10 L/min).
- 1 L/min is typical for neonates.
- Heat exchanger.
- Countercurrent warm water bath.

Bridge

- ECMO equivalent of an arteriovenous fistula (AV) fistula.
- Usually clamped, but is opened periodically to prevent clotting.
- If venous drainage and return to patient limbs of circuit are clamped, unclamping the bridge allows the ECMO pump to run while the patient is "off" ECMO.

During an ECMO circuit emergency
- Clamp the venous line above the bridge.
- Unclamp the bridge.
- Clamp the arterial line above the bridge.

Medications on ECMO
- Lasix, fentanyl, and phenobarbital are highly bound to the membrane.
- Morphine clearance is decreased.
- Heparin clearance is increased.

Complications
- Air embolism.
- Cardiac tamponade.
- Tension pneumothorax.
- Tension hemothorax.
- Circuit disseminated intravascular coagulation.
- Clot in the circuit.
- Bleeding.

Further reading

Bahrami KR. ECMO for neonatal respiratory failure. *Semin Perinatol.* 2005; 29(1):15–23.

Coté CJ, Lerman J, Anderson BJ. *Coté and Lerman's A Practice of Anesthesia for Infants and Children*, 5th edition. Philadelphia, PA: Elsevier, 2013; 1427–8.

Davis PJ. *Smith's Anesthesia for Infants and Children*, 8th edition. Philadelphia: Elsevier, 2011; 1257–8.

Frenckner B. Respiratory failure and extracorporeal membrane oxygenation. *Semin Pediatr Surg.* 2008; 17(1):34–41.

Gaffney AM, Wildhirt SM, Griffin MJ, Annich GM, Radomski MW. Extracorporeal life support. *BMJ.* 2010; 341:c5317.

Part A: Basic concepts in pediatric anesthesiology

Chapter 105

Medical genetics
General concepts

Vidya Chidambaran and Senthilkumar Sadhasivam

Pharmacogenetics

- Pharmacogenetics (PGx) is defined as the study of genetic variations affecting drug response.
- History
  - 1950s–1960s: Genetic basis established for glucose-6-phosphate dehydrogenase deficiency, succinylcholine apnea, isoniazid hepatotoxicity, and malignant hyperthermia.
  - The Human Genome Project (1990–2004) elucidated in a landmark publication of the 2.85 billion nucleotides that make up the human genome.
- Human genome is diploid – has 2×23 chromosomes.
- Gene – basic unit of genetic information (20–25,000 genes).
  - Locus – location of a gene.
  - Allele – one variant form of a gene at a particular locus.
  - Genotype: The two genes at each locus constitute the individual's genotype at the locus.
  - Phenotype: The expression of a genotype is termed a phenotype.
  - Haplotype is a combination of closely linked alleles which tend to be inherited together.
- The most common type of allelic variation is the single nucleotide polymorphism (SNP); this occurs when two alternative bases appear at an appreciable frequency in a population (> 1%). Other variations are called mutations (incidence < 1%) which may be duplication, deletion, insertion, translocation, or inversion of DNA segments.
  - SNPs are frequent, occurring in approximately 1:100–1:1,000 bases.
  - Variations may have no consequence (silent mutations) while others alter the phenotype of the organism.
- Genetic information from nuclear DNA gets transcribed to RNA in the cytoplasm; this is then translated to protein formation. Variations in the genetic sequence affect protein formation and function, including enzymes, drug transporters, and receptors; and hence, influence pharmacokinetics and pharmacodynamics of drugs.

Handbook of Critical Incidents and Essential Topics in Pediatric Anesthesiology, ed. David A. Young and Olutoyin A. Olutoye. Published by Cambridge University Press. © Cambridge University Press 2015.

- Only 30,000 human genes code for several million unique proteins. This is because of post-translational modifications which include various reversible and irreversible phenomena.

Anesthesia and genomics

- Prolonged succinylcholine action is associated with two common variants of the butylcholinesterase gene (*BChE*) that code for defective pseudocholinesterases. Malignant hyperthermia, a life-threatening hypermetabolic response to volatile anesthetics and succinylcholine, is associated with mutations of the ryanodine receptor gene (*RYR1*).
- Increased desflurane anesthetic requirements have been associated with red hair phenotype, coded by variations of the *Melanocortin 1 receptor* gene.
- Deaths reported after codeine in a breast-fed infant of an ultrarapid metabolizer phenotype mother and in children after tonsillectomy have been attributed to presence of *CYP2D6* variants causing increased conversion of prodrug codeine to active morphine.
- Effect of the G allele of the μ-opioid receptor gene (*OPRM1*) causes decreased opioid response and increased analgesic requirements after surgery and in cancer patients.
- Increased bleeding after therapy with warfarin and non-steroidal anti-inflammatory agents have been associated in variants of the *CYP2C9* gene.
- SNP of the muscarinic acetylcholine receptor 3 subtype (*CHRM3*) gene, dopamine receptor DRD2 and serotonin receptors 5-HT3A and 5-HT3B have been found to increase risk for postoperative nausea and vomiting.
- Genetic variants of P-glycoprotein have been associated with increased risk for opioid side effects such as postoperative nausea and respiratory depression.

Genetic diseases in children

- Pediatric anesthesiologists often encounter children with challenging genetic disorders, who often have higher perioperative morbidity and mortality due to specific anatomic, physiologic, and metabolic abnormalities. Knowledge of associated anomalies and anesthesia-associated risk is important for their optimal care. The etiology of these disorders may be:
    - Single gene (autosomal dominant (AD) or recessive (AR) or X-linked): Marfan syndrome is AD; mucopolysaccharidoses such as Hurler syndrome are inherited as an AR condition while Hunter syndrome is X-linked recessive and Duchenne muscular dystrophy is inherited as an X-linked recessive condition with deficient dystrophin synthesis. Some conditions like Ehlers–Danlos syndrome and epidermolysis bullosa (EB) may be either AD/AR or X-linked, and for the latter, the severity may depend on the type of genetic defect, that is, autosomal recessive dystrophic EB affecting the type VII collagen is a more severe form.
    - Chromosomal (deletions, trisomy): Down syndrome is the most commonly encountered trisomy (chromosome 21) while an example of a deletion disorder is the *cri du chat* (cat's cry) syndrome (-5p).
    - Multifactorial or sporadic: Klippel–Feil syndrome, Goldenhar syndrome, and VACTERL (Vertebral anomalies, Anal atresia, Cardiac defects, Tracheo-esophageal

fistula, Radial anomalies, and Limb defects) syndrome do not have an identified pattern of inheritance.
  - The presence of associated genetic mutations may also affect disease presentation, e.g., in spinal muscle atrophy (SMA), type 1, which is severe, involves deletion in the spinal motor neuron *SMN1* gene; activity of *SMN2* gene can mitigate the effects and results in presentation of milder forms of the disease (SMA type 2 and 3).
  - Epigenetics also plays a role in genomic imprinting, that is, genes may be expressed differently depending on inheritance. Prader Willi and Angelman syndromes are often caused by an identical deletion on the long arm of chromosome 15. However, when the deletion is inherited from the child's father, Prader Willi syndrome results, and if from the mother, then Angelman syndrome results.
- Knowledge of the underlying genetics and mechanism of disease paves the way for prenatal and pre-anesthetic diagnostic and treatment options. Now it is possible to diagnose Down syndrome prenatally with the triple test (alpha-fetoprotein, unconjugated estriol, and human chorionic gonadotropin), and other genetic disorders such as epidermolysis bullosa.

Further reading

Butler MG, Hayes BG, Hathaway MM, Begleiter ML. Specific genetic diseases at risk for sedation/anesthesia complications. *Anesth Analg*. 2000; 91(4):837–55. PubMed PMID: 11004035. Epub 2000/09/27. eng.

Chidambaran V, Ngamprasertwong P, Vinks AA, Sadhasivam S. Pharmacogenetics and anesthetic drugs. *Curr Clin Pharmacol*. 2012; 7(2):78–101. PubMed PMID: 22432844. Epub 2012/03/22. eng.

Denborough MA, Forster JF, Lovell RR, Maplestone PA, Villiers JD. Anaesthetic deaths in a family. *Br J Anaesth*. 1962; 34:395–6. PubMed PMID: 13885389. Epub 1962/06/01. eng.

Gregory GA, Andropoulos DB. *Gregory's Pediatric Anesthesia*, 5th edition. Hoboken: Wiley-Blackwell, 2012; 993–1000.

Kelly LE, Rieder M, van den Anker J, Malkin B, Ross C, Neely MN, et al. More codeine fatalities after tonsillectomy in North American children. *Pediatrics*. 2012; 129(5):e1343–7. PubMed PMID: 22492761.

Rosenberg H, Rueffert H. Clinical utility gene card for: malignant hyperthermia. *European Journal of Human Genetics: EJHG*. 2011; 19(6). PubMed PMID: 21248738. Pubmed Central PMCID: 3110041. Epub 2011/01/21. eng.

Part A   Basic concepts in pediatric anesthesiology

Chapter 106

Medical genetics
Down syndrome
Julia Chen

Etiology and clinical features

Etiology
- Most common chromosomal abnormality resulting from trisomy 21, translocation of chromosome 21, or chromosome 21 mosaicism.
- Estimated prevalence 1:800.

Clinical features
- Craniofacial and airway features include: microbrachycephaly, short neck, low set ears, microdontia, mandibular hypoplasia, broad flat nose, macroglossia, tracheal and subglottic stenosis.
    - Contributing factors for obstructive sleep apnea include: narrow nasopharynx, hypertrophic tonsils and adenoids, and generalized hypotonia.
- Cervical spine disorders
    - Atlantoaxial instability occurs at higher rates and is related to ligamentous laxity or skeletal anomalies.
- Cardiovascular defects
    - Cardiovascular defects are common in Down syndrome patients (40–50%); defects include ventricular septal defects, atrioventricular canal defects, and Tetralogy of Fallot.
    - Predisposition to development of pulmonary hypertension either from cardiac lesions or chronic hypoxemia.
- Other clinical features
    - Developmental delay.
    - Hypotonia.
    - Gastrointestinal disease including duodenal atresia, annular pancreas, and esophageal atresia.
    - Thyroid disease including congenital and compensated hypothyroidism.

Handbook of Critical Incidents and Essential Topics in Pediatric Anesthesiology, ed. David A. Young and Olutoyin A. Olutoye. Published by Cambridge University Press. © Cambridge University Press 2015.

- Increased risk for acute myeloid leukemia (AML) and acute lymphocytic leukemia (ALL).

Anesthetic considerations

Airway/Pulmonary

- Cervical spine injury
  - Screening radiographs for asymptomatic patients are no longer routinely recommended; however, some organizations may recommend cervical spine radiographs prior to entering grade school or sports participation.
  - Patients with neurological symptoms should have radiologic evaluation and neurosurgical evaluation prior to elective procedures.
  - Caution should be taken to avoid unnecessary flexion, rotation, and extension of the neck, particularly during airway manipulation and patient positioning.
- Upper airway obstruction
  - Increased risk for airway obstruction during inhalation induction and mask ventilation.
  - Patients with obstructive sleep apnea may require supplemental breathing support postoperatively (continuous positive airway pressure, oral airway, oxygen) and may also require prolonged monitoring as well as postoperative admission.
- Post-extubation stridor
  - An appropriately sized endotracheal tube and correct use of the endotracheal tube cuff decreases the risk of post-extubation stridor; it is strongly recommended to use a tracheal tube at least one-half size smaller than estimated and to titrate air in the tracheal tube cuff to obtain an audible leak of approximately 20 cmH$_2$O.
  - Treatment of stridor includes dexamethasone, humidified oxygen, and nebulized racemic epinephrine.
- Respiratory symptoms
  - Patients are more likely to have recurrent respiratory infections and reactive airway disease.

Cardiovascular

- Preoperative evaluation should include cardiac history; anesthetic plan, and management should incorporate understanding of cardiac defects.
  - Consideration for infective endocarditis (IE) prophylaxis if appropriate.
  - Increased risk of conduction defects in patients with history of prior cardiac repair (e.g., right bundle branch block).
- Increased incidence of bradycardia and hypotension after inhalation induction that is independent of preexisting cardiovascular defects.

Thyroid disease
Patients with symptoms of hypothyroidism should have thyroid function studies prior to anesthesia for an elective procedure as well as pharmacologic therapy to create a clinically euthyroid state.

Vascular access
Arterial and venous catheterization in Down syndrome patients may be especially challenging secondary to small vessel size, vascular hyperreactivity, skin and fat abnormalities.

Further reading
Bull MJ; Committee on Genetics. Health supervision for children with Down syndrome. *Pediatrics*. 2011; 128(2):393–406.

Davis PJ, Cladis FP, Motoyama EK. *Smith's Anesthesia for Infants and Children*, 8th edition. Philadelphia: Elsevier Mosby, 2011; 19–20.

Gregory GA, Andropoulos DB. *Gregory's Pediatric Anesthesia*, 5th edition. Hoboken: Wiley-Blackwell, 2012; 304, 331–332, 357, 782–3, 920, 995–6, 1026–27, 1250.

Part A Basic concepts in pediatric anesthesiology

Chapter 107

Medical genetics
Other conditions
Shakeel Siddiqui

- A syndrome is the occurrence of more than one recognizable phenotypical trait that occurs in a specific association, that has characteristic features, and originates from a genetic cause.
- An association is a constellation of several recognizable phenotypical traits, either without a known genetic cause or with a variety of genetic causes.

CHARGE association syndrome
- The letters in the acronym stand for Coloboma, Heart defect, Atresia choanae, Retarded growth and development, Genital hypoplasia, and Ear anomalies/deafness.
- Incidence of CHARGE syndrome is 1:10,000 live births. A leading gene is the chromodomain-helicase-DNA binding protein 7 (*CHD7*) gene on the long arm of chromosome 8. Mutations of this gene are found in 60–65% of patients with the syndrome. Over 150 mutations have been discovered.
- Major features seen in most CHARGE patients are the 4C's:
  - Coloboma of iris/retina, microphthalmia (80% of patients); Choanal atresia/stenosis (unilateral or bilateral); Cranial nerve anomalies – olfactory tract, facial paralysis, sensory neural deafness, incoordination of swallowing; characteristic ear anomalies – Cup-shaped ear (80–100%).
- Distinctive CHARGE facies and features – sloping forehead and flattened tip of nose; growth and developmental delay.
- Minor features seen less frequently in CHARGE syndrome and less specific:
  - Cardiac malformations (75–80%), most often conotruncal defects; Tetralogy of Fallot, aortic arch anomalies and atrioventricular canal defects, genital hypoplasia including micropenis and cryptorchidism; cleft lip and palate; tracheo-esophageal fistula.
- Anesthetic considerations
  - Common procedures performed include choanal atresia repair, cardiac surgery, plastic surgery repair of ear anomalies and cochlear implants.
  - Airway management may be difficult. Coexisting mental retardation and developmental delay with autism spectrum disorders may make care more challenging

Handbook of Critical Incidents and Essential Topics in Pediatric Anesthesiology, ed. David A. Young and Olutoyin A. Olutoye. Published by Cambridge University Press. © Cambridge University Press 2015.

VACTERL/VATER syndrome

- This syndrome includes Vertebral anomaly, Anal atresia, Tracheo-esophageal fistula, Esophageal atresia and Radial as well as renal dysplasia (VATER).
- Tracheo-esophageal fistula is accepted as essential for diagnosis, along with at least one other major defect in five additional categories.
- Limb anomalies are observed in about 10%, and 30–50% of children have cardiac malformations: ventricular septal defect, atrial septal defect, and Tetralogy of Fallot (hence L and C in VACTERL).
- Vertebral anomalies occur in 25% of patients: hemivertebrae, fused/butterfly vertebrae, or extra vertebrae.
- Renal anomalies occur in 20% of patients: these include horseshoe kidney, renal agenesis, vesicoureteral reflux, hypospadias, dysplastic kidney, and/or cryptorchidism.
- Atresias of the gastrointestinal tract are present in 15% of patients, commonly anal atresias.

Micrognathia syndromes

Pierre Robin sequence

- Pierre Robin sequence (PRS): micro/retrognathia, glossoptosis, and cleft palate.
- Incidence 1:8,500 live births.
- Mildly affected patients need minimal interventions; severely affected patients manifest airway symptoms early.
- Significantly affected neonates require prone positioning for adequate ventilation, nasal continuous positive airway pressure (CPAP), endotracheal intubation or tracheostomy.
- Feeding difficulties are common and feeding gastrostomy may be required.
- Airway surgery including cleft palate repair, veloplasty, and mandibular operations are often necessary.

Treacher Collins syndrome

- Autosomal dominant disorder of bilateral facial development.
- Affects 1:50,000 live births.
- Genetic developmental disorder of first and second branchial arches.
- Characterized by hypoplasia of the maxilla, zygoma, and mandible; external and middle ear defects, and sensorineural deafness.
- Anesthetic considerations
  - Patients often require bony/soft tissue, external ear, orbital and zygomatic facial reconstruction, and mandibular advancement.
  - Difficulties in airway management for the anesthesiologist arise from mandibular hypoplasia and the high arched palate.

Goldenhar syndrome

- Oculo-auriculo-vertebral syndrome (hemifacial microsomia).
- Developmental disorder of first and second branchial arches.
- Affects 1:5,600 live births, frequently unilateral.

- Malformations/hypoplasia of external and middle ear with sensorineural hearing loss, mandibular hypoplasia, eye abnormalities; vertebral anomalies including cervical spine malformations are often present.
- Congenital heart disease occurs in approximately 33% of patients, commonly septal and conotruncal defects.
- Developmental delay and autism spectrum disorders may occur.
- Anesthetic concerns
    - Mandibular hypoplasia results in possible difficult intubation.

Cardiac syndromes

Di-George (velocardiofacial) syndrome
- Microdeletion of chromosome 22.
- Incidence: 1:2,000 live births.
- Incidence of cardiac defects is 70% (i.e., truncus arteriosus, interrupted aortic arch and tetralogy of Fallot, conotruncal anomalies, pulmonary stenosis, and ventricular septal defect).
- Central nervous system involvement: hypocalcemic tetany, developmental delay.
- Airway defects: cleft palate, micrognathia, choanal atresia, laryngobronchomalacia and velopharyngeal incompetence, small mouth and short philtrum.
- Anesthetic considerations
    - Direct laryngoscopy and intubation can be challenging.
    - Extubation may also be difficult due to velopharyngeal insufficiency. Choanal atresia makes placement of nasal airway and nasogastric tube difficult.
    - Hyperventilation may worsen hypocalcaemia.

Williams syndrome
- Incidence: 1:10,000 live births.
- Spontaneous occurrence or autosomal dominant pattern.
- "Elfin" facies, periorbital puffiness, flat nasal bridge, long philtrum, full cheeks, and full lower lip.
- Developmental delay, hypercalcemia, hypotonia, joint laxity, and hypertension.
- Cardiac defects are present in approximately 75% of patients: supravalvular aortic stenosis and peripheral pulmonary artery stenosis.
- Elastin arteriopathy: cerebral artery stenosis, abdominal aortic aneurysm, obstructed coronaries.
- Anesthetic considerations
    - Thorough preoperative evaluation of the cardiovascular system is strongly recommended.
    - Peripheral pulmonic stenosis is often present during infancy but improves over time.

Noonan syndrome

- Incidence: 1:1,000–2,500 live births.
- Occurs sporadically, or as autosomal dominant inheritance.
- Hypertelorism with downslanting palpebral fissures, low-set, posteriorly rotated ears, short webbed neck, pectus excavatum.
- Central nervous system: Arnold Chiari malformations, myopia, ptosis, and mild mental retardation.
- Cardiovascular: hypertrophic cardiomyopathy, pulmonary stenosis, atrial septum defect/ventricular septal defects, left ventricular hypertrophy, patent ductus arteriosus.
- Pulmonary restrictive lung disease, cryptorchidism, lymphedema.
- Gastroesophageal reflux may also be present.
- Anesthetic considerations
    - Acute subcutaneous edema causes difficult peripheral intravenous access, short webbed neck and micrognathia may make intubation difficult. Keep patient well hydrated and heart rate in low to normal range for management of cardiomyopathy. Severe kyphoscoliosis may preclude epidural placement.

Epidermolysis bullosa

- Epidermolysis bullosa (EB) is a disease of the epidermis/dermis and mucous membranes that leads to formation of bullae.
- Three major types
    - EB simplex – epidermis is affected.
    - Junctional EB – basement membrane is involved.
    - Dystrophic EB – dermis is primarily involved.
- Repeated formation and breakage of bullae leads to blisters that heal with atrophic scars and development of contractures.
- Oral, pharyngeal, and esophageal blistering leads to contractures of mouth and tongue. Painful blisters leads to decreased oral intake and poor nutrition, esophageal strictures, and dental caries. Acute pharyngeal bullae may cause airway obstruction or hemorrhage.
- Anesthetic considerations
    - Avoid friction and shearing forces. Airway management is best performed with a well-lubricated mask or supraglottic airway device.
    - Adhesives should be avoided when securing monitors, intravenous lines or airway devices. Clip-on pulse oximetry probes should be used and EKG electrodes applied without adhesive portion. Non-invasive blood pressure cuffs should not have direct contact with skin; skin should be wrapped prior to application of blood pressure cuff.
    - Succinylcholine should be avoided due to fasciculations and existing contractures.

Further reading

Gregory GA, Andropoulos DB. *Gregory's Pediatric Anesthesia*, 5th edition. Hoboken: Wiley-Blackwell, 2012; 993–100.

System-based topics in pediatric anesthesiology

Chapter 108

Respiratory system
Anatomy and physiology

Vanessa A. Olbrecht and Senthilkumar Sadhasivam

Fetal development and anatomy

- The fetal lungs begin to form within the first few weeks of embryonic development. The respiratory tract is derived from the endodermal tissue layer.
- By 16 weeks of gestation, the bronchiolar system down to the terminal bronchioles is formed. If pulmonary expansion is inhibited during this stage of development, such as with the presence of a congenital diaphragmatic hernia, pulmonary hypoplasia occurs.
- By 26–28 weeks of gestation, the vascular network surrounding the terminal air sacs is sufficient for gas exchange.
- Alveoli develop postnatally and, while the number of alveoli that will be present into adulthood is present by 18 months of age, the lungs continue to mature until 8–10 years of age.
- Type II pneumocytes, the cells responsible for surfactant production, begin to appear at 24–26 weeks of gestation.
- Breathing activities occur *in utero* and are a part of normal fetal development.

Physiology

- At birth, the neonate must generate a strong negative force (–40 to –80 cmH$_2$O) to effectively transform the fluid-filled lungs to lungs filled with air. Fluid within the lungs is primarily removed via the upper airways; remaining fluid in the lungs is removed through the capillaries and lymphatics during the first few days of neonatal life.
- During this neonatal transition, as the lungs fill with air, pulmonary vascular resistance decreases, allowing pulmonary blood flow to increase and gas exchange to begin. At the same time, systemic vascular resistance increases dramatically, leading to the switch from a fetal to neonatal circulation system.
- Since infants have a considerably increased metabolic requirement when compared to older children and adults on a per kg basis, their corresponding ventilatory requirement is also increased. Due to these circumstances, oxygen desaturation occurs more rapidly in infants than adults during short periods of hypoventilation from any cause (e.g., apnea, airway obstruction). When compared with adults on a per kg basis, neonates have the same tidal volume and functional residual capacity. In contrast, when

Handbook of Critical Incidents and Essential Topics in Pediatric Anesthesiology, ed. David A. Young and Olutoyin A. Olutoye. Published by Cambridge University Press. © Cambridge University Press 2015.

compared with adults on a per kg basis, neonates have increased minute ventilation, alveolar ventilation, and oxygen consumption.
- Infants are more prone to lung collapse due to increased compliance of the chest wall. Increased compliance of the infant's chest wall is secondary to a cartilaginous (non-calcified) rib cage and reduced muscular tone. These factors exacerbate the potential for airway collapse and rapid oxygen desaturation.
- Neonates and infants are more prone to airway obstruction as their absolute airway diameters are smaller when compared to an adult. Neonates and infants also have increased risk for developing subglottic edema due to this decreased diameter.
- Neonates are much less sensitive to the respiratory stimulating effects of a rising partial pressure of carbon dioxide ($PaCO_2$). Hypoxia decreases rather than increases their drive to breathe. Co-administration of anesthetic medications may increase the risk of respiratory depression, particularly in patients born prematurely.
- Periodic breathing, defined by breathing that is interrupted by apnea lasting < 10 seconds with no associated cyanosis or bradycardia, can be seen in normal, full-term neonates and is almost uniformly present in preterm infants; no therapy is required.
- Central apnea, defined as a cessation of breathing for 15 seconds or longer, or shorter pauses associated with cyanosis and/or bradycardia, is common in preterm infants secondary to immature neural respiratory control centers.
- Due to the risk of postoperative apnea in infants, most centers recommend postoperative observation for preterm infants less than 50–60 weeks post-conceptual age and full-term infants less than 44 weeks post-conceptual age following the delivery of any anesthetic (e.g., surgery, MRI).
- Risk factors for postoperative apnea include: decreased post conceptual age, hypoxemia, hypothermia, and anemia (hematocrit less than 30). Caffeine and/or theophylline may be helpful in decreasing the risk of post-operative apnea in premature infants.
- Acute life-threatening events (ALTE) are defined by a sudden episode of color change (cyanosis/pallor), tone change (limpness or sometimes stiffness), and apnea which requires immediate resuscitation to restore ventilation to the child. The incidence of such events can be as high as 3% and can occur in previously healthy, full-term neonates.
- During general anesthesia, infants and neonates are particularly vulnerable to developing laryngospasm which may lead to life-threatening airway obstruction, hypoxemia and possibly cardiorespiratory arrest.

Further reading

Davis PJ, Cladis FP, Motoyama EK. *Smith's Anesthesia for Infants and Children*, 8th edition. Philadelphia: Elsevier, 2011; 22–73.

Coté CJ, Lerman J, Anderson BJ. *Coté and Lerman's A Practice of Anesthesia for Infants and Children*, 5th edition. Philadelphia, PA: Elsevier, 2013; 11–18.

Part B System-based topics in pediatric anesthesiology

Chapter 109

Respiratory system
Medical conditions

Vanessa A. Olbrecht and Senthilkumar Sadhasivam

Bronchopulmonary dysplasia

- Bronchopulmonary dysplasia (BPD), also known as chronic lung disease, is a chronic disease of the lung parenchyma and small airways. BPD is thought to be caused by the release of inflammatory mediators (cytokines); this overall lung inflammation unfavorably influences pulmonary maturation. Risk factors associated with the development of BPD include prematurity, prolonged mechanical ventilation, ventilator-associated lung injury, chorioamnionitis, and persistence of a patent ductus arteriosus (PDA).
- BPD is rarely seen in the full-term infant but can occur in the setting of prolonged mechanical ventilation and associated ventilator-induced lung injury.
- BPD is defined as oxygen dependence at more than 28 days after birth and is characterized as mild, moderate, or severe depending on oxygen requirements and if ventilator support is required. BPD is characterized by a restrictive lung disease pattern as well as decreased vascular surface area.
- Pulmonary hypertension and cor pulmonale may be sequelae of severe BPD and are associated with significant morbidity and mortality.
- Clinical symptoms of BPD include: increased work of breathing, wheezing, rhonchi, prolonged expiratory time, air trapping, hyperinflation, and diminished exercise tolerance (e.g., poor feeding).
- Hypoxemia in BPD results from a combination of several factors including broncho-bronchiolar hyperreactivity, ventilation and perfusion (V/Q) mismatch, hypoventilation, and right-to-left shunting; in severe BPD, pulmonary hypertension and cor pulmonale may be present.
- Infants who have mild disease may improve over time and may eventually become asymptomatic. Airway hyperreactivity may still persist even if a child is clinically asymptomatic with "resolved" disease.
- Infants with severe BPD may have normal to near-normal oxygen saturation values on room air due to hypoxic pulmonary vasoconstriction. Following induction of general anesthesia, these children may experience rapid oxygen desaturation as their compensatory hypoxic pulmonary vasoconstriction is attenuated secondary to the effects of inhaled anesthetic agents. Hypoxemia and hypercarbia may also develop due to the relatively increased mechanical ventilatory settings required in patients with decreased pulmonary compliance.

Handbook of Critical Incidents and Essential Topics in Pediatric Anesthesiology, ed. David A. Young and Olutoyin A. Olutoye. Published by Cambridge University Press. © Cambridge University Press 2015.

- The use of antenatal steroids, surfactant therapy, and lung protective strategies during mechanical ventilation has led to a significant decrease in the incidence and severity of BPD. Lung protective strategies include permissive hypercapnia, lower peak ventilator settings, and goal setting to include lower acceptable oxygen saturation values.
- Treatment for BPD is mainly supportive and involves the use of medical therapies and protective ventilatory strategies. Bronchodilators such as albuterol and ipratropium bromide can be used to help decrease airway resistance and improve air flow. Diuretics are used to assist with pulmonary mechanics. Corticosteroids may be beneficial in decreasing airway inflammation.
- Anesthetic management in these patients can be quite challenging as bronchospasm, pulmonary hypertension, central airway malacia, and V/Q mismatch are common. During management, positive airway pressures (e.g., PEEP) can be useful to help prevent collapse of both large and small airways as well as to help maintain functional residual capacity (FRC).

Sleep-disordered breathing/obstructive sleep apnea

- Breathing during sleep is associated with a decrease in tidal volume and respiratory rate. Hypoxic and hypercapnic ventilatory drives are also decreased and upper airway resistance is increased. In children with underlying pulmonary or upper airway dysfunction, these changes can result in significant abnormalities, whereas in the normal child these physiologic changes are rarely of significant clinical concern.
- Sleep apnea is one of most common causes of sleep-disordered breathing. Sleep apnea may be central, obstructive or mixed. The incidence of obstructive sleep apnea (OSA) is increasing, this has been strongly associated with the epidemic increase of childhood obesity. OSA is more common in patients aged 2–8 years; this is the period in which the tonsils and adenoids are relatively increased in size compared with the upper airway.
- Neurologic and behavioral symptoms are commonly found in children with sleep-disordered breathing; failure to thrive may develop. Sudden infant death syndrome (SIDS) has been associated with infantile sleep apnea.
- Over time, severe, untreated sleep apnea may lead to cardiovascular disease including pulmonary and systemic hypertension, cor pulmonale, and heart failure.
- The gold standard for diagnosis involves overnight polysomnography, but clinical symptoms of daytime somnolence, snoring, and gasping during sleep may also guide clinicians towards the diagnosis.
- Symptomatic management includes continuous positive airway pressure (CPAP) and weight loss; in cases in which symptoms are being caused by enlarged tonsils and/or adenoids, adenotonsillectomy may be curative.
- Children with OSA experience a higher risk for perioperative morbidity and mortality. Children with OSA are sensitive to opioids, anesthetics, and other central depressants. Careful titration of perioperative medications, vigilant post-anesthesia care unit monitoring, strong consideration for postoperative observation, and appropriate instructions upon hospital discharge are necessary to ensure superior safety for children with OSA.

Further reading

Coté CJ, Lerman J, Anderson BJ. *Coté and Lerman's A Practice of Anesthesia for Infants and Children*, 5th edition. Philadelphia, PA: Elsevier, 2013; 748–9.

Davis PJ, Cladis FP, Motoyama EK. *Smith's Anesthesia for Infants and Children*, 8th edition. Philadelphia: Elsevier, 2011; 74–6, 791–6.

Patino M, Sadhasivam S, Mahmoud M. Obstructive sleep apnoea in children. *British Journal of Anaesthesia*. December 2013 PGA Special Issue.

Part B System-based topics in pediatric anesthesiology

Chapter 110

Respiratory system
Reactive airway disease/cystic fibrosis

Vanessa A. Olbrecht and Senthilkumar Sadhasivam

Reactive airway disease

- Asthma is the most common respiratory and chronic disease found in children. It is one of the most frequent reasons children seek medical care; up to 10% of children in the United States are affected by asthma. Asthma is a condition that has significant anesthetic implications. Patients should ideally receive all preoperative asthma medications prior to surgery.
- Asthma is characterized by chronic inflammation of the airways leading to reversible airway obstruction. This chronic inflammation is mediated by several cell types, including mast cells, eosinophils, neutrophils, and T lymphocytes.
- Asthma primarily affects the medium and small airways and can be triggered by many stimuli including allergens, pollution, cold, exercise, infections, and tobacco smoke. Asthma can also be triggered in the perioperative setting by pain, stress, and airway instrumentation.
- The primary pathologic finding is airway obstruction secondary to smooth muscle spasm (bronchospasm), mucosal edema, hypersecretion, and mucus plugging. This airway obstruction is usually reversible, either spontaneously or with pharmacologic (e.g., beta-2 agonist) agents.
- Asthma is divided into two categories depending upon the age of onset. Early-onset asthma is defined by the development of reactive airway disease before 3 years old; it is generally non-allergic and is usually triggered by viral respiratory tract infections. Later-onset asthma, which develops after the age of 3 years, tends to be more often associated with allergies and tends to correlate with a positive family history of asthma. Children who develop early-onset asthma are more likely to be free of symptoms by the time they reach 6 years of age as compared to those who develop asthma later in childhood.
- During an asthma exacerbation, ventilation and perfusion (V/Q) mismatching develops. Over the course of the exacerbation, air trapping, hyperinflation, hypoxemia, diaphragmatic fatigue, hypercapnia, and respiratory failure may occur.
- Signs and symptoms of an asthma exacerbation include: wheezing, cough, chest tightness, shortness of breath, respiratory distress/failure, tachypnea, cyanosis, hypoxemia, and tachycardia.

Handbook of Critical Incidents and Essential Topics in Pediatric Anesthesiology, ed. David A. Young and Olutoyin A. Olutoye. Published by Cambridge University Press. © Cambridge University Press 2015.

- From a physiologic perspective, asthma is associated with impaired (and prolonged) expiration rather than compromised inspiration.
- In chronic disease, airway remodeling occurs, leading to airway fibrosis and fixed airway obstruction that may result in unresponsiveness to pulmonary bronchodilators.
- The development of severe respiratory acidosis during an exacerbation indicates imminent respiratory collapse and is an indication for endotracheal intubation and mechanical ventilation.
- Patients with asthma are medically managed and six different classes of medications are used: corticosteroids, leukotriene inhibitors, beta-adrenergic agonists (short- and long-acting), phosphodiesterase inhibitors (theophylline), mast cell stabilizers (cromolyn), and anticholinergics.
- Intraoperative bronchospasm and asthma exacerbations are typically managed by increasing anesthetic depth, administering inhaled beta-2 adrenergic agonists, utilizing protective ventilatory strategies to avoid barotrauma, and avoiding histamine-releasing medications such as morphine and atracurium. Avoid desflurane which may irritate the airway and increase airway reactivity. Consideration for deep extubation should occur since it may reduce airway reactivity. Severe and refractory cases of bronchospasm may require the administration of low dose epinephrine, high doses of inhaled anesthetic agents, anticholinergic agents, helium-oxygen gas mixtures, and magnesium sulfate.

Cystic fibrosis

- Cystic fibrosis (CF) is a disease caused by an autosomal recessive mutation. The most common mutation of CF results in the loss of phenylalanine at position 508 (d508) on the CF transmembrane conductance regulator (CFTR) protein resulting in decreased volume of airway surface liquid. Reduced airway surface liquid results in decreased ciliary function and mucociliary transport. Decreased mucociliary transport results in stasis of secretions which increases the risk for pulmonary infections and adverse events such as bronchospasm.
- CF is a multisystem disease characterized by pulmonary, hepatic, and pancreatic dysfunction.
- The gold standard for diagnosis is the sweat chloride test. Neonatal screening is routinely performed in the United States.
- Pulmonary dysfunction is the most common cause of morbidity and mortality. The predicted mean age of survival is steadily increasing from 32 years in 2000 to 37 years in 2008. Inability to produce airway secretions results in dehydration, thickening of respiratory secretions and impaired ciliary beating. Impaired ciliary beating results in decreased mucociliary transport, stasis of respiratory secretions, chronic infections (including pulmonary and sinus), airway inflammation, and destruction of airway elastin.
- Longstanding chronic pulmonary infections result in bronchiolitis characterized by airway hyperreactivity, as well as bronchiectasis, atelectasis, and potential for pneumothorax development.
- Hemoptysis, cor pulmonale and respiratory failure are terminal findings and occur in the end-stage of the disease. Patients with severe CF generally require lung transplantation.

- Children presenting with CF often have small airway obstruction, hyperinflation, and V/Q mismatch; airway hyperreactivity is also common.
- Treatments include: nutritional therapy via the use of vitamins, supplemental pancreatic enzymes and dietary supplements; antibiotics; inhaled therapies; and aggressive airway clearance such as high-frequency chest wall compression vest therapies.
- General anesthesia may result in accumulation of lower airway secretions and increased airway reactivity; both previously mentioned conditions can be detrimental to a patient with CF. Prior to anesthetizing a patient with CF, it is important to ascertain their baseline pulmonary function. Anesthetic management should include provisions for patients having increased airway reactivity. The postoperative management should include aggressive airway clearance therapies and adequate pain control so that coughing is not inhibited. Coughing is a key component in the clearance of airway secretions.

Further reading

Coté CJ, Lerman J, Anderson BJ. *Coté and Lerman's A Practice of Anesthesia for Infants and Children*, 5th edition. Philadelphia, PA: Elsevier, 2013; 233–5.

Davis PJ, Cladis FP, Motoyama EK. *Smith's Anesthesia for Infants and Children*, 8th edition. Philadelphia: Elsevier, 2011; 74–8.

Part B System-based topics in pediatric anesthesiology

Chapter 111 Cardiovascular system
Anatomy and physiology
Premal M. Trivedi and Pablo Motta

Fetal circulation

- Blood flow *in utero*
    - The placenta is the organ of oxygenation and ventilation *in utero*.
    - Umbilical vein: delivers oxygenated and nutrient-rich blood to the fetal heart.
    - Two umbilical arteries: removes desaturated blood and metabolic waste and delivers them to the placenta.
    - Pulmonary vascular resistance (PVR) is high as the lungs are collapsed and fluid-filled.
    - Systemic vascular resistance (SVR) is low due to the placenta.
- Three shunts facilitate oxygen delivery:
    - Ductus venosus
        - Allows 50% of umbilical vein blood flow to bypass the liver and enter the inferior vena cava (IVC).
    - Foramen ovale
        - Allows the relatively highly oxygenated IVC blood to stream preferentially to the left atrium.
        - Results in the brain receiving most of the oxygenated blood.
    - Ductus arteriosus
        - Desaturated blood from the superior vena cava (SVC) preferentially enters the right ventricle (RV).
        - Allows the RV to eject to the descending aorta rather than to the high resistance pulmonary vasculature.
- Both ventricles contribute to systemic output.
    - Fetal circulation works in parallel.
- Volume and pressure loading in the heart is markedly different *in utero*.
    - Right atrial pressure (RAP) > left atrial pressure (LAP).
    - Right ventricular volume > left ventricular volume.
        - Right atrium receives systemic venous return + umbilical venous return.
        - Left atrium receives minimal pulmonary venous return + volume shunted across the foramen ovale.

Handbook of Critical Incidents and Essential Topics in Pediatric Anesthesiology, ed. David A. Young and Olutoyin A. Olutoye. Published by Cambridge University Press. © Cambridge University Press 2015.

- Right ventricular afterload > left ventricular afterload.
- Fetal hemoglobin (HgbF)
    - Composed of 2 alpha and 2 gamma subunits ($\alpha_2\gamma_2$).
    - Has a greater affinity for oxygen than adult hemoglobin (HgbA).
        - HgbF has a P50 of 19 mmHg for oxygen (PO_2) vs. HgbA of 27 mmHg in adults.
        - Facilitates oxygen transfer from mother to fetus.
        - Oxyhemoglobin curve is left-shifted.
    - Maximal oxygen tension *in utero*: 30–35 mmHg (70–80% saturation).
    - Tissue oxygen delivery is maintained by increased 2,3-diphosphoglycerate (DPG) and higher hemoglobin.

Transitional circulation

- Changes with birth
    - Expansion of the lungs: PVR decreases, pulmonary blood flow increases, and arterial oxygen tension increases.
        - Pulmonary venous return increases, resulting in increased LAP.
        - Ductus arteriosus functionally constricts.
    - Removal of the placental circulation
        - Venous return to the right atrium decreases with umbilical vein ligation.
        - Portal pressures decrease: triggering closure of the ductus venosus.
        - SVR increases.
    - Net effects:
        - LAP > RAP
            - Functional closing of the foramen ovale.
        - RV afterload decreases.
        - LV afterload increases.
- Although PVR and PAP are lower than *in utero*, they remain elevated.
    - Any condition that exacerbates PVR can cause persistence of the fetal circulation.
    - Certain congenital heart lesions require persistence of the fetal circulation to maintain life (ductal-dependent lesions).

Persistent fetal circulation

- Pathophysiology
    - PVR remains markedly elevated, exceeding SVR.
        - Promotes right-to-left shunting across the ductus arteriosus and foramen ovale.
        - Cyanosis and acidosis are exacerbated, further increasing PVR.
- Conditions that predispose to persistent fetal circulation
    - Prematurity.
    - Pulmonary disease.
    - Hypoxemia.

- Hypercarbia.
- Congenital heart disease.
- Sepsis.
- Acidosis.
- Hypothermia.

Patent ductus arteriosus with left-to-right shunting

- In premature patients, significant overcirculation and heart failure may occur.
- May serve as a nidus for endocarditis in older patients.
- Closure can be achieved via:
  - Indomethacin (decreases prostaglandin levels), used in neonates.
  - Surgical ligation via a left thoracotomy.
  - Coiling or ductal occluder placement.

The neonatal myocardium

- Structurally immature.
  - Fewer myocytes
    - Cell division continues until ~ 6 months.
  - Fewer, less organized myofibrils containing fewer contractile elements.
  - Incompletely developed sarcoplasmic reticulum and T tubules.
    - More dependent on calcium flux through the sarcolemma, and thus on serum calcium levels.
  - Reduced number of mitochondria and signaling pathways.
- These structural differences result in a less compliant heart with limited preload and contractility reserve.
- Increased systemic oxygen demands require an equally matched cardiac output.
  - Neonatal cardiac output is 2–3 times that of an adult (per kg basis).
  - At baseline, neonates are functioning near their maximum heart rate (HR) and stroke volume (SV) in order to meet oxygen demands.
    - Volume can be used to increase SV, but excessive amounts may decrease SV and cause pulmonary congestion.
    - Cardiac output is augmented primarily by increases in HR.
- Neonates are more susceptible to volatile agent-induced myocardial depression.

Innervation of the heart

- Sympathetic innervation is incomplete in the neonatal heart.
- Parasympathetic tone predominates until ~ 6 months of life.
  - Clinically observed as a tendency towards bradycardia in response to noxious stimuli and a decrease in response to exogenous catecholamines.

Normal physiologic variables

- Heart rate can vary widely in the first few months.
    - 50% of healthy newborns demonstrate some type of transient heart block.
- Blood pressure increases over the first 6 weeks to a mean systolic of 95 mmHg, and then remains stable to 6 years of life (Table 111.1).

Table 111.1 Normal ranges of blood pressure and heart rate for healthy patients based on age.

Age	Mean HR	Mean systolic	Mean diastolic
Premature	120–170	55–75	35–45
0–3 months	100–150	65–85	45–55
3–6 months	90–120	70–90	50–65
6–12 months	80–120	80–100	55–65
1–3 years	70–110	90–105	55–70
3–6 years	65–110	95–110	60–75
6–12 years	60–95	100–120	60–75
> 12 years	55–85	110–135	65–85

Adapted from Coté CJ et al. *A Pratice of Anesthesia for Infants and Children*. 5th Ed. Philadelphia: Saunders; 2013.

Further reading

Andropoulos DB. *Anesthesia for Congenital Heart Disease*, 2nd edition. Hoboken: Wiley-Blackwell, 2010; 55–7.

Coté CJ, Lerman J, Anderson BJ. *Coté and Lerman's A Practice of Anesthesia for Infants and Children*, 5th edition. Philadelphia, PA: Elsevier, 2013; 15.

Gregory GA, Andropoulos DB. *Gregory's Pediatric Anesthesia*, 5th edition. Hoboken: Wiley-Blackwell, 2012; 102–104.

Part B: System-based topics in pediatric anesthesiology

Chapter 112

Cardiovascular system
Medical conditions
Premal M. Trivedi and Pablo Motta

Acquired heart disease

Infectious diseases

- **Endocarditis:** infection of the endocardium
  - Pathogenesis
    - Bacterial seeding of damaged endothelium or exposed prosthetic grafts.
    - Endothelial injury occurs due to turbulent blood flow.
    - Causative bacteria are related to recent procedures or patient risk factors:
      - *Streptococcus viridans*: dental procedures.
      - Enterococci: genitourinary or gastrointestinal procedures.
      - *Staphylococcus aureus*: most common agent in postoperative endocarditis and intravenous drug users.
      - HACEK organisms (*Haemophilus, Actinobacillus, Cardiobacterium, Eikenella,* and *Kingella*): common in neonates and immunosuppressed patients.
  - Diagnosis is based on the modified Duke criteria and is confirmed when there is pathologic evidence along with compatible echocardiographic findings (e.g., oscillating intracardiac mass, abscess, dehiscence of a prosthetic valve).
  - Endocarditis prophylaxis is indicated in procedures that can induce bacteremia in patients with history of cardiac disease.
    - Unrepaired cyanotic congenital heart disease (CHD) including palliative shunts and conduits.
    - Completely repaired CHD with prosthetic material or device, during the first 6 months after the procedure.
    - Repaired CHD with residual defects at the site or adjacent to the site of a prosthetic patch or prosthetic device (inhibits endothelialization).
    - Cardiac transplantation recipients who develop a cardiac valvulopathy.
- **Myocarditis:** infection of the myocardium
  - Pathogenesis
    - Myocardial injury secondary to cell-mediated immunologic reaction.
    - Etiology:

Handbook of Critical Incidents and Essential Topics in Pediatric Anesthesiology, ed. David A. Young and Olutoyin A. Olutoye. Published by Cambridge University Press. © Cambridge University Press 2015.

- Infectious: viral agents (adenovirus, coxsackie B and echoviruses) are the most common.
- Non-infectious: immune-mediated (e.g., Kawasaki disease), collagen vascular disease, and toxic myocarditis (drugs, toxin or anoxic agents).
  - Clinical manifestations
    - Acute: fulminant heart failure.
    - Chronic: progressive congestive heart failure.
- **Pericarditis:** inflammation of the parietal and visceral surfaces of the pericardium
  - Pathogens:
    - Most common are viral infectious agents.
    - Bacterial infection (rare):
      - Tuberculosis.
      - Rheumatic fever.
  - Clinical manifestations: onset/severity is dependent on the speed of pericardial fluid accumulation and underlying myocardial function. Slow onset effusions are better tolerated.
  - Electrocardiogram: low voltage QRS complex with ST segment elevation.
  - Echocardiogram: pericardial effusions appear as an echo-free space between the epicardium and the pericardium.
  - Anesthetic considerations and management: see Pericardial disease, below.

Cardiomyopathies

- Definition: cardiomyopathy (CM) is disease of the heart muscle not associated with congenital, valvular, coronary disease, and/or systemic disorders.
- Classification is based on anatomical and functional features.
  - Dilated CM: characterized by decreased contractility with poor systolic function and ventricular dilation.
    - Etiology
      - Viral myocarditis.
      - Drugs (e.g., anthracyclines).
      - Metabolic: abnormalities of fatty acid, amino acid, glycogen, mucopolysaccharide metabolism, mitochondria and genetic disorders.
      - Chronic arrhythmias.
      - Coronary artery abnormalities.
    - Echocardiogram: Biventricular dilation with atrial enlargement.
  - Hypertrophic CM: characterized by septal and left ventricular hypertrophy, a small ventricular cavity, and diastolic dysfunction with preserved systolic function.
    - Etiology: inherited as an autosomal dominant trait.
    - Echocardiogram: thickened left ventricle and/or interventricular septum, normal contractility and reduced relaxation.
    - May result in sudden death during induction of anesthesia if undiagnosed.
  - Restrictive CM: characterized by restriction to diastolic filling due to a myocardial infiltrative process.

- Etiology
  - Amyloidosis.
  - Hemochromatosis.
  - Glycogen storage disease.
  - Mucopolysaccharidosis.
  - Sarcoidosis.
  - Endomyocardial fibrosis.
- Echocardiogram: preserved systolic function with restrictive relaxation pattern.

Pericardial disease

- **Pericarditis:** described above
- **Constrictive pericarditis:** rare in children
  - Etiology: multifactorial; usually occurs as cardiac involvement of other disease states:
    - Uremia secondary to end-stage renal disease.
    - Juvenile rheumatoid arthritis.
    - Septic arthritis.
    - Drug-induced effects (e.g., procainamide and chemotherapeutic agents such as anthracyclines).
  - Clinical manifestations: increased jugular venous pressure, hepatomegaly with ascites, and diastolic pericardial knock.
  - Electrocardiogram: low voltage QRS complex with T wave flattening or inversion.
  - Echocardiogram
    - Thickened visceral and parietal pericardium.
    - Dilated inferior vena cava and hepatic vein.
    - Paradoxical septal motion.
    - Diastolic dysfunction pattern.
  - Management: treatment of predisposing condition or in severe cases, pericardial stripping on cardiopulmonary bypass
- **Cardiac tamponade**
  - Etiology
    - Congenital heart disease.
    - Iatrogenic: following cardiac catheterization procedures.
    - Trauma.
  - Pathophysiology: fluid accumulation in pericardial space results in reduced ventricular filling and hemodynamic compromise.
  - Clinical manifestations
    - Diastolic dysfunction with elevated right heart pressures.
    - Equalization of diastolic pressures.
    - Decreased cardiac output and blood pressure.
    - Pulsus paradoxus.

- Echocardiogram
    - Collapse of the right atrium in late diastole.
    - Compression of right ventricular free wall.
- Anesthetic considerations
    - Avoid hypotension, vasodilation, and bradycardia by administration of volume and/or inotropes before induction.
    - Avoid positive pressure ventilation until effusion has been drained.
    - Sedation with ketamine and/or etomidate and local anesthesia can be employed while effusion is partially drained in order to relieve tamponade physiology before inducing general anesthesia.
- Management: Surgical options for recurrent effusion include:
    - Pericardial window via a subxyphoid approach.
    - Partial pericardiectomy.
    - Full pericardiectomy via sternotomy.

Intracardiac masses

- **Cardiac tumors:** rare in the pediatric population
    - Types
        - Rhabdomyoma: most common (> 50%); commonly occurs in a ventricle, may be multiple in number (in patients with tuberous sclerosis).
        - Other types include:
            - Fibroma (ventricular, solitary).
            - Teratoma (intrapericardial, close to the great arteries).
            - Myxoma (atrial, more common in adults).
    - Clinical manifestations: nonspecific, varies with tumor location, and includes: chest pain, arrhythmias, conduction anomalies, and inflow or outflow obstruction.
    - Echocardiogram: confirms the presence, extent, location, and hemodynamic compromise of the mass.
    - Anesthetic considerations:
        - Maintain euvolemia; hypovolemia may exacerbate inflow or outflow obstruction.
        - Defibrillation pads should be placed prior to induction as lethal arrhythmias may occur in this group of patients.

Further reading

Andropoulos DB. *Anesthesia for Congenital Heart Disease*, 2nd edition. Hoboken:Willey-Blackwell, 2010; 489.

Wilson W, Taubert KA, Gewitz M. Prevention of Infective Endocarditis Guidelines From the American Heart Association. A Guideline From the American Heart Association Rheumatic Fever, Endocarditis, and Kawasaki Disease Committee, Council on Cardiovascular Disease in the Young, and the Council on Clinical Cardiology, Council on Cardiovascular Surgery and Anesthesia, and the Quality of Care and Outcomes Research Interdisciplinary Working Group. *Circulation*. 2007; 116(15):1736–54.

Part B System-based topics in pediatric anesthesiology

Cardiovascular system
Valvular disorders/rhythm disorders
Premal M. Trivedi and Pablo Motta

Valvular disorders

Regurgitant lesions
Regurgitant lesions impose an increased volume burden on the chambers proximal and distal to the regurgitant valve, leading to chamber dilation and ultimately heart failure.

- **Mitral regurgitation (MR)**
  - Etiology
    - Congenital
      - Mitral valve prolapse.
      - Cleft mitral valve: isolated, or may occur in patients with atrioventricular (AV) canal defects.
    - Acquired
      - Endocarditis.
      - Rheumatic heart disease.
      - Annular dilation secondary to dilated cardiomyopathy.
  - Findings on echocardiogram
    - Systolic flow reversal in the pulmonary veins.
    - Prominent flail mitral valve or ruptured papillary muscle.
- **Tricuspid regurgitation (TR)**
  - Etiology
    - Congenital
      - Ebstein anomaly: apical displacement of the tricuspid septal leaflet.
    - Acquired
      - Endocarditis.
      - Carcinoid tumor.
      - Rheumatic disease.
      - Annular dilation secondary to right ventricular remodeling.
  - Findings on echocardiogram

Handbook of Critical Incidents and Essential Topics in Pediatric Anesthesiology, ed. David A. Young and Olutoyin A. Olutoye. Published by Cambridge University Press. © Cambridge University Press 2015.

- Dense triangular tricuspid regurgitation jet with early peaking.
- Severe hepatic systolic flow reversal.

- **Aortic insufficiency (AI)**
  - Etiology
    - Congenital
      - Bicuspid aortic valve.
    - Acquired
      - Valvulitis secondary to inflammatory disease (e.g., Kawasaki disease).
      - Endocarditis.
    - Ascending aorta dilation (e.g., Marfan syndrome).
  - Findings on echocardiogram
    - Abnormal flail defect.
    - Steep decelerating jet (pressure half time < 200 ms).
    - Prominent holodiastolic descending aortic flow reversal.

- **Pulmonic insufficiency (PI)**
  - Etiology
    - Acquired
      - Consequence of tetralogy of Fallot repair or balloon valvuloplasty for pulmonary stenosis.
  - Findings on echocardiogram
    - Steep decelerating wide jet.
    - Markedly increased pulmonic systolic flow.

- **Anesthetic considerations for regurgitant lesions**
  - Maintain sinus rhythm.
  - Maintain heart rate at upper limits of normal or at fast rate.
  - Decrease left ventricular afterload for MR and AI to decrease regurgitation.
  - Decrease right ventricular afterload for TR and PR: avoid hypercarbia, hypoxemia and acidosis.
  - Maintain contractility.

Stenotic lesions

Stenotic lesions impose an increased afterload on the emptying chamber, leading to pressure overload and remodeling, ultimately resulting in heart failure.

- **Mitral stenosis (MS)**
  - Etiology
    - Congenital
      - Usually associated with other obstructive left-sided lesions.

- Acquired
  - Rheumatic disease.
- Findings on echocardiogram.
  - Severe MS = mean gradient > 10 mmHg.

- **Tricuspid stenosis (TS)**
  - Etiology
    - Congenital form is rare.
    - Acquired
      - Rheumatic disease.
      - Systemic lupus erythematosus.
      - Carcinoid syndrome.
  - Findings on echocardiogram
    - Significant TS
      - Mean gradient ≥ 5 mmHg.

- **Aortic stenosis (AS)**
  - Etiology
    - Congenital
      - Undeveloped commissures.
      - Unicuspid or bicuspid valve.
      - Supravalvar AS (Williams syndrome).
  - Findings on echocardiogram
    - Severe AS
      - Peak velocity > 4 m/s.
      - Mean gradient > 40 mmHg.
      - Indexed aortic valve area < 0.6 cm^2/m^2.

- **Pulmonic stenosis (PS)**
  - Etiology
    - Congenital
      - Often isolated.
      - Unicuspid or bicuspid valve.
  - Findings on echocardiogram
    - Severe PS.
    - Peak velocity > 4 m/s.
    - Peak gradient > 64 mmHg.

- **Anesthetic considerations for stenotic lesions**
  - Maintain sinus rhythm
    - Avoid tachycardia – slow heart rate is better.
  - Keep filling pressure normal
    - Chambers are relatively non-compliant.

- Preserve contractility.
- Avoid systemic vasodilation and hypotension.

Rhythm disorders

- **Sinus node dysfunction:** alternating periods of bradycardia and tachycardia.
  - Etiology
    - Common in procedures with extensive atrial baffling.
  - Treatment
    - Pacemaker implantation with atrial anti-tachycardia pacing.
- **Junctional rhythm:** regular rhythm but lacks a P wave as the impulse originates in the bundle of His (QRS is indistinguishable from that of normal sinus rhythm).
  - Etiology
    - Related to surgical manipulation and atrial dissection.
  - Treatment
    - Temporary atrial pacing if symptomatic.

Conduction disorders

- **Atrioventricular (AV) block**
  - 1st degree
    - Fixed PR interval prolongation (all P waves are followed by a QRS wave).
    - Treatment
      - Observation unless symptomatic (rarely).
  - 2nd degree
    - Mobitz I: progressive lengthening of the PR interval leading to a dropped ventricular beat.
    - Mobitz II: dropped ventricular beats without warning – may progress to 3rd-degree AV block.
  - 3rd degree (complete AV block)
    - Complete AV dissociation.
    - Etiology
      - Congenital.
      - Acquired secondary to surgical injury.
    - Treatment
      - Permanent pacemaker.

Supraventricular arrhythmias

- **Supraventricular tachycardia (SVT):** most common arrhythmia in children characterized by a narrow complex tachycardia.

- Treatment
    - Compensated or hemodynamically stable patient: adenosine and/or vagal maneuvers.
    - Hemodynamic compromise: synchronized direct-current cardioversion.
- **Junctional tachycardia:** occurs due to an increase in the automaticity of junctional tissue.
    - **Accelerated junctional rhythm:** narrow complex tachycardia with no preceding P wave (usually retrograde).
        - Treatment: temporary overdrive pacing reestablishes normal sinus rhythm.
    - **Junctional ectopic tachycardia (JET):** narrow complex tachycardia with no preceding P wave. Heart rate > 95% predicted for age (> 170 bpm). Related to surgical dissection and occurs in the immediate postoperative period.
        - Treatment
            - Correct electrolytes.
            - Avoid and/or stop catecholamines.
            - Amiodarone.
            - Temporary atrial pacing at rates 10–20 bpm > JET rate.
            - Core temperature cooling (to 34 or 35°C).
- **Reentrant supraventricular tachycardia.**
    - **Atrial flutter:** negative sawtooth P wave pattern with atrial rates > 300 bpm.
        - Etiology: congenital heart disease (CHD) with extensive atrial suturing (e.g., Senning or Mustard operations) and/or atrial dilation (e.g., Fontan).
        - Treatment
            - Adenosine: promotes AV block.
            - Rate control (e.g., β-blockers).
            - Cardioversion if hemodynamically compromised.
    - **Atrial fibrillation:** rare in the pediatric population, characterized by very rapid atrial rates (400–700 bpm) with variable ventricular response. Management similar to atrial flutter. Anticoagulation is indicated for chronic atrial fibrillation due to the risk of emboli.
    - **Atrioventricular reentrant tachycardia (AVRT):** most common form of SVT in infancy and childhood.
        - Etiology: accessory pathway between the atrium and ventricle.
        - Two types:
            - "Orthodromic": atrial impulse is conducted down the AV node and returns retrograde through the accessory pathway (narrow QRS).
            - "Antidromic": atrial impulse is conducted down the accessory pathway to the ventricle which returns retrograde through the AV node (wide QRS complex).
    - **Atrioventricular nodal reentrant tachycardia (AVNRT):** the reentry circuit is *within* the AV node.
        - Treatment of AVRT and AVNRT
            - Cardioversion if patient is hemodynamically unstable.

- AVNRT: AV nodal blockers (adenosine, β-blockers, calcium channel blockers).
- AVRT: Cautious use of AV nodal blockers as they can promote accessory pathway conduction leading to malignant arrhythmias.
- Transcatheter ablation.

Ventricular arrhythmias

- **Ventricular tachycardia (VT):** three or more premature ventricular contractions in a row, at a rate 20% higher than the normal sinus rhythm. Sustained VT is defined as lasting > 10 seconds.
  - EKG: AV dissociation and QRS morphology of bundle branch block.
  - Types:
    - Monomorphic ventricular tachycardia: only one type of QRS complex.
    - Polymorphic ventricular tachycardia: multiple different types of QRS complexes.
      - Torsades de pointes: polymorphic VT with varying QRS morphologies manifested as positive and negative oscillations.
  - Etiologies
    - Metabolic: hypoxia, acidosis and/or electrolyte imbalance.
    - Channelopathies (Long QT syndrome, Brugada syndrome).
    - Cardiomyopathies.
    - Perioperative myocardial ischemia.
  - Treatment
    - Hemodynamically stable
      - Amiodarone: 5 mg/kg over 5–10 minutes, may repeat × 2 to maximum of 15 mg/kg.
      - Lidocaine: 1–2 mg/kg bolus dose; 20–50 µg/kg/min infusion.
      - Procainamide: 10–15 mg/kg bolus dose; 20–80 µg/kg/min infusion.
      - Beta-blockers e.g., esmolol (250–500 µg/kg bolus dose and 50–300 µg/kg/min infusion) or propanolol (0.01–0.1 mg/kg loading dose).
      - Torsades de pointes: magnesium sulfate: 25–50 mg/kg over 30–60 minutes.
    - Hemodynamically unstable patient: defibrillation
      - External defibrillation: (initial dose 2 J/kg for the transthoracic approach, increase to 4 J/kg if unsuccessful.
- **Ventricular fibrillation:** asynchronous ventricular depolarizations that do not generate cardiac output.
  - EKG: low amplitude irregular deflections without identifiable QRS complexes.
  - Lethal if untreated – medical emergency.
  - Treatment
    - Defibrillation (initial dose 2 J/kg for the transthoracic approach).
    - Increase to 4 J/kg if unsuccessful.
    - Follow Pediatric Advanced Life Support protocols.
    - Amiodarone and lidocaine may make defibrillation more successful.

Further reading

Andropoulos DB. *Anesthesia for Congenital Heart Disease*, 2nd edition. Chichester, UK: Wiley-Blackwell, 2010; 398–414.

ASE Guidelines at www.asecho.org/clinical-information/guidelines-standards/ last accessed November 14, 2013.

Part B System-based topics in pediatric anesthesiology

Chapter 114

Cardiovascular system
Pulmonary hypertension/heart failure
Premal M. Trivedi and Pablo Motta

- Heart failure is defined by the clinical picture of edema, respiratory distress, growth failure, and feeding or exercise intolerance.
- Accompanying symptoms include circulatory, neurohormonal, and molecular abnormalities.
- Responsible for ~12,000 pediatric hospital admissions per year.

Classification of heart failure

- The Modified Ross Heart Failure Classification, analogous to the New York Heart Failure Classification in adults, has been used to assess severity of heart failure in the pediatric population.
    - Class I: asymptomatic.
    - Class II: mild tachypnea or diaphoresis with feeds in infants, or dyspnea on exertion in older children.
    - Class III: marked tachypnea or diaphoresis with feeds in infants, prolonged feeding times with growth failure, or marked dyspnea on exertion.
    - Class IV: tachypnea, retractions, grunting, or diaphoresis at rest.

Cardiovascular causes of heart failure

- Most common cause is congenital heart disease (~60%).
    - Volume overload
        - Left-to-right shunting: ventricular septal defect, patent ductus arteriosus, atrioventricular canal defect.
        - Atrioventricular or semilunar valve insufficiency: cleft mitral valve, aortic insufficiency due to a bicuspid aortic valve, pulmonary insufficiency following Tetralogy of Fallot repair.
    - Pressure overload
        - Neonatal coarctation of the aorta.
        - Critical aortic stenosis.
        - Severe pulmonary stenosis.

Handbook of Critical Incidents and Essential Topics in Pediatric Anesthesiology, ed. David A. Young and Olutoyin A. Olutoye. Published by Cambridge University Press. © Cambridge University Press 2015.

- Single ventricles, ductal-dependent
  - Hypoplastic left heart syndrome.
  - Pulmonary atresia.
  - Tricuspid atresia.
- Cardiomyopathy (~20%)
  - Dilated cardiomyopathy
    - Multiple etiologies
      - Idiopathic.
      - Viral myocarditis.
        - Leading cause of acute heart failure in patients with a structurally normal heart.
      - Mitochondrial or genetic disorders.
      - Abnormalities in fatty acid, amino acid, glycogen, and mucopolysaccharide metabolism.
      - Anthracycline toxicity.
      - Ischemia secondary to coronary artery anomalies.
      - Muscular dystrophy.
  - Hypertrophic cardiomyopathy.
  - Restrictive cardiomyopathy
    - Associated with myocardial infiltrative processes.
    - Diastolic dysfunction.
    - Elevated atrial and pulmonary pressures.
  - Left ventricular noncompaction cardiomyopathy
    - Diagnosed based on the spongy, trabeculated appearance of the left ventricle (LV) on echocardiogram.
  - Arrhythmogenic right ventricular cardiomyopathy.
- Pulmonary hypertension.

Pulmonary hypertension

- Defined as a mean pulmonary artery pressure (PAP) > 25 mmHg at rest, or a pulmonary vascular resistance index (PVRI) > 3 Wood units.
- Associated with increased perioperative risk.
- Characterized by a progressive pulmonary vasculopathy resulting in right heart failure if untreated.
- Etiology
  - Pulmonary arterial hypertension (PAH)
    - Idiopathic.
    - Familial.
    - Associated with:
      - Congenital heart disease.
      - Collagen vascular disease.

- Portal hypertension.
- Human immunodeficiency virus (HIV).
- Pulmonary veno-occlusive disease.
- Persistent pulmonary hypertension of the newborn.
- Pulmonary hypertension with left heart disease
  - Systolic or diastolic dysfunction.
  - Valvular heart disease.
- Pulmonary hypertension with lung disease or hypoxemia
  - Chronic obstructive pulmonary disease.
  - Interstitial lung disease.
  - Sleep-disordered breathing.
- Pulmonary hypertension due to thromboembolic disease.
- Miscellaneous
  - Sarcoidosis.
  - Mechanical compression (tumor, adenopathy, mediastinitis).
  - Histiocytosis X.

Mechanisms of cardiovascular risk in pulmonary hypertension

- Acute pulmonary hypertensive crisis
  - Precipitated by an acute rise in pulmonary vascular resistance (PVR) and PAP, or acute systemic hypotension.
  - Factors that exacerbate PVR include:
    - Noxious stimuli.
    - Hypoxemia.
    - Alveolar hypoxia.
    - Hypercapnia.
    - Hypothermia.
    - Acidosis.
  - Pathophysiology
    - The acute increase in PAP/PVR induces a strain on the right ventricle (RV), increasing RV end-diastolic volume and pressure.
    - Decrease in RV stroke volume leads to a decrease in LV stroke volume.
    - The enlarged RV may also displace the septum towards the LV, further impairing LV stroke volume.
    - The resulting hypotension decreases RV coronary perfusion and worsens RV function.
    - Clinically, this manifests as desaturation, decrease in end tidal carbon dioxide ($ETCO_2$), hypotension, tachycardia, and signs of RV strain/ischemia on EKG.
    - In the presence of an atrial septal defect or patent foramen ovale (PFO), right-to-left shunting may occur, preserving cardiac output at the expense of cyanosis.

- Management
    - Increase FiO$_2$ to 100%.
    - Institute inotropic support.
    - Start inhaled nitric oxide (iNO) at 20–40 parts per million (ppm).
    - Eliminate noxious stimuli.
    - Treat acidosis if present.
    - Correct hypothermia.
- Chronic pulmonary hypertension
    - The RV hypertrophies over time and ultimately dilates and fails.
    - Maintaining coronary perfusion pressure will prevent ischemia.

General perioperative considerations in patients with pulmonary hypertension

- Continue current medications patient may be taking for pulmonary hypertension.
- For elective procedures, avoid prolonged periods of fasting to avoid hypovolemia.
- Consider the need for additional equipment or monitoring for the patient.
    - Five-lead EKG to monitor for strain/ischemia.
    - Arterial line.
    - Central access.
    - Confirm availability of inhaled nitric oxide.
    - Ensure inotropes, pressors, and vasodilators are readily available.
- Anesthetic technique and agents
    - No specific technique – general anesthesia or sedation – has been shown to be more beneficial than another.
    - Avoid noxious stimuli, hypoxemia, hypercapnia, and acidosis.
    - Positive-pressure ventilation should be used cautiously to provide the most appropriate tidal volume for the patient.
        - Too large a tidal volume can diminish venous return and increase PVR.
        - Too small a tidal volume will also increase PVR and cause hypercapnia.

Further reading

Andropoulos DB. *Anesthesia for Congenital Heart Disease*, 2nd edition. Hoboken: Wiley-Blackwell, 2010; 528–9.

Coté CJ, Lerman J, Anderson BJ. *Coté and Lerman's A Practice of Anesthesia for Infants and Children*, 5th edition. Philadelphia, PA: Elsevier, 2013; 359–60.

Friesen RH, Williams GD. Anesthetic management of children with pulmonary arterial hypertension. *Paediatr Anaesth.* 2008; 18(3):208–16.

Hsu DT, Pearson GD. Heart Failure in Children Part I: History, Etiology, and Pathophysiology. *Circ Heart Fail.* 2009; 2(1):63–70.

Shukla A, Almodovar MC. Anesthesia considerations for children with pulmonary hypertension. *Pediatr Crit Care Med.* 2010; 11(2 Suppl):S70–3.

Nervous system
Anatomy and physiology
Yang Liu

Anatomy

- The intracranial compartments contain:
    - Brain and interstitial fluid (80%).
    - Cerebrospinal fluid (CSF) (10%).
    - Blood (10%).
- The fontanelles
    - Infants at birth have many fontanelles which close at different times:
        - Anterolateral fontanelle: 3 months.
        - Posterior fontanelle: 3 to 6 months.
        - Anterior fontanelle: 10 to 18 months.
        - Posterior-lateral fontanelles: 2 years of age.
    - A full fontanelle may be a sign of increased intracranial pressure.
    - A depressed fontanelle can indicate dehydration or aggressive drainage of CSF.
    - Early closure of sutures and fontanelles results in craniosynostosis.
- Intracranial compartments
    - The brain is 10–15% of the body weight at birth, grows rapidly throughout the first year of life, and reaches adult weight by 12 years.
    - The supratentorial compartment includes the anterior and middle cranial fossa which contains the cerebral hemispheres and diencephalon.
        - Diencephalon comprises the thalamus, hypothalamus, epithalamus, and subthalamus.
    - A differential pressure between the two cerebral hemispheres may lead to herniation of the brainstem and other vital structures.
    - The infratentorial compartment, often described as the posterior cranial fossa, contains the cerebellum and brainstem.
    - The cerebellum mainly regulates posture, muscle tone, and coordination.
    - Increased pressure within the posterior fossa may lead to herniation of the cerebellar tonsils through the foramen magnum.
- The spinal canal compartment contains the spinal cord and the CSF.

Handbook of Critical Incidents and Essential Topics in Pediatric Anesthesiology, ed. David A. Young and Olutoyin A. Olutoye. Published by Cambridge University Press. © Cambridge University Press 2015.

- The spinal cord ends at the intervertebral level of L3 at birth and rises to adult level of L1–L2 by the age of 8 years.
- The dural sac shortens from S3 at birth to S1 by 1 year of age.
- Vascular anatomy
    - The brain receives blood supply via two sets of paired arteries – the internal carotid arteries and the vertebral arteries.
    - At the base of the brain, the carotid and vertebrobasilar arteries form a circle of communicating arteries known as the circle of Willis.
    - Collateral flow in the circle of Willis prevents cerebral ischemia and infarction if one of the main arteries is occluded.
    - The superior sagittal sinus is composed of dural venous sinuses and is the most prominent of the venous sinus drainage systems of the brain. It is located in the sagittal plane within the midline of the cerebral vault.
    - The anterior spinal artery supplies the ventral two-thirds of the spinal cord. The dorsal one-third is supplied by the posterior spinal artery. There is no collateral flow between these arteries.
    - Venous drainage from the spinal cord is usually by three anterior and three posterior spinal veins.

Neurophysiology

- Cerebral blood flow (CBF)
    - The CBF of children aged 6 months to 4 years is twice that of the adult (50 mL/100 g/min).
    - Adequate cerebral blood flow must be maintained to ensure a constant delivery of oxygen and substrates and also to remove the waste products of metabolism.
    - Manipulation of the CBF helps to control intracranial pressure (ICP).
    - The CBF is one of the variables that can be directly modified by anesthesiologist.
        - Volatile agents and hypercarbia increase cerebral blood flow.
- Cerebral autoregulation
    - Allows CBF to remain constant over a wide range of cerebral perfusion pressures (CPP).
    - Is decreased by volatile agents in a dose-dependent manner.
    - The CBF is dependent on a number of factors that can change the cerebral perfusion pressure and the radius of cerebral blood vessels.
    - Cerebral perfusion pressure (CPP)
        - Perfusion of the brain is dependent on CPP and the pressure gradient between the arteries and the veins (mean arterial pressure – ICP or central venous pressure (CVP)).
    - The radius of cerebral arterial blood vessels
        - The radius of cerebral arterial blood vessels is regulated by cerebral metabolism, carbon dioxide and oxygen, autoregulation, and neurohumoral factors.
        - Carbon dioxide (CO_2) is the most powerful vasodilator to the cerebral vessels.

- The relationship between $PaCO_2$ and CBF is almost linear between a $PaCO_2$ of 20 mmHg and 80 mmHg.
- An increased radius (vasodilation) leads to an increase in cerebral blood volume which in turn increases ICP and therefore reduces CPP.
  - Cerebral autoregulation may be impaired in some pathological conditions such as in patients with hypertension, brain tumors, subarachnoid hemorrhage, stroke, or head injury.
  - The brain cannot tolerate any mass effect due to the low elasticity of the skull and dura. Therefore any increase in brain mass (tumor) or volume of skull (hemorrhage or obstruction to flow of CSF) will result in a rapid rise in intracranial pressure.

Further reading

Davis PJ. *Smith's Anesthesia for Infants and Children*, 8th edition. Philadelphia: Mosby, Inc., 2011; 713–18.

Gregory GA, Andropoulos DB. *Gregory's Pediatric Anesthesia*, 5th edition. Hoboken: Wiley-Blackwell, 2012; 117–38.

Part B: System-based topics in pediatric anesthesiology

Chapter 116

Nervous system
Medical conditions
Yang Liu

Hydrocephalus

- Common causes of hydrocephalus in pediatric patients include:
  - Intraventricular hemorrhage in premature infants.
  - Infection – meningitis.
  - Brain tumor.
  - Arnold Chiari malformation.
  - Aqueduct atresia and stenosis.
  - Dandy-Walker malformation.
- Hydrocephalus may cause:
  - Increased intracranial pressure.
  - Progressive enlargement of the head.
  - Seizures.
  - Developmental delay.
  - Brain herniation.
  - Death.
- Classification
  - Nonobstructive or communicating hydrocephalus is associated with impaired cerebrospinal fluid (CSF) absorption.
  - Obstructive hydrocephalus.

Arachnoid cyst

- CSF-filled sacs which may be located anywhere along the central nervous system (CNS).
- Majority of the cysts form outside the temporal lobe of the brain in the middle cranial fossa.
- Symptoms depend on the location and size of the cyst.

Handbook of Critical Incidents and Essential Topics in Pediatric Anesthesiology, ed. David A. Young and Olutoyin A. Olutoye. Published by Cambridge University Press. © Cambridge University Press 2015.

Arnold Chiari malformation
- Part of the cerebellum is located below the foramen magnum.
- May occur as a result of structural defects during fetal development or excessive drainage of CSF from the lumbar or thoracic region.
- Classification
    - Type I: extension of the cerebellar tonsils into the foramen magnum.
    - Type II: extension of both cerebellar and brainstem tissue into the foramen magnum.
        - Usually accompanied by myelomeningocele and hydrocephalus.
    - Type III: the cerebellum, medulla and the fourth ventricle protrude through the foramen magnum.
    - Type IV: an incomplete or underdeveloped cerebellum exists.
- Arnold Chiari malformations may also be associated with syringomyelia, tethered cord syndrome, spinal curvature, or hereditary syndromes.

Brain tumors
- Most common solid tumors of childhood.
- Brain tumors can be classified according to their location.
    - Supratentorial tumors
        - Astrocytomas.
        - Craniopharyngiomas.
        - Germ cell tumors.
        - Optic pathway and hypothalamic glioma.
    - Infratentorial tumors (comprise about half of all brain tumors in children)
        - Medulloblastomas – most common type of childhood brain tumor.
        - Cerebellar astrocytomas.
        - Ependymomas.
        - Brainstem glioma.
- Symptoms
    - Headaches and visual deficits are the most common presenting symptoms.
    - Other symptoms may include seizure, personality and behavior changes, somnolence, weakness or numbness, etc.
    - Posterior fossa tumors in children are often associated with hydrocephalus.

Vascular malformations
- In the neonatal period, vein of Galen malformations (VGAMs), dural sinus malformations, and pial arteriovenous shunts are the predominant vascular lesions.
- After 2 years of age, arteriovenous malformations (AVMs), cavernomas, aneurysms, and dural arteriovenous shunt may be encountered.
- Prenatal magnetic resonance imaging (MRI) or ultrasound may diagnose high-flow AVMs.

- Arteriovenous malformations (AVMs)
    - Most common cause of spontaneous intracerebral hemorrhage in children.
    - May cause arterial steal and/or venous congestion.
    - Common clinical findings include intracranial hemorrhage, neurologic deficits, headaches, and seizures.
- Vein of Galen malformations (VGAMs)
    - A single artery or multiple arteries deliver blood directly into an enlarged and primitive vein of Galen.
    - High-flow shunts can lead to cardiac insufficiency and failure.
    - Many patients present with hydrocephalus.
- Moyamoya disease
    - An occlusive disease of unknown origin.
    - Presents with "puff of smoke" appearance on cerebral angiography.
    - Classically involves the supraclinoid internal carotid arteries.
    - Most children present with transient ischemic attacks or cerebral infarctions.

Craniosynostosis

- Craniosynostosis consists of premature fusion of one (simple) or more cranial sutures (complex), often resulting in craniofacial abnormalities.
- Multiple suture synostoses are more commonly associated with Crouzon syndrome or Apert syndrome.
- The frequencies of the various types of craniosynostosis are sagittal 50–58%, coronal 20–29%, metopic 4–19%, and labdoid 2–4%.

Spinal dysraphism

- Spina bifida
    - Myelomeningocele
        - Most common type of spina bifida.
        - All patients have radiographic evidence of Chiari II malformation and about 85% have shunt-dependent hydrocephalus.
        - Symptoms may include loss of bladder or bowel control, lack of sensation and paralysis of the legs.
    - Spina bifida occulta.
    - Meningoceles.
- Occult spinal dysraphism (OSD)
    - Characterized by thickened or fatty filum terminale, intramedullary lipoma, lipomyelomeningocele, etc.
    - May result in tethering of the spinal cord and possible neurological and bladder/bowel function deficits.

Spinal cord tumors

- Extradural tumors – chordomas and sarcomas.
- Intradural extramedullary tumors – neurofibromas and meningiomas.
- Intramedullary spinal cord tumors.

Cranial trauma

- Major causes of head injuries in children include falls, recreational activities, non-accidental trauma, and motor vehicle accidents.
- Classification
    - Skull fracture.
    - Epidural hematoma.
    - Subdural hematoma.
    - Intracerebral hemorrhage.

Spine injury

- Pediatric spine injuries are not very common.
- The cervical spine is the most commonly injured portion when injury does occur.

Further reading

Coté CJ, Lerman J, Anderson BJ. *Coté and Lerman's A Practice of Anesthesia for Infants and Children*, 5th edition. Philadelphia, PA: Elsevier, 2013; 510–30.

Gregory GA, Andropoulos DB. *Gregory's Pediatric Anesthesia*. 5th edition. Hoboken: Wiley-Blackwell, 2012; 540–68.

Part B System-based topics in pediatric anesthesiology

Chapter 117

Nervous system
Seizure disorder/cerebral palsy/autism

Amanda K. Brown and Rhonda A. Alexis

Seizure disorder

- An abrupt interruption of brain function causing involuntary motor, sensory, or autonomic disturbance.
- Partial seizures are isolated to one cerebral hemisphere while general seizures are global.
- Etiology: idiopathic or secondary to metabolic disturbances, trauma, anoxia or infection.
- Categories are defined by age of onset and pattern.
- Categories of seizures include neonatal, febrile, infantile, benign childhood epilepsy, juvenile myoclonic, and generalized tonic-clonic.
- Status epilepticus:
  - Sustained seizure event extending 30 minutes or more.
  - Progressive hypoxia and acidosis that may lead to neurologic injury or death.
  - No discernable cause has been elicited.
  - Management:
    - Respiratory and cardiovascular support including resuscitation may be required.
    - Treatment of any underlying metabolic disturbances.
    - First-line therapy commonly includes benzodiazepines; long-term anti-epileptic medications are typically initiated after a thorough neurologic evaluation.
- Anesthetic management
  - Requires knowledge of anticonvulsants and drug interactions.
  - Anticonvulsant therapy accelerates clearance of nondepolarizing muscle relaxants resulting in the need for frequent redosing during surgery.
  - Risk profiles of individual therapies should be reviewed; carbamazepine and valproic acid may cause hepatotoxicity and bone marrow suppression.
  - Some therapies raise additional anesthetic concerns. Use of ACTH or corticosteroids for infantile seizures may cause adrenal corticosteroid suppression and hypokalemia.
  - Anesthetic agents may potentiate therapy-induced drowsiness.
  - Treatment of recalcitrant seizures may include a ketogenic diet.

Handbook of Critical Incidents and Essential Topics in Pediatric Anesthesiology, ed. David A. Young and Olutoyin A. Olutoye. Published by Cambridge University Press. © Cambridge University Press 2015.

- Metabolic acidemia may occur from ketosis intraoperatively.
- Fluid management may require ongoing carbohydrate restriction.
- Anesthetic selection may affect seizure thresholds.
  - Myoclonic movements have been reported with etomidate and sevoflurane; use of these agents is acceptable.
  - Sevoflurane elicits a pattern of epileptogenicity concordant with the seizure pattern of an affected individual; this effect is not clinically significant.
  - Ketamine and etomidate both sustain evoked seizure activity during electroconvulsive therapy (ECT); however both have been used to treat status epilepticus.
  - Use of meperidine promotes accumulation of its proconvulsant metabolite normeperidine.
  - Hypocarbia lowers the seizure threshold.
- Surgical management
  - Surgery is often therapeutic, with either implantation of a vagal nerve stimulator or resection of the epileptogenic foci.
  - Vagal stimulation blunts paroxysmal epileptiform activity. Aberrant side effects include vocal cord disruption, bronchoconstriction, and bradycardia.
  - Resection of the epileptogenic foci may require partial temporal lobectomy. An awake craniotomy may also be performed in order to preserve core brain functions such as speech.
  - Alternatively, the epileptogenic foci may be mapped electrically via surgically placed cortical grids.
  - Bradycardia and sinus arrest have been reported during surgical resection with manipulation of the amygdala and insular cortex.

Cerebral palsy

Disorder of movement and posture evolving from a static motor encephalopathy, often attributed to gestational asphyxia.

- Approximately 11% of babies delivered prematurely between 24–27 weeks gestation have cerebral palsy.
- Classification: spastic or extrapyramidal.
- Spastic type: characterized by clonus and increased tone. Pattern of distribution is varied but may include quadriplegia.
- Extrapyramidal type: characterized by clonus and rigidity with variable tone. Subtypes include choreoathetotic, ataxic or hypotonic versions.
- Indications for surgery commonly include: hip dysplasia, dental restorations, seizure surgeries, gastric tube placement, and limb contractures.
- Anesthetic management
  - Evaluate degree of compromise.
  - Judicious use of oral anxiolytics is recommended as they may exacerbate upper airway obstruction.
  - Consider use of an antisialagogue as increased oral secretions may be present.

- ○ Respiratory insufficiency may develop from bulbar dysfunction and recurrent aspiration.
- ○ Existing altered thoracic development may reduce functional residual capacity.
- ○ Cerebral palsy is not an absolute contraindication to the use of succinylcholine.
- ○ Minimal anesthetic (MAC) requirements are reduced and the risk for opioid-induced respiratory depression is increased.
- ○ Anesthetic sensitivity may be exacerbated by hypothermia. Rapid heat loss may occur due to reduced muscle mass and inadequate hypothalamic control.
- ○ Neuraxial blockade has been shown to further reduce anesthetic requirements and improve postoperative pain control.

Autism

- Neurologic disorder characterized by impaired social interaction and communication.
- Stereotypical behavior occurs demonstrating restrictive and repetitive activities.
- Etiology is unclear, but a strong familial component and concordance in monozygotic twins has been demonstrated.
- Higher incidence is observed in males, and in individuals with Down syndrome, Cornelia de Lange syndrome, tuberous sclerosis, and Fragile X syndrome.
- Management
    - ○ Pharmacotherapy may be initiated to modify behavior.
    - ○ Neuroleptic medications may modify aggressiveness and hyperactivity.
    - ○ Psychostimulants and selective serotonin receptor inhibitors (SSRIs) may be incorporated to improve functionality.
    - ○ A concerted effort between the anesthesiologist and patient caregivers may enable patient cooperation.
    - ○ Continuation of neuroleptic therapy on day of surgery and adjuvant premedications may be required.

Further reading

Coté CJ, Lerman J, Anderson BJ. *Coté and Lerman's A Practice of Anesthesia for Infants and Children*, 5th edition. Philadelphia, PA: Elsevier, 2013; 490.

Gregory GA, Andropoulos DB. *Gregory's Pediatric Anesthesia*, 5th edition. Hoboken: Wiley-Blackwell, 2012; 560–2.

Part B: System-based topics in pediatric anesthesiology

Chapter 118

Renal system
Anatomy and physiology
Julia Chen

Developmental anatomy

- Development of kidneys begins in the fetus during the 5th week and the kidneys assume an abdominal, retroperitoneal position during the 9th week.
    - Urine production begins during the 10th week and contributes to amniotic fluid volume.
    - Oligohydramnios can lead to pulmonary hypoplasia, facial and skeletal anomalies.
- Nephron development begins during the 8th week with completion of development by 36 weeks.
    - Each kidney has approximately one million nephrons.
    - Kidneys do not contribute to excretion of waste products until after birth.
    - Premature infants with fewer nephrons may be susceptible to glomerular hypertrophy.
- Developmental abnormalities of the kidney and urinary tract include: hypoplastic kidneys, renal ectopia, renal agenesis, and urinary tract duplication.

Renal physiology

- Glomerular filtration
    - Glomerular filtration is the process for filtering undesirable fluids and solutes from the plasma across the glomerular membrane.
    - The glomerular membrane is a highly specialized network of capillaries and ducts.
    - Glomerular filtration begins in the fetus during the 9th week and reaches adult capability by age 1–2 years.
    - Glomerular filtration rate (GFR) is determined by renal blood flow, perfusion pressure, hydrostatic and oncotic pressures.
        - Renal blood flow is autoregulated over a wide range of blood pressures and is under the influence of multiple hormones.
        - The kidneys receive approximately 25% of the cardiac output.
        - GFR can be estimated by a formula which incorporates the height of the child and serum creatinine.
        - GFR may be useful in calculating adjusted drug dosages and monitoring the status of renal function.

Handbook of Critical Incidents and Essential Topics in Pediatric Anesthesiology, ed. David A. Young and Olutoyin A. Olutoye. Published by Cambridge University Press. © Cambridge University Press 2015.

- Fluid and electrolyte balance
  - Sodium reabsorption occurs throughout the nephron.
    - Sodium balance is affected by multiple hormones including aldosterone, angiotensin II, atrial natriuretic peptide, and renin.
  - Potassium excretion occurs at the distal convoluted tubule and collecting ducts.
    - Aldosterone increases the activity of the Na-K-ATPase enzyme and increases luminal membrane permeability of potassium; the net effect is increased secretion of potassium into the urine.
    - Causes of hyperkalemia include transcellular shifts of potassium, decreased excretion of potassium (renal failure), and increased potassium intake.
  - Serum osmolality is regulated by arginine vasopressin (AVP) and is also referred to as antidiuretic hormone (ADH).
    - AVP is released by the posterior pituitary in response to increases in extracellular osmolality, increases in extracellular sodium concentration, or reduction in intravascular fluid volume.
    - AVP acts at the collecting ducts to increase water reabsorption.
    - Water reabsorption also occurs passively via solute reabsorption (proximal tubule) and osmotic gradients (descending loop of Henle).
  - Compared to older children and adults, neonates have limited ability to conserve sodium, to excrete potassium, and are also less efficient at water conservation and excretion.
- Acid–base balance
  - Bicarbonate reabsorption occurs at the proximal tubule and is regenerated at the distal nephron.
  - Neonates have reduced ability to handle acid loads and reabsorb bicarbonate.

Further reading

Barash PG. *Clinical Anesthesia*, 7th edition. Philadelphia: Lippincott Williams & Wilkins, 2013; 1401–4.

Coté CJ, Lerman J, Anderson BJ. *Coté and Lerman's A Practice of Anesthesia for Infants and Children*, 5th edition. Philadelphia, PA: Elsevier, 2013; 555–6.

Davis PJ, Cladis FP, Motoyama EK. *Smith's Anesthesia for Infants and Children*, 8th edition. Philadelphia: Elsevier Mosby, 2011; 116–23.

Gregory GA, Andropoulos DB. *Gregory's Pediatric Anesthesia*, 5th edition. Hoboken: Wiley-Blackwell, 2012; 159–64.

Part B System-based topics in pediatric anesthesiology

Chapter 119

Renal system
Medical conditions
Julia Chen

Acute kidney injury

- Acute kidney injury (AKI) is the acute deterioration in glomerular filtration rate and overall kidney function; the rate of urine output may also be reduced.
- AKI is commonly classified as either prerenal, renal, or post-renal.
    - Prerenal is the most common perioperative category of AKI and results from decreased renal perfusion. Etiologies include: hypovolemia, hypotension, decreased renal blood flow, and vascular occlusion.
    - Renal causes of AKI are the result of intrinsic renal disease. Common causes include: glomerulonephritis, interstitial nephritis, and acute tubular necrosis (hypoxic/ischemic injury, toxins, drugs).
    - Post-renal causes of AKI are due to congenital or acquired obstruction of the urinary tract (e.g., kinked urinary catheter tubing).
    - Evaluation of AKI includes history, physical examination, laboratory evaluation (blood urea nitrogen, serum creatinine, electrolytes, and urinalysis), and may include renal imaging.
        - Prerenal AKI is associated with a fractional excretion of sodium (FE_{Na}) < 1% in children (< 2.5% in infants) and a blood urea nitrogen to creatinine ratio greater than 20.
        - Renal AKI related to acute tubular necrosis is suggested by FE_{Na} > 2% and a blood urea nitrogen to creatinine ratio in the normal range of 10–15; the serum creatinine level may also be increased.
        - Urinary casts may assist with diagnosis (granular casts in prerenal azotemia and red cell casts in glomerulonephritis).
        - Renal ultrasound may also support the etiology of AKI (e.g., dilation of urinary tract).
- Management of AKI
    - Management of AKI includes treatment of the underlying cause, improving renal function, and optimization of fluids and electrolytes.
    - Optimizing renal perfusion for suspected prerenal etiologies may include volume resuscitation while urinary catheter irrigation may be indicated for postrenal causes.

Handbook of Critical Incidents and Essential Topics in Pediatric Anesthesiology, ed. David A. Young and Olutoyin A. Olutoye. Published by Cambridge University Press. © Cambridge University Press 2015.

- ○ Renal replacement therapy (hemodialysis, peritoneal dialysis, continuous replacement therapy) may be indicated for patients with severe AKI.
    - Accepted indications include: severe hyperkalemia, severe metabolic acidosis, volume overload resistant to diuretics, and symptomatic uremia (i.e., pericarditis, encephalopathy).
- ○ Low dose dopamine has not been shown to change outcome in patients with AKI and is not routinely recommended.

Chronic kidney disease

- Chronic kidney disease (CKD) refers to an irreversible decline in kidney function. CKD can be progressive and often progresses to end-stage renal disease requiring renal replacement therapy and/or transplantation.
- CKD can present in infancy (congenital anomalies, perinatal asphyxia), childhood (dysplasia, polycystic kidney disease, focal segmental glomerulosclerosis, membranoproliferative glomerulonephritis), and adolescence (deterioration of renal function in acquired and inherited disease, sickle cell disease, systemic lupus erythematosus, diabetes mellitus, vasculitis, malignancy).
- Complications of CKD include fluid imbalance, electrolyte disorders (hyperkalemia, metabolic acidosis), anemia, bleeding related to platelet dysfunction, hypertension (volume overload, alterations in the renin-angiotensin-aldosterone system), renal osteodystrophy, and growth impairment.

Anesthetic considerations for patients with renal dysfunction

- Preoperative
    - ○ Evaluation of patients with renal dysfunction should include:
        - History and physical examination: type of renal disease, presence of complications/comorbid conditions related to renal dysfunction, current urine output, review of medications.
        - Renal replacement therapy: Patients on intermittent hemodialysis should ideally be dialyzed the day before surgery whereas patients on peritoneal dialysis can be dialyzed up to the day of surgery.
        - Laboratory evaluation should include: serum electrolytes (especially evaluate for hyperkalemia, hypocalcemia, hypomagnesemia) and hemoglobin (assess degree of anemia).
- Intraoperative
    - ○ Renal dysfunction can alter the pharmacokinetics and pharmacodynamics of anesthetic drugs.
        - Drugs that depend on renal excretion for elimination should be used with caution and in reduced doses (e.g., gentamicin, pancuronium).
        - Highly protein-bound drugs may exhibit pronounced effects due to reduced protein binding.
        - Active metabolites of morphine and meperidine can accumulate in patients with renal dysfunction and result in respiratory depression and seizures, respectively.

- Isoflurane and desflurane do not directly impair renal function as long as renal perfusion pressure is maintained.
- Sevoflurane at prolonged low gas flows has been associated with the formation of compound A; compound A has been shown to be nephrotoxic in some animal studies but no detrimental effects on renal function have been demonstrated in humans.
○ Patients with CKD may have delayed gastric emptying and may be at increased risk for pulmonary aspiration of gastric contents.
- Judicious administration of succinylcholine is indicated in patients with preexisting hyperkalemia since succinylcholine administration can increase serum potassium 0.5–1 mEq/L.
○ Induction agents
- Propofol may cause hypotension particularly in patients who are hypovolemic, such as those recently completing hemodialysis.
- The hypertensive effects of ketamine may be undesirable in patients with preexisting hypertension.
- Patients on chronic hypertensive agents and diuretics may be prone to hypotension; induction agents should be carefully titrated to desired effects.
- Patients with renal dysfunction commonly have instability of blood pressure values throughout the surgical procedure; the immediate availability of vasoactive medications is strongly recommended.
○ Fluid administration
- Cautious administration of fluids should occur to avoid complications related to hypovolemia or hypervolemia.
- Avoid potassium-containing solutions such as lactated Ringer's solution which may exacerbate hyperkalemia.
○ Vascular access
- Maintain a strong indication to place central and arterial lines since these vessels may be future sites for long-term vascular access and arteriovenous shunts.
- Utilize proper positioning and protection of extremities with existing arteriovenous shunts.
- Postoperative
○ Postoperative concerns include optimizing fluid management, control of hypertension, electrolyte management, metabolic acidosis, and resuming renal replacement therapy.

Further reading

Barash PG. *Clinical Anesthesia*, 7th edition. Philadelphia: Lippincott Williams & Wilkins, 2013; 1408–13.

Coté CJ, Lerman J, Anderson BJ. *Coté and Lerman's A Practice of Anesthesia for Infants and Children*, 5th edition. Philadelphia, PA: Elsevier, 2013; 556–67.

Gregory GA, Andropoulos DB. *Gregory's Pediatric Anesthesia*, 5th edition. Hoboken: Wiley-Blackwell, 2012; 164–67, 693–7.

Part B — System-based topics in pediatric anesthesiology

Chapter 120

Gastrointestinal system
Anatomy and physiology

Amanda K. Brown and Rhonda A. Alexis

Anatomy and embryology

- The peritoneal cavity initially develops as an open structure communicating with the yolk sac.
- Regression of this open communication to the umbilical cord is not completed until the 12th week of development.
- Peritoneal midgut contents develop extra-embryonically within the umbilicus until the 10th week.
- Extra-embryonic rotation of gastrointestinal structures, completed upon invagination, contributes to proper development and function as described below.
- Failed regression may lead to umbilical and omphalomesenteric duct patency, presenting with conditions ranging from an umbilical hernia to omphalocele.
- In contrast, gastroschisis is associated with proper umbilical development but is also associated with a full-thickness defect in the anterior wall which allows visceral herniation.
- The digestive system arises from endoderm with mesodermal structures creating a support matrix to the abdominal cavity.
- Cavitation of endodermal structures is an essential developmental event; failure or errant progression may lead to intestinal atresia.
- Intestinal development is segmented by vascular architecture into three segments.
    - Celiac artery → foregut.
    - Superior mesenteric artery → midgut.
    - Inferior mesenteric artery → hindgut.
- The foregut encapsulates the gastrointestinal system from the mouth through duodenum, including the liver and pancreas.
    - The pharyngeal development of the foregut is remarkable for its contribution to the development of the upper and lower respiratory tract. The laryngotracheal groove on the pharynx evolves into the respiratory diverticulum.
    - Hepatic development also proceeds from the foregut.
    - The midgut extends from the jejunum through the proximal two-thirds of the transverse colon.

Handbook of Critical Incidents and Essential Topics in Pediatric Anesthesiology, ed. David A. Young and Olutoyin A. Olutoye. Published by Cambridge University Press. © Cambridge University Press 2015.

- - Rapid intestinal growth through the 10th week of development requires extra-embryonic extrusion, the components of which are midgut structures.
  - Anomalous rotation with invagination causes intestinal obstruction and may compromise vascular supply, placing the neonatal gut at risk for ischemia.
- The hindgut proceeds from the left colic flexure through the upper anal canal. Developmental continuity with the lower anal canal, an ectodermal structure, commonly gives rise to gastrointestinal malformations and atresias.

Physiology

- The gastrointestinal tract must accomplish ingestion, digestion, nutrient absorption, and waste excretion.
- These physiologic achievements require enzymatic secretion, gastric acidification, intraluminal fluid secretion, and reabsorption.
- Peristalsis aids digestion and prevents excessive enzymatic and bacterial flora accumulation; this action impedes overgrowth by pathogenic bacteria.
- The gastrointestinal system serves an important role in immunity both as a barrier presented by the tight junctions of the endothelium, and in its immune response capacity through secretion of immunoglobin A (IgA).
- Emesis or diarrhea can rapidly disrupt fluid balance, leading to dehydration and compromised gut perfusion.
- Enteral feedings of the neonatal gut promote gut function and appropriate floral colonization.

Further reading

Coté CJ, Lerman J, Anderson BJ. *Coté and Lerman's A Practice of Anesthesia for Infants and Children*, 5th edition. Philadelphia, PA: Elsevier, 2013; 17.

Gregory GA, Andropoulos DB. *Gregory's Pediatric Anesthesia*, 5th edition. Hoboken: Wiley-Blackwell, 2012; 148–58.

Part B System-based topics in pediatric anesthesiology

Gastrointestinal system
Medical conditions
Amanda K. Brown and Rhonda A. Alexis

Gastro-esophageal reflux

- Reflux of gastric contents occurs due to decreased lower esophageal sphincter tone.
- Physiologic maturity of the sphincter may not occur until approximately 15 months of age, leading to postprandial reflux.
- Both prematurity and neurologic deficits potentiate gastro-esophageal sphincter dysfunction. Severe reflux can be injurious to the esophagus and may result in pulmonary aspiration, chronic cough, wheezing, and lung infections. Surgical management may be required for refractory cases (laparoscopic fundoplication). This procedure is increasingly being performed in children to ameliorate reflux-induced lung injury.

Intussusception

- Common cause of gastrointestinal obstruction characterized by bowel telescoping, usually occurs proximal to the ileocecal valve.
- The highest incidence is in children less than 1 year of age.
- Meckel's diverticulum is a common etiology. Acute intussusception results in paroxysmal abdominal pain with bloody stools; chronic intussusception clinically mimics gastroenteritis.

Atresia

- Atretic bowel may involve any part of the gastrointestinal tract but most commonly involves the duodenum, esophagus, and anus.
- Duodenal atresia is commonly accompanied by other anomalies: trisomy 21, congenital heart defects, malrotation, biliary atresia, and annular pancreas.
- Bilious vomiting occurs within 24 hours of birth.
- Radiographic examination reveals a "double bubble" sign due to gastric and duodenal dilation.

Esophageal atresia

- Esophageal atresia (EA) rarely occurs in isolation and is usually associated with tracheo-esophageal fistula (TEF).

Handbook of Critical Incidents and Essential Topics in Pediatric Anesthesiology, ed. David A. Young and Olutoyin A. Olutoye. Published by Cambridge University Press. © Cambridge University Press 2015.

- Most common combination involves a blind esophageal pouch and a distal esophageal fistula communicating with the trachea just above the carina.
- The VACTERL (vertebral, anorectal, cardiac, tracheo-esophageal, renal, limb anomalies) spectrum should be sought when TEF/EA is present.

Malrotation and volvulus

- Incomplete rotation of abdominal contents from the yolk sac back into the abdomen results in bowel malrotation.
- Affected infants present with abdominal distension and bilious vomiting in the neonatal period.
- Aberrant rotation can stress the superior mesenteric artery, cause atresia or ischemia and lead to volvulus.
- These disorders comprise some of the surgical emergencies encountered in the first 2 months of life, commonly requiring exploration to rule out bowel ischemia.

Pyloric stenosis

- Characterized by hypertrophy of the antrum and pylorus causing gastric outlet obstruction.
- Non-bilious projectile vomiting occurring before 12 weeks of age.
- Resulting volume depletion leads to a hypochloremic, hypokalemic, metabolic alkalosis.
- Adequate preoperative hydration is mandatory; confirmation of adequate hydration is by normalization of serum chloride and bicarbonate prior to surgical repair.
- Suctioning of gastric contents is recommended prior to induction, allowing for a modified rapid sequence induction, thereby avoiding precipitous oxygen desaturation.
- Normalization of cerebrospinal fluid alkalosis lags behind that of serum; therefore, infants are more sensitive to even modest amounts of opioids. Many providers avoid the routine administration of opioids to these patients.

Appendicitis

- Presents with periumbilical pain localized to the right lower quadrant.
- Etiology is thought to be secondary to luminal obstruction with bacterial overgrowth.
- Obstruction may progress to perforation, development of peritonitis, and abscess formation.

Meckel diverticulum

- Patent omphalomesenteric duct located at the distal ileum.
- Occurs in 2% of the population and is symptomatic in a minority, presenting as painless rectal bleeding, obstruction, or Littre's hernia.

Necrotizing enterocolitis

- Necrotizing enterocolitis (NEC) is a disease of prematurity and small birth weight, with a 10% incidence in infants less than 1.5kg.

- A precipitating stress event compromises bowel perfusion, results in enteric infection, and overwhelms the neonatal immune system.
- Gross abdominal distension heralds evolving intestinal ischemia with pneumatosis on plain radiography.
- Neonatal sepsis carries high morbidity and mortality, with resultant anemia, coagulopathy, myocardial depression, and liver insufficiency.
- Early management is medical, but bowel perforation mandates surgical intervention.
- These patients may be critically ill and require volume resuscitation, blood products, vasoactive medications, and increased mechanical ventilatory support.

Inguinal and umbilical hernia

- Hernia repair is the most frequent general surgical procedure performed in the first year of life.
- Indirect inguinal hernias occur due to patency of the processus vaginalis (30% of term infants), with a higher percentage in preterm infants.
- Right-sided hernias are predominant but bilateral disease may be occult, prompting laparoscopic evaluation of the contralateral side.
- Umbilical hernias are skin-covered umbilical ring defects containing abdominal contents.
- Umbilical defects are common in premature infants.
- Defects less than 1 cm often regress, but larger ones may require surgical repair.

Abdominal tumors

Neuroblastoma

- Extracranial solid tumor of the postganglionic sympathetic nervous system, usually diagnosed < 4 years.
- 50% are adrenal in origin.
- Paraneoplastic effects include hypertension from excessive neuroendocrine secretion, and watery diarrhea from vasoactive intestinal peptide syndrome (VIP).

Wilm's tumor (nephroblastoma)

- Often present prior to age 6 as an abdominal mass originating in the kidney.
- Hypertension and hematuria are characteristic signs.
- Associated with concomitant anomalies of genitourinary system.

Hirschsprung's disease

- Congenital absence of ganglia extending from anus to varying lengths of colon.
- Loss of intrinsic innervation causes regional spasm and constipation.
- Acute enterocolitis and intestinal obstruction can develop.

Further reading

Coté CJ, Lerman J, Anderson BJ. *Coté and Lerman's A Practice of Anesthesia for Infants and Children*, 5th edition. Philadelphia, PA: Elsevier, 2013; 764.

Davis PJ. *Smith's Anesthesia for Infants and Children*, 8th edition. Philadelphia: Mosby, Inc., 2011; 750-1.

Dominguez KM, Moss RL. Necrotizing enterocolitis. *Clin Perinatol*. 2012; 39(2):387–401.

Part B System-based topics in pediatric anesthesiology

Chapter 122

Hepatic system
Anatomy and physiology
Yang Liu

Anatomy

- The liver is the largest organ in the body.
- It contains about 13% of the body's blood supply at any given moment.
- A unique feature of the liver is its dual blood supply.
   - Approximately 30% of hepatic blood flow is oxygenated blood from the hepatic artery.
   - The portal vein delivers about 70% of hepatic blood and carries nutrients absorbed from the gastrointestinal tract.
   - In the fetus, the ductus venosus shunts oxygenated blood from the umbilical vein to the right atrium through the immature liver.
- The liver has two main lobes, right and left, both of which are made up of thousands of lobules.
- Central veins of the hepatic lobule receive blood from the portal venule and hepatic arteriole.
- The hepatic duct transports bile produced by the liver cells to the gallbladder and duodenum.
- The biliary system includes the gallbladder, bile ducts, and cells from inside the liver.

Physiology

- Hepatic hematopoiesis develops *in utero* at 5 to 6 weeks gestation.
- Liver function is immature in the neonate, resulting in slower metabolism of many medications and a longer duration of action.
- The liver carries out many other important functions:
   - Carbohydrate metabolism.
   - Amino acid metabolism.
   - Lipid metabolism.
   - Production and excretion of bile.
   - Synthesis of clotting factors and components (factors II, V, VII, IX, and X).
   - Synthesis of serum proteins (albumin, globulins, and fibrinogen).
   - Energy storage (glycogen) and regulation of serum glucose.

Handbook of Critical Incidents and Essential Topics in Pediatric Anesthesiology, ed. David A. Young and Olutoyin A. Olutoye. Published by Cambridge University Press. © Cambridge University Press 2015.

- Biotransformation of drugs and toxins.
- Blood circulation.
- Hepatic drug metabolism:
  - Liver transforms lipid-soluble drugs into water-soluble metabolites for renal and biliary excretion.
  - Drug biotransformation and metabolism primarily occur by hydroxylation and conjugation.
  - Cytochrome P450 (CYP) system is the primary family of liver enzymes for drug metabolism.
  - The CYP enzyme system can be divided into three distinct families – CYP1, CYP2, and CYP3 – which further divide into many subfamilies.
  - There is a wide range of variability in the enzymatic activity across all CYP families.
  - The concentration and activity of each enzyme can be enhanced or inhibited by certain drugs or environmental toxins.
  - Approximately 5% of white-skinned individuals lack CYP2D6 activity.
  - Plasma pseudocholinesterase is a group of protein enzymes synthesized by the liver. Pseudocholinesterase deficiency results in delayed metabolism of compounds such as succinylcholine, mivacurium, and ester-based local anesthetics (cocaine, procaine, 2,3-chloroprocaine, tetracaine).
- The biliary system creates, stores, and releases bile into the duodenum.
  - Bile is a complex secretory product synthesized by the liver.
  - It provides an excretory route for many endogenous and exogenous substances such as bilirubin and cholesterol.
  - It assists in the absorption and digestion of lipids from the intestine.
  - The gallbladder stores and concentrates bile acids for further secretion into the proximal small intestine.

Hepatic drug metabolism and anesthesia

- Inhalation anesthetics
  - Poorly metabolized in humans with varying percentages of drug undergoing biotransformation: halothane: 20%; enflurane: 2–4%; sevoflurane: 2–5%; isoflurane: 0.2%; and desflurane: 0.02%.
  - Halothane, sevoflurane, and enflurane can inhibit protein synthesis and secretion.
  - Halothane exposure is associated with halothane hepatitis. Other inhalation anesthetics have also been associated with liver injury.
- Sedatives
  - The commonly used sedatives – midazolam, propofol and ketamine – all undergo hepatic metabolism. However, 88% of propofol is eliminated, primarily via the kidneys.

- About 95% of midazolam is bound to albumin. Decreased hepatic albumin synthesis results in decreased plasma levels of albumin and an exaggerated pharmacodynamic effect of midazolam.

- Opioids
  - Elimination of opioids is prolonged in neonates due to a reduced capacity of hepatic glucuronidation.
  - Codeine is metabolized to morphine by the CYP2D6 enzyme. A deficiency of this enzyme results in little or no analgesic effect from codeine. In patients with *CYP2D6* gene duplication or an ultra-rapid metabolizing allele, respiratory depression or death may result from exaggerated effects of morphine.

- Local anesthetics
  - The amide local anesthetics (e.g., lidocaine, bupivacaine, and ropivacaine) are degraded in the liver by cytochrome P-450 enzymes.
  - The ester local anesthetics (e.g., procaine, 2,3-chloroprocaine, and tetracaine) are hydrolyzed by plasma pseudocholinesterase which is produced by the liver.

- Neuromuscular blocking drugs
  - Succinylcholine is hydrolyzed by plasma pseudocholinesterase.
  - About 75% of most aminosteroid nondepolarizing muscle relaxants (e.g., vecuronium, rocuronium) are bound to plasma proteins, primarily albumin.
  - Pancuronium primarily undergoes renal excretion while only 12–22% of rocuronium is excreted through the kidney.

Further reading

Coté CJ, Lerman J, Anderson BJ. *Coté and Lerman's A Practice of Anesthesia for Infants and Children*, 5th edition. Philadelphia, PA: Elsevier, 2013; 590–3.

Gregory GA, Andropoulos DB. *Gregory's Pediatric Anesthesia*, 5th edition. Hoboken: Wiley-Blackwell, 2012; 139–48.

Piñeiro-Carrero VM. Liver. *Pediatrics*. 2004; 113:1097.

Part B: System-based topics in pediatric anesthesiology

Chapter 123: Hepatic system
Medical conditions
Paul A. Stricker

Congenital disorders

- Biliary atresia
  - Most common cause of liver transplantation in children, a disorder of progressive inflammation and destruction of extrahepatic bile ducts.
- Choledochal cysts
  - Treated with surgical excision and Roux-en-Y anastomosis.
- Metabolic diseases
  - Cystic fibrosis
    - Affects liver and pancreas (in addition to lungs) and is a cause of liver failure in adolescents.
  - Alpha-1 antitrypsin deficiency
    - Homozygotes at risk for progressive hepatic fibrosis and failure (in addition to pulmonary emphysema).
  - Porphyria
    - Hepatic-type porphyrias can cause progressive hepatic failure requiring transplantation.
  - Tyrosinemia
    - Inborn error of amino acid tyrosine metabolism; liver transplantation is curative for those who fail medical management.
  - Wilson disease
    - Autosomal recessive disorder that leads to copper accumulation, resulting in progressive hepatic failure and central nervous system dysfunction.

Cholelithiasis

- Hemolytic anemias (spherocytosis, sickle cell disease) represent common causes of cholelithiasis in children.
- Obesity: increasingly becoming a more common cause.

Handbook of Critical Incidents and Essential Topics in Pediatric Anesthesiology, ed. David A. Young and Olutoyin A. Olutoye. Published by Cambridge University Press. © Cambridge University Press 2015.

Infectious conditions
- Hepatitis A, B, C.
- Epstein–Barr virus.

Autoimmune hepatitis
- Most often causes chronic liver disease and is managed with immunosuppressant or immunomodulatory therapy. Less commonly can present as fulminant hepatic failure.

Acute hepatotoxicity
- Occurs from ingested toxins or is drug-induced.

End-stage liver disease
- Portal hypertension, with splenomegaly, ascites, and esophageal/porto-systemic varices.
- Cardiovascular system: total hypervolemia, central hypovolemia, decreased systemic vascular resistance with arteriovenous shunting and increased cardiac output.
- Pulmonary system: arterial hypoxemia, impaired hypoxic pulmonary vasoconstriction, V/Q mismatch, restrictive ventilatory patterns.
- Reduced synthetic function
  - Hypoalbuminemia exacerbates ascites from portal hypertension.
  - Coagulopathy occurs from decreased clotting factor production.
- Hematopoietic
  - Anemia.
  - Thrombocytopenia from decreased production of thrombopoietin.
- Reduced metabolic and endocrine function
  - Increased risk for hypoglycemia from impaired gluconeogenesis and reduced glycogen stores.
  - Impaired drug metabolism with altered pharmacokinetics.
  - Nutritional defects from altered bile production impacting intestinal absorption.
- Neurologic system: hepatic encephalopathy from increased ammonia and cerebral edema.
- Renal system: renal dysfunction progressing to the high mortality hepatorenal syndrome.

Further reading

Coté CJ, Lerman J, Anderson BJ. *Coté and Lerman's A Practice of Anesthesia for Infants and Children*, 5th edition. Philadelphia, PA: Elsevier, 2013; 599–601.

Davis PJ, Cladis FP, Motoyama EK. *Smith's Anesthesia for Infants and Children*, 8th edition. Philadelphia: Elsevier Mosby, 2011; 906–14.

Gregory GA, Andropoulos DB. *Gregory's Pediatric Anesthesia*, 5th edition. Hoboken: Wiley-Blackwell, 2012; 683–5.

Part B System-based topics in pediatric anesthesiology

Chapter 124

Endocrine system
Anatomy and physiology
Tae W. Kim

Introduction

- The endocrine system is composed of specialized organs in the body which are capable of hormone biosynthesis and secretion, feedback regulation, hormone receptor binding, and initiation of intracellular signaling. These hormones are capable of circulating in the bloodstream to effect changes in other parts of the body, or acting locally.
- There are five types of hormone derivatives: steroids, biogenic amines, small neuropeptides, large proteins, and vitamins. The hormones are receptor specific causing change in the target cells either through cell-surface membrane or intracellular receptors.
- The endocrine system is responsible for helping to maintain homeostasis within the body, mainly through utilizing negative feedback loops. Major functions of the endocrine system include growth and maturation, regulation of the body's metabolism, electrolyte and fluid equilibrium, and reproduction. Endocrine glands that are clinically relevant to the practice of anesthesia are the hypothalamus, pituitary, thyroid, parathyroid, and adrenal glands.

Anatomy

- Hypothalamus
    - Located between the thalamus and brainstem forming the ventral part of the diencephalon.
    - Composed of distinct nuclei.
    - Link between the nervous and endocrine systems.
- Pituitary
    - Pea-sized structure below the hypothalamus.
    - Pituitary and hypothalamus together control growth, development, metabolism, and homeostasis.
    - Two morphologically and functionally distinct glands.
        - Adenohypophysis – anterior pituitary.
        - Neurohypophysis – posterior pituitary.

Handbook of Critical Incidents and Essential Topics in Pediatric Anesthesiology, ed. David A. Young and Olutoyin A. Olutoye. Published by Cambridge University Press. © Cambridge University Press 2015.

- Thyroid
  - Comprised of two lateral lobes connected by an isthmus overlying the trachea below the larynx.
- Parathyroid
  - Four glands located in pairs on the posterior aspect of the superior and inferior poles of the thyroid gland.
- Adrenal
  - Comprised of an outer cortex and inner medulla; located on the upper pole of each kidney.

Physiology

- Hypothalamus
  - Regulation of metabolic and autonomic systems through hormonal and neural inputs.
  - Regulates the anterior pituitary by releasing hormones, which also inhibit those that suppress anterior pituitary hormones.
  - Hormones regulated by the hypothalamus: thyrotrophic-releasing hormone, dopamine, growth hormone-releasing hormone, somatostatin, gonadotropin-releasing hormone, corticotropin-releasing hormone, oxytocin, vasopressin.
- Pituitary
  - Anterior pituitary
    - Human growth hormone – regulates body growth and metabolism.
    - Thyroid-stimulating hormone – regulates thyroid function.
    - Follicle-stimulating hormone (FSH), luteinizing hormone (LH) – stimulates secretion of estrogen and progesterone, maturation of oocytes, secretion of testosterone and sperm production.
    - Prolactin – stimulates milk production in the mammary glands.
    - Adrenocorticotropic hormone (ACTH) – stimulates adrenal cortex to secrete glucocorticoids.
    - Melanocyte-stimulating hormone (MSH) – affects skin pigmentation.
  - Posterior pituitary
    - Does not synthesize its own hormones, acts as a storage site.
    - Stores and secretes oxytocin as well as antidiuretic hormone produced by hypothalamus.
    - Oxytocin regulates uterine contractions during delivery and milk release during breastfeeding.
    - Antidiuretic hormone increases water permeability in the distal renal tubules and collecting ducts.
- Thyroid
  - Regulates metabolism, growth, and development.
  - Large storage capacity for hormones.

- Produces three hormones:
    - Thyroxine or tetraiodothyronine (T_4).
    - Triiodothyronine (T_3) – produced from conversion of T_4.
    - Calcitonin – decreases calcium levels in the blood.
- T_3 and T_4 are synthesized from iodine and tyrosine under negative feedback control from the hypothalamus.
- Only 1% of thyroid hormones are biologically active.

- Parathyroid
    - Produces three forms of parathyroid hormone (PTH) or parathormone.
    - Released from secretory granules in response to decreased serum ionized calcium.
    - Three mechanisms to increase calcium:
        - Calcium reabsorption in proximal convoluted tubule.
        - Bone resorption through increased osteoclast activity.
        - Renal conversion of 25-hydroxyvitamin D to active metabolite, calcitriol (increases absorption of calcium and phosphate from the GI tract and bone resorption).
    - Secretion of PTH inhibited by hyperphosphatemia, profound hypomagnesemia or hypermagnesemia, and increased 1,25-dihydroxyvitamin D (calcitriol).
    - Hypocalcemia may result in tetany, hypotension, dysrhythmias.

- Adrenal cortex
    - Mineralocorticoids (zona glomerulosa)
        - Affects fluid and mineral homeostasis.
        - Controlled by ACTH and renin–angiotensin system, stimulates aldosterone synthesis.
        - Aldosterone accounts for 95% of activity, sodium reabsorption.
    - Glucocorticoids (zona fasciculata)
        - Affects glucose homeostasis, helps regulate body metabolism and stress response.
        - Cortisol accounts for 95% of activity.
        - Reduces inflammation and is essential for immune function.
    - Androgens (zona reticularis) – dehydroepiandrosterone (DHEA), sulfated conjugate, DHEA-S.

- Adrenal medulla
    - Chromaffin cells
        - Under direct control of autonomic nervous system.
        - Catecholamines derived from tyrosine through process of hydroxylation and decarboxylation.
        - Produces epinephrine (80%), norepinephrine, and dopamine.
        - Active in "fight or flight" response, and maintains hemodynamics.

Further reading

Coté CJ, Lerman J, Anderson BJ. *Coté and Lerman's A Practice of Anesthesia for Infants and Children*, 5th edition. Philadelphia, PA: Elsevier, 2013; 533–54.

Goldman L, Schafer AI. *Goldman's Cecil Medicine*, 24th edition. Philadelphia: Elsevier, 2012; 1423–31.

Hines RL, Marschall KE. *Stoelting's Anesthesia and Co-Existing Disease*, 6th edition. Philadelphia: Churchill Livingstone, 2012; 376–406.

Rhoades RA, Bell DR. *Medical Physiology Principles of Clinical Medicine*, 4th edition. Philadelphia: Lippincott Williams & Wilkins, 2012; 581–668.

Part B System-based topics in pediatric anesthesiology

Chapter 125

Endocrine system
Medical conditions
Tae W. Kim

Introduction

Anesthesia for patients with endocrine disorders requires a thorough understanding of the condition and the effects of anesthesia. In particular, this chapter reviews potentially life threatening conditions associated with hyper- or hypoactivity of the specific endocrine gland. The dramatic and sudden changes in physiology brought on by the endocrinopathy are outlined, as well as the anesthetic management.

Hyperthyroid (thyrotoxicosis)

- Graves disease (diffuse toxic goiter)
    - Common cause in childhood.
    - Autoimmune disorder.
    - Autoimmune disorder – Thyroid-stimulating immunoglobulins bind TSH receptors.
    - Excess T_4 and T_3, low Thyroid stimulating hormone.
- Clinical manifestations
    - Diffuse goiter.
    - Proptosis.
    - Heat intolerance.
    - Diarrhea.
    - Weight loss.
    - Tachycardia.
- Treatment options
    - Antithyroid medications (methimazole or propylthiouracil)
        . 25% of children suffer adverse effects.
        . Minor – increased liver enzymes, neutropenia, rash, lymphadenopathy.
        . Major – agranulocytosis, liver failure.
    - Thyroidectomy.
    - Radioactive iodine.
    - Relapse likely after 2–3 years of treatment.
    - Radioactive ablation (less risk) or surgery for definitive treatment.
    - β-adrenergic blockade for hemodynamic stability.

Handbook of Critical Incidents and Essential Topics in Pediatric Anesthesiology, ed. David A. Young and Olutoyin A. Olutoye. Published by Cambridge University Press. © Cambridge University Press 2015.

- Perioperative management
  - Euthyroid for elective procedures.
  - Beta-blockers are the first-line agents for rapid control of the hypermetabolic state.
  - Lugol solution (saturated potassium iodine) inhibits synthesis of thyroid hormones and can also be used for control but is administered orally.
  - Preoperative
    - Neck examination for potential difficult airway and review of diagnostic studies.
    - Patients may be relatively hypovolemic with the potential for hypotension on induction.
  - Intraoperative
    - No specific anesthetic technique has been shown to be superior.
    - Choice of anesthetic drug should have minimal cardiovascular effects; metabolism of drugs may be accelerated.
    - Regional anesthesia if indicated, is beneficial for ablating sympathetic response.
  - Postoperative
    - Complications from thyroidectomy include: damage to laryngeal nerve, tracheal compression (hematoma) and hypoparathyroidism (stridor, laryngospasm, tingling).

Thyroid storm

- Clinical manifestations
  - Predisposing factors: surgery, undertreated or no treatment of hyperthyroidism.
  - May mimic presentation of malignant hyperthermia.
  - Differentiated from MH by:
    - Less severe acidosis.
    - No increase in creatine kinase.
- Treatment
  - Parental β-blockers (decrease conversion T_4 to T_3).
  - Propylthiouracil (inhibits new hormone synthesis, decreases conversion T_4 to T_3).
  - Symptomatic treatment.
  - Mortality 20–30% if untreated.

Hypothyroidism

- Occurrence: most common thyroid disorder.
- Etiology
  - Worldwide – iodine deficiency.
  - United States – autoimmune, if not malnourished from iodine deficiency.
  - Pituitary or hypothalamic insufficiency secondary to tumor or surgery.
- Thyroid function test
  - TSH is the most sensitive test for diagnosing primary thyroid function.
  - TSH may be increased (primary) or decreased (secondary).
  - Thyroxine (T_4) and triiodothyronine (T_3) are both decreased.

- Clinical manifestations
  - Short stature.
  - Fatigue.
  - Cold intolerance.
  - Weight gain.
  - Constipation.
  - Hoarse voice.
  - Developmental delay due to missed diagnosis as neonate.
- Treatment
  - Goal is to normalize TSH and T_4.
  - T_4 response to levothyroxine takes approximately one week.
  - TSH equilibration occurs over 4–6 weeks.
- Perioperative management
  - Preoperative
    - Review preexisting testing of thyroid function (e.g., TSH level).
    - Ensure patient is clinically euthyroid for elective procedures.
    - Children with unknown hypothyroid status should have a detailed history of thyroid treatment, risk factors and comorbidities, such as autoimmune disorders (diabetes type I, celiac disease) or genetic syndromes (trisomy 21, Turner syndrome).
    - Patients with subclinical or mild hypothyroidism may proceed with procedures if thyroid replacement has already been initiated.
    - Moderate to severe hypothyroid patients, consider postponing surgery due to:
      - Decreased cardiac function.
      - Diminished breathing capacity.
      - Increased sensitivity to anesthetic agents.
  - Intraoperative
    - Patient at increased risk for respiratory depression from anesthetic drugs.
    - Patient at increased risk for hemodynamic instability because of diminished cardiac function.
    - Gastric emptying may be delayed.
    - Increased risk for developing hypothermia, hypoglycemia, and hyponatremia.
  - Postoperative
    - Potential for increased sensitivity to sedating drugs: use non-opioid analgesics for postoperative pain control if possible.

Myxedema coma

- Profound form of hypothyroidism.
- Results in life-threatening coma and heart failure.
- Consider diagnosis in patients with unexplained hemodynamic instability, difficulty weaning from ventilator or delirium.
- Mainstay of therapy is the intravenous administration of thyroid hormones such as T_3 (triiodothyronine).
- Cardiopulmonary support such as mechanical ventilation may also be required.

- Monitoring for excessive sympathetic stimulation (i.e., tachycardia, myocardial ischemia) from the administration of thyroid hormones is strongly recommended.
- Additional therapy may include glucose administration, stress dose steroids and correction of electrolyte disorders.
- Supportive therapy such as active warming may also be required.

Neonatal hypothyroidism

- Cause of preventable mental retardation.
- Common causes include thyroid dysgenesis or agenesis.
- Neonatal screening for TSH is standard of care.
- Screening ineffective for central hypothyroidism.

Adrenal insufficiency

- Normal endogenous cortisol secretion is 6–8 mg/m^2/day.
- Most common cause: autoimmune adrenal insufficiency.
- Secondary insufficiency: due to ACTH deficiency.
- Iatrogenic – depending on duration and dose of glucocorticoid.
- Testing for adrenal insufficiency
    - Primary adrenal insufficiency
        - ACTH stimulation test demonstrates an increase in the cortisol level.
    - Hypothalamic–pituitary axis (HPA) insufficiency
        - Absence ACTH levels or response to stimulation test.
        - Response to ACTH stimulation test may imply only tonic ACTH secretion and not ability to secrete a greater amount during stress.
    - Iatrogenic adrenal suppression
        - Results from prolonged administration of exogenous glucocorticoids.
        - High dose steroids for 7–10 days; does not significantly suppress HPA.
        - High dose steroids for 3–6 weeks require a taper over 1–2 weeks for recovery of the HPA.
        - Long-term, high doses may require up to 6–9 months for complete recovery of HPA function.
    - Perioperative management
        - Replacement depends on age, body size, and complexity of surgical procedure.
        - Stress glucocorticoid dosing is 3–10 times replacement dose.
        - Hydrocortisone is one of the commonly utilized medications for replacement (2 mg/kg immediately pre-op and every 6 hours on day of surgery *or* 25 mg/m^2 pre-op, 50 mg/m^2 continuous infusion intra-op and 50 mg/m^2 continuous infusion post-op for remainder of first 24 hr).

Further reading

Coté CJ, Lerman J, Anderson BJ. *Coté and Lerman's A Practice of Anesthesia for Infants and Children*, 5th edition. Philadelphia, PA: Elsevier, 2013; 547–55.

Davis PJ, Cladis FP, Motoyama EK. *Smith's Anesthesia for Infants and Children*, 8th edition. Philadelphia: Elsevier Mosby, 2011; 1104–10.

Part B: System-based topics in pediatric anesthesiology

Chapter 126

Endocrine system
Diabetes mellitus/diabetes insipidus/SIADH

Tae W. Kim

Introduction
Diabetes mellitus and diabetes insipidus are different forms of endocrinopathies.
- Diabetes mellitus
  - Diabetes mellitus is differentiated into type I or II.
  - The etiology can be genetic or iatrogenic as in the case of exogenous steroid therapy.
  - Associated comorbidities in diabetes mellitus patients include Cystic fibrosis, Prader-Willi syndrome, Down syndrome, Turner syndrome, and Cushing syndrome.
  - Type I diabetics are insulin-dependent for glucose control.
  - Type II diabetics are managed with diet and exercise, as well as insulin oral agents such as metformin. Metformin decreases hepatic glucose production and increases insulin sensitivity in peripheral tissues.
- Diabetes insipidus
  - Diabetes insipidus (DI) is caused by a deficiency of antidiuretic hormone, arginine vasopressin, which acts on the distal tubule and collecting ducts of the kidney to promote reabsorption of water.
  - Central DI may result from iatrogenic causes, surgery/trauma, disorders of the hypothalamus or pituitary, neoplasms affecting vasopressin neurons or fiber tracts and autoimmune or infectious diseases.
  - Nephrogenic DI (renal tubular unresponsiveness to arginine vasopressin) is due to genetic mutations such as to the vasopressin receptor; this condition may be effectively managed utilizing hydrochlorothiazide and nonsteroidal anti-inflammatory medications.
- Syndrome of inappropriate antidiuretic hormone secretion (SIADH) results from an excess amount of antidiuretic hormone relative to the amount necessary to maintain intravascular volume.

Diabetes mellitus
- Type I
  - Pathophysiology – hyperglycemia results from immune-mediated destruction of pancreatic β-cells causing an absolute deficiency of insulin.

Handbook of Critical Incidents and Essential Topics in Pediatric Anesthesiology, ed. David A. Young and Olutoyin A. Olutoye. Published by Cambridge University Press. © Cambridge University Press 2015.

- Type II
  - Pathophysiology – hyperglycemia results from the combination of insulin resistance, insulin deficiency, and excessive glucagon secretion.
- Effects of surgical stress
  - Surgical stress results in hyperglycemia
    - Increased levels of epinephrine, glucagon, cortisol, and growth hormone.
    - Stimulation of glycogenolysis and gluconeogenesis.
    - Increased lipolysis and ketogenesis.
    - Inhibition of glucose uptake and utilization.
- Preoperative management
  - Coordinate with endocrinologist for specific insulin dosing recommendations.
  - Ideally schedule as first case of the day to minimize fasting period.
  - Preoperative glucose control
    - Goal is to maintain normoglycemia: 100–200 mg/dL.
    - Administer regular insulin for glucose levels ≥250 mg/dL.
    - Evaluate for comorbid conditions such as gastroparesis, autonomic neuropathy, renal dysfunction, and myocardial ischemia.
  - Preoperative instructions
    - Hold rapid or short-acting insulin preparations on morning of surgery.
    - Perform preoperative blood glucose check.
    - Administer 50% of intermediate (NPH)/full dose of long-acting insulin dose on morning of surgery.
    - Administer dextrose-containing intravenous solutions if insulin administered in preoperative setting.
    - Hold metformin for 24 hours to decrease potential for lactic acidosis.
    - Sulfonylureas and thiazolidinediones to be held on morning of surgery.
- Intraoperative management
  - Inhalation agents are acceptable and may be beneficial by inhibiting insulin secretion.
  - Regional analgesia inhibits the hyperglycemic response by reducing the neuroendocrine stress response.
  - Glucose-containing fluid is optional for surgery ≤ 1 hour.
  - Glucose infusions in addition to maintenance fluids should be considered for procedures > 1 hour.
  - Insulin pumps may remain enabled for minor procedures < 2 hours.
  - Intravenous insulin infusions should be considered for procedures > 2 hours.
  - Intravenous insulin infusion and major surgery lasting ≥ 2 hours.
    - D5½NS or D5 LR for maintenance fluid.
    - Adjust insulin infusion for glucose goal of 100–200 mg/dL.
  - Key strategy is to monitor blood glucose at least every hour and adjust fluids/insulin accordingly.
- Postoperative management
  - Check blood glucose levels frequently in post-anesthesia care unit (every 1–2 hours) until stabilized.

- Resume preoperative insulin regimen after regular oral intake has been achieved.
- Continue insulin infusion and frequent glucose checks if prolonged recovery/critical condition/patient not eating.
- Hold metformin for 48 hours if IV contrast administered and check renal function prior to restarting medication.

• Adverse effects of hyperglycemia
- Impaired wound healing, decreased tensile strength.
- Impaired neutrophil function.
- Osmotic diuresis resulting in polydypsia, polyuria, hypovolemia.
- Diabetic ketoacidosis (DKA)
    - Laboratory findings include: hyperglycemia (>300 mg/dL), glucosuria, ketonuria, and ketoacidosis (pH <7.30, HCO_3^- <15 mEq/L).
    - Severe volume depletion may be present.
    - Precipitated by cessation of insulin therapy or new onset stress, such as infectious process.
    - Management centers on insulin administration, volume resuscitation, and correction of metabolic and electrolyte disorders (e.g., hypokalemia).

Diabetes insipidus

• Etiology
- Vasopressin deficiency (neurogenic DI) – craniopharyngioma, surgical trauma, encephalitis, genetic (autosomal dominant).
- Vasopressin insensitivity/resistance (nephrogenic DI) – pyelonephritis, amyloidosis, sarcoidosis, genetic (X-linked recessive).
- Primary polydipsia – psychogenic

• Pathophysiology
- Neurogenic DI results from inadequate production of antidiuretic hormone (ADH).
- Lack of ADH results in polyuria, polydypsia, hypovolemia, hypernatremia and hyperosmolality.

• Laboratory tests
- Serum sodium is elevated (> 145 mmol/L).
- Polyuria (> 4 mL/kg/hr).
- Plasma osmolality is elevated (> 300 mOsm/L).
- Urine osmolality is reduced (< 300 mOsm/L).
- Urine specific gravity is reduced (< 1.005).

• Perioperative management
- Neurogenic DI is typically managed by using a vasopressin analogue for replacement such as desmopressin (DDAVP).
- Minor surgery – administer daily routine dose of DDAVP.
- Major surgery – first case of the day, 50% evening dose of DDAVP.

- Standard monitors, arterial line, ± central venous line, urinary catheter.
- Consider initiating intraoperative vasopressin infusion with D5NS to replace insensible losses if DI develops.
  - New onset DI
    - Common scenario during pituitary or hypothalamic tumor resections; this may occur intraoperatively or postoperatively.
    - Initial presentation is polyuria (> 4 mL/kg/hr).
    - Laboratory analysis should be obtained for serum sodium, serum osmolality, urine specific gravity.
    - Vasopressin infusion should be initiated if laboratory and clinical suspicion for DI is present (start with 0.0015 unit/kg/hr and double every 15 to 30 minutes; titrate to a urine output <2 ml/kg/hr).
- Postoperative management
  - Urine output should not be used to guide fluid therapy.
  - Admit patient to ICU for further monitoring and therapy.
  - Continue vasopressin infusion and strict monitoring of fluid input/output.
  - Frequent analysis of serum sodium, osmolality, and hourly urine output.
  - Stop vasopressin infusion when weaned off or transitioned back to DDAVP.

Syndrome of inappropriate antidiuretic hormone secretion

- Syndrome of inappropriate antidiuretic hormone secretion (SIADH) results from a relative excess amount of antidiuretic hormone (ADH).
- Positive pressure ventilation can increase ADH secretion.
- Excess ADH secretion can occur due to the following neurologic conditions:
  - Infections (meningitis).
  - Tumor (brain tumor, pituitary resection).
  - Trauma (subarachnoid hemorrhage).
- Severity of condition based on the absolute serum sodium concentration (<125 mEq/L) and rate of decrease (>0.5 mEq/L/hr)
- Clinical findings include headache, nausea, vomiting, muscle cramps, lethargy, restlessness, disorientation and depressed reflexes
- Laboratory values
  - Hyponatremia (<132 mEq/L).
  - Decreased serum osmolality (< 280 mOsm/L).
  - Increased urine osmolality (> 200 mOsm/L).
  - Increased urine specific gravity (> 1.005).
  - Increased urine sodium (> 20 mmol/L).
- Treatment
  - Fluid restriction for mild cases (50% of maintenance rate).
  - Consider hypertonic (3%) saline for severe cases but increase sodium gradually to reduce risk of central pontine myelinolysis (CPM).

Further reading

Coté CJ, Lerman J, Anderson BJ. *Coté and Lerman's A Practice of Anesthesia for Infants and Children*, 5th edition. Philadelphia, PA: Elsevier, 2013; 533–47.

Davis PJ, Cladis FP, Motoyama EK. *Smith's Anesthesia for Infants and Children*, 8th edition. Philadelphia: Elsevier Mosby, 2011; 1099–104.

Part B System-based topics in pediatric anesthesiology

Chapter 127

Endocrine system
Thyroid disorders/adrenal disorders
Tae W. Kim

Introduction
The thyroid and adrenal glands both play a major role in the homeostasis of the human body. Each gland is capable of synthesizing and excreting hormones into the bloodstream to affect distant target organs, causing alterations in metabolic and autonomic balance. The etiologies for many of these changes are multifactorial and are categorized as intrinsic or extrinsic in nature.

Thyroid disorders
- Intrinsic – autoimmune-related, associated disorder of the pituitary or hypothalamus.
- Extrinsic – iodine deficiency.
- Pathophysiology
  - Changes in hormone levels
    - Thyrotropin-releasing hormone (TRH).
    - Thyroid-stimulating hormone (TSH).
    - Thyroxine (T_4) conversion to triiodothyronine (T_3).
  - Failure of feedback mechanism.
- Testing
  - Serum TSH.
  - Serum total or free T_4.
  - Serum T_3.
- Hyperthyroidism
  - Most common form is diffuse toxic goiter (i.e., Graves disease).
    - Autoimmune-mediated, circulating antibodies mimic effects of thyroid-stimulating hormone.
    - Increased triiodothyronine (T_3), thyroxine (T_4) or with decreased or absent TSH.
    - Highest incidence in adolescence.
    - More common in girls (5X) than boys.

Handbook of Critical Incidents and Essential Topics in Pediatric Anesthesiology, ed. David A. Young and Olutoyin A. Olutoye. Published by Cambridge University Press. © Cambridge University Press 2015.

- Congenital hyperthyroidism is additional etiology of hyperthyroidism which is a transient condition seen in neonates.
    - Due to placental transfer of thyroid-stimulating antibodies from mothers with Graves disease.
- Common clinical findings include irritability, tremors, palpitations, exophthalmos, goiter, hyperhidrosis.
- Thyroid storm represents unique hyperdynamic state: severe tachycardia, hyperthermia and restlessness potentially resulting in delirium, coma and death.
- Treatment options
    - Antithyroid medications: methimazole, propylthiouracil, radioiodine iodine-131.
    - Beta blockade for cardiovascular effects.
    - Thyroidectomy after converting to a clinically euthyroid state.

- Hypothyroidism
    - Primary hypothyroidism is etiology in 95% of cases.
    - Most common cause is autoimmune (chronic thyroiditis or Hashimoto thyroiditis).
    - Progressive destruction of thyroid gland.
    - Decreased circulating concentrations of T_3 and T_4, increased TSH.
    - Subclinical form with only increased thyroid-stimulating hormone concentration present in 5% of American population.
    - Iatrogenic causes from medical or surgical treatment (e.g., thyroidectomy, pituitary tumor resection).
    - Moderate to severe form may be characterized by diminished cardiac function, respiratory drive and increased sensitivity to anesthetic agents.
    - Emergent surgery may require treatment with intravenous thyroid hormones (T_3 or T_4) with or without glucocorticoids.

- Perioperative management
    - Hyperthyroid patients should be clinically euthyroid prior to elective surgery.
        - Beta-blockers should be utilized to control hyperdynamic states and inhibit peripheral conversion of T_4 to T_3.
    - Hypothyroid patients with severe myxedema coma, pericardial effusion, or cardiac failure should receive replacement hormone therapy.
        - Antithyroid medications such as propylthiouracil and methimazole decrease thyroid hormone synthesis.
        - Attention should be given for sensitivity to anesthetic drugs, prolonged muscle weakness, and delayed emergence.
        - Refractory hypotension may suggest acute primary adrenal insufficiency.

Adrenal disorders

- Extrinsic – tuberculosis, adrenal hemorrhage.
- Intrinsic – autoimmune, multiple endocrine neoplasia (MEN) syndrome, congenital adrenal hyperplasia, pheochromocytoma.
- Pathophysiology – disruption of hypothalamic–pituitary–adrenal (HPA) axis, the following conditions may occur or hormone production may be impaired:

- Hypothalamus
  - Corticotrophin-releasing hormone (CRH).
- Pituitary – adrenocorticotropic hormone (ACTH) deficiency
  - Pituitary agenesis or hypoplasia, septo-optic dysplasia, infiltrative disease, tumors (craniopharyngiomas), cranial irradiation, chemotherapy.
  - ACTH – diurnal pattern, increase with trauma, acute illness, high fever, hypoglycemia.
- Adrenal
  - Primary adrenal disorder.
  - Secondary – hypothalamic–pituitary insufficiency.
  - Absence of ACTH.
  - Atrophy of adrenal gland.

- Testing
  - Measure serum cortisol and plasma ACTH.
  - ACTH stimulation test.

- Adrenal insufficiency
  - Iatrogenic – results from chronic steroid use.
  - HPA suppression is transient following steroid use for 2 weeks or less, longer periods of steroid use may result in prolonged suppression for 6 to 9 months.
  - Patients with prolonged duration of steroid therapy or a diagnosis of adrenal insufficiency (i.e., critically ill patients) require perioperative steroid administration.

- Pheochromocytoma
  - 10% to 20% of all cases occur in pediatric the population; average age 11 years old.
  - Autosomal dominant trait, associated with von Hippel–Lindau syndrome or multiple endocrine neoplasia (MEN) type II or III.
  - 10% of tumors are bilateral, 10% extra-adrenal, < 10% malignant.
  - Primarily involve catecholamine-producing chromaffin cells of adrenal medulla, which mainly produce norepinephrine.
  - Other sites of chromaffin cells: abdominal sympathetic chain near aorta, at inferior mesenteric artery or aortic bifurcation, neck, mediastinum, and wall of bladder or ureters.
  - Signs and symptoms: paroxysmal hypertension (most common), headaches, palpitations, sweating – all four account for >90% of presenting signs in patients.
  - Hypermetabolic state: weight loss, in spite of increased caloric intake, polyuria, polydipsia, and abdominal pain.
  - Presentation may be confused with diabetes, renal vascular disease, hyperthyroidism, coarctation of the aorta, cerebral disorders, other catecholamine-secreting tumors such as neuroblastoma.

- Diagnostic evaluation
  - Test for increased levels of catecholamines
    - Plasma-free metanephrines – sensitivity 99%.
    - Urine catecholamine concentrations are directly proportional to circulating levels.

- 24-hour urine collection for primary catecholamines and their metabolites, 3-methoxy 4-hydroxy vanillyl-mandelic acid (VMA) and metanephrine, specificity 95%.
  - Imaging studies
    - MRI, computerized tomography (CT) and nuclear imaging to locate catecholamine-producing mass.
    - Magnetic resonance angiography (MRA) and venography (MRV) – may be required to detect vascular supply of mass.
    - Echocardiography to assess anatomy and ventricular function.
- Coexisting disease
  - Cardiac: hypertrophic cardiomyopathy, left ventricular hypertrophy, EKG changes (e.g., repolarization abnormalities, nonspecific ST-T wave changes, QTc interval prolongation).
  - Associated endocrinopathies related to MEN type II or III.
  - Neurofibromatosis – intracardiac tumor or laryngeal neurofibroma.
- Preoperative stabilization
  - First initiate alpha blockade (e.g., oral phenoxybenzamine) to attenuate vasoconstriction effects from catecholamines.
  - After alpha blockade attained, administer β-blockers (e.g., oral propranolol) to control heart rate.
  - Assess fluid and electrolyte status, such as hemoglobin, hematocrit, potassium, calcium, glucose and renal function.
- Intraoperative management
  - Consider preoperative anxiolysis to reduce sympathetic tone.
  - Avoid agents associated with increased sympathetic activity such as ketamine, pancuronium, ephedrine, desflurane, morphine, meperidine and droperidol.
  - Obtain and have immediately available fast-acting, short duration vasopressors such as esmolol, nitroprusside, nicardipine.
  - Consider regional technique; for use after tumor resection is completed.
  - Vasopressin or phenylephrine (may observe resistance due to preexisting alpha blockade) for refractory hypotension.
  - Strongly consider placing an arterial line and perhaps central venous access.

Further reading

Coté CJ, Lerman J, Anderson BJ. *Coté and Lerman's A Practice of Anesthesia for Infants and Children*, 5th edition. Philadelphia, PA: Elsevier, 2013; 547–53, 579–82.

Davis PJ, Cladis FP, Motoyama EK. *Smith's Anesthesia for Infants and Children*, 8th edition. Philadelphia: Elsevier Mosby, 2011; 1110–11.

Kohl BA, Schwartz S. Preoperative medical consultation: a multidisciplinary approach surgery in the patient with endocrine dysfunction. *Anesthesiol Clin.* 2009; 27(4):687–703.

Part B System-based topics in pediatric anesthesiology

Chapter 128
Hematology system
Anatomy and physiology
Shakeel Siddiqui

Development of hematopoietic system
- Hematopoiesis occurs in three steps within the fetus:
  - Mesoblastic erythropoiesis occurs in the yolk sac at 10–14 days of life.
  - Hepatic erythropoiesis occurs at 6–8 weeks gestation and diminishes at 20–24 weeks.
  - Myeloid erythropoiesis starts in the second trimester and continues throughout life.
- The sterile environment of the fetus does not require neutrophils.
- 85% of cells are erythroid with no neutrophils in hepatic phase (compared to 40% erythroid and 15% neutrophils in bone marrow).

Granulocytopoiesis
- Neutrophils are not observed until the second trimester although some cells with phagocytic properties are present in early fetal life.
- Granulocytes are a very minor component of fetal cells until the 24th week of gestation.

Thrombopoiesis
- Megakaryoblasts develop from committed progenitor cells.
- Long strips of cytoplasm peel off the cytoplasm to form platelets.

Erythropoiesis
- Stimulated solely by erythroid growth factors from the fetus.
- Erythropoietin (EPO) has the most regulatory role in erythropoiesis and is produced by accessory cells which stimulate transformation of erythroid precursors to mature red blood cells.
- Initially EPO is produced in the liver and, by the third trimester to the first week of postnatal life, production site shifts to the kidney.

Hemoglobin
- Embryonic hemoglobin (Hgb): In the early human embryo, embryonic hemoglobin dominates the circulation. It disappears in the 3rd month of fetal life.

Handbook of Critical Incidents and Essential Topics in Pediatric Anesthesiology, ed. David A. Young and Olutoyin A. Olutoye. Published by Cambridge University Press. © Cambridge University Press 2015.

- Fetal Hgb: Predominant Hgb from 24 weeks of life (90%) but gradually decreases to 70% at birth and rapidly falls to trace concentrations by 6–12 months of life.
- Adult Hgb: First observed at 16–20 weeks of gestation and increases by 5–10% at 24 weeks. It steadily increases throughout fetal life to birth levels of 30% and by 6–12 months it is the only major Hgb.

Development and physiology of hemostasis

- All fetal coagulation factors are produced independently of the mother; fibrinogen formation starts as early as 5½ weeks of gestational age and fetal blood is capable of clot formation at 11 weeks.
- Despite the upregulation of coagulation factors at birth, vitamin K-dependent factors (II, VII, IX, and X) in the neonate are only 50% of adult values; this leads to a slightly prolonged prothrombin time (PT) and international normalized ratio (INR).
- The contact factors: high molecular weight kallikrein (HMWK), prekallikrein, and factors XI and XII are also approximately 50% of adult values.
- The reduced contact factors account for a disproportionally prolonged activated partial thromboplastin time (aPTT).
- The reduced concentration of factors at birth is best explained by reduced synthesis of factors by the liver. However, the levels rapidly increase, reaching approximately 80% of adult values by 6 months of age.
- At birth, plasma proteins C and S are 35% of adult values. The concentration of protein C does not reach adult levels until adolescence.
- Neonatal levels of antithrombin (AT) are 50% of adult values; they reach adult levels by 6 months of age.

Hematologic physiology in the neonate

- Preterm infants reach their lowest hemoglobin level (7–9 g/dL) at 3–6 weeks and for full-term infants the lowest level is 9–11 g/dL at 8–12 weeks.
- The neonate has relative polycythemia, reticulocytosis, and leukocytosis. Infants experience physiological anemia at 2–3 months of age.
- Hemoglobin values reach adults levels by 1 year of life (Table 128.1).

Table 128.1 Hematology values at different ages.

	Preterm 28–32 wk	Preterm 32–36 wk	Term infant	1-year-old	Child	Adult
Hemoglobin (g/dL)	12.9	13.6	16.8	12	13	15
Hematocrit (%)	40.9	43.6	55	36	38	45
Platelet count (/mm^3)	255,000	260,000	300,000	300,000	300,000	300,000
Prothrombin time (sec)	15.4	13	13	11	11	12
International normalized ratio (INR)	—	1	1	1	1	1
Activated partial thromboplastin time (sec)	108	53.6	42.9	30	31	28
Fibrinogen (mg/dL)	256	243	283	276	279	278
Bleeding time (min)	—	3.5	3.5	6	7	5

All values are means.
Adapted from Coté, Lerman and Anderson, *A Practice of Anesthesia for Infants and Children*, 5th edition; p. 178.

Blood volume

Circulating blood volume in preterm infants can be as much as 100 mL/kg; and in a term infant: 80 mL/kg. The blood volume stabilizes at 70–80 mL/kg in adolescence. In an obese child the blood volume is about 60–65 mL/kg.

Further reading

Coté CJ, Lerman J, Anderson BJ. *Coté and Lerman's A Practice of Anesthesia for Infants and Children*, 5th edition. Philadelphia, PA: Elsevier, 2013; 178, 410.

Gregory GA, Andropoulos DB. *Gregory's Pediatric Anesthesia*, 5th edition. Hoboken: Wiley-Blackwell, 2012; 225–9.

Part B System-based topics in pediatric anesthesiology

Hematology system
Medical conditions
Shakeel Siddiqui

Hemolytic anemia

Hemolytic syndromes are a group of disorders in which there is lysis of erythrocytes leading to anemia. The most significant types are due to intracellular defects.

Hereditary spherocytosis

- Hereditary spherocytosis (HS) is the most common inherited chronic hemolysis disorder.
- Autosomal dominant pattern in 75% of patients.
- Pathophysiology includes abnormalities of erythrocyte membrane proteins ankyrin and beta spectrin.
- The shape of the red blood cell is spherical instead of the normal biconcave shape, resulting in altered stability. Deformity leads to loss of flexibility and premature rupture.
- Damaged erythrocytes are sequestered into splenic capillaries and the combination of extravascular and intravascular hemolysis leads to extramedullary erythropoiesis and splenomegaly.
- Clinical features include hyperbilirubinemia (unconjugated bilirubin), increased lactate dehydrogenase, and thrombocytopenia resulting from hypersplenism.
- Mild disease affects 20% of children. Approximately 5% have severe HS (hemoglobin < 8 g/dL) requiring transfusion, especially during acute viral infections.
- There are several significant perioperative considerations (Table 129.1).

Table 129.1 Perioperative anesthetic implications for the patient with hereditary spherocytosis.

Preoperative
Determine the hemoglobin and platelet values
Inquire about blood product transfusion history
Intraoperative
Administer appropriate antibiotic coverage
Recognize potential for significant blood loss (i.e., splenectomy and cholecystectomy)
Cautious use of regional anesthesia, intramuscular medications, nasogastric tubes, etc. (if thrombocytopenia is present)
Postoperative
Consider evaluation of hemoglobin and platelet values

Handbook of Critical Incidents and Essential Topics in Pediatric Anesthesiology, ed. David A. Young and Olutoyin A. Olutoye. Published by Cambridge University Press. © Cambridge University Press 2015.

- Cholecystectomy and splenectomy are common surgical procedures performed in children affected with HS.

Glucose-6-phosphate dehydrogenase deficiency

- Glucose-6-phosphate dehydrogenase (G6PD) deficiency is one of the most common enzyme deficiencies.
- It is an X-linked recessive disease and is most prevalent in geographic areas where malaria is endemic.
- G6PD deficiency causes hemolysis in the presence of oxidative stressors.
- Pathology: pathognomonic finding is the presence of Heinz bodies in the peripheral blood smear. Other features include normocytic anemia, increased reticulocyte count, and elevated bilirubin.
- Patients appear jaundiced clinically.
- Anesthetic considerations
    - There are several significant perioperative considerations (Table 129.2).
    - Avoid known activating medications as they may cause hemolysis from production of methemoglobin (Table 129.3).

Table 129.2 Perioperative anesthetic implications for the patient with G6PD deficiency.

Preoperative
Determine history of hemolysis and precipitating factors
Determine hemoglobin value

Intraoperative
Avoidance of known activating medications
Avoidance of agents that increase methemoglobin

Postoperative
Follow urine output closely particularly if hemolysis is present

Table 129.3 Activating medications that may precipitate hemolysis in G6PD deficiency.

Antibiotics
Sulfonamides
Co-trimoxazole (Bactrim, Septrin)
Dapsone
Chloramphenicol
Nitrofurantoin

Antimalarials
Chloroquine
Hydroxychloroquine
Primaquine
Quinine

Other Medications
Aspirin
Sulfasalazine

Table 129.3 (cont.)

Methyldopa
Hydralazine
Procainamide
Quinidine
Chemicals
Methylene blue

Hemoglobinopathies

Thalassemia

- Genetic disorder characterized by disruption of the normal 1:1 ratio of α to β polypeptide chains.
- The pathophysiology in thalassemia results from both hemolysis and ineffective erythropoiesis.
- This results in symptoms that range from chronic hemolytic anemia to fetal death (hydrops fetalis).
- This condition may be misdiagnosed as iron deficiency anemia due to hypochromic, microcytic anemia that occurs; however this anemia does not respond to iron supplementation.
- Complications include abnormal bone growth, alloimmunization from recurrent transfusion, infections, cardiomyopathy, endocrine dysfunction, splenomegaly, and thromboembolism.
- Treatment of severe disease includes blood transfusions, chelation therapy, vitamin D, hormone therapy, and stem cell transplantation.
- Common indications for surgery include long-term vascular access placement, cholecystectomy, and splenectomy.
- Anesthetic considerations: see Table 129.4.

Table 129.4 Perioperative considerations for the patient with thalassemia.

Preoperative
Determine hemoglobin level
Transfusion of crossmatched blood if indicated
Evaluate cardiac function
Evaluate hepatic function
Pre-splenectomy antibiotics if indicated
Intraoperative
Cautious positioning of extremities
Vigilance for post-splenectomy hypertension
Consider prophylaxis for thromboembolism
Postoperative
Consider continuation of thromboembolism prophylaxis

Thrombocytopenia

- Platelets are an essential component of the coagulation cascade with a lifespan of about 7–10 days.
- Mainly distributed in a 2:1 ratio in the blood.
- Causes of thrombocytopenia can be subdivided into primary and secondary disorders.

Idiopathic thrombocytopenic purpura

- Idiopathic thrombocytopenic purpura (ITP) is a benign self-limited disorder affecting children with an incidence of 4/100,000.
- Pathophysiology includes presence of antiplatelet antibodies in plasma and increased megakaryocytes in bone marrow.
- Platelet autoantibodies exist alone or as immune complexes of immunoglobulin G, specific for platelet membrane glycoproteins IIb/IIIa and Ib/IX.
- Clinical laboratory findings include platelet counts of < 10,000–20,000/mm^3 and an increased incidence of intracranial hemorrhage (0.1–0.9%).
- Corticosteroid therapy often inhibits phagocytosis of antibody-coated platelets in spleen and inhibits antibody production.
- Antimetabolites, notably vincristine, and intravenous immunoglobulins block reticuloendothelial receptors in Rh-positive patients.
- Splenectomy is reserved for acute life-threatening events or patients refractory to medical therapy.
- Anesthetic implications for patients with ITP: see Table 129.5.

Table 129.5 Anesthetic considerations for the patient with idiopathic thrombocytopenia purpura.

Preoperative

Determine hemoglobin and platelet values

Determine plan for platelet transfusion including transfusion trigger (i.e., platelet count < 50,000/mm^3)

Discontinue all platelet-inhibiting medications (e.g., ibuprofen)

Intraoperative

Consider administering corticosteroid stress dose

Cautious use of regional anesthesia, intramuscular medications, nasogastric tubes, etc.

Postoperative

Follow regular hemoglobin and platelet counts

Consider continuation of corticosteroid coverage

Further reading

Coté CJ, Lerman J, Anderson BJ. *Coté and Lerman's A Practice of Anesthesia for Infants and Children*, 5th edition. Philadelphia, PA: Elsevier, 2013; 187–8.

Gregory GA, Andropoulos DB. *Gregory's Pediatric Anesthesia*, 5th edition. Hoboken: Wiley-Blackwell, 2012; 236–40.

Part B System-based topics in pediatric anesthesiology

Chapter 130

Hematology system
Sickle cell disease/von Willebrand/ hemophilia

Tae W. Kim

Sickle cell disease

- Hemoglobin A is replaced by hemoglobin S.
- Affects 1:375 African-Americans (sickle cell trait present in 8% of African-American population).
- Multiple types of crisis: vaso-occlusive, sequestration, aplastic, hemolytic.
- Genetics
    - Inherited autosomal recessive disorder of chromosome 11.
    - Substitution of valine for glutamic acid.
    - Homozgous state, SS, confers sickle cell disease (70%).
    - HbSC disease (20%).
    - HbSβ disease (10%).
    - Heterozygous state, AS, confers sickle cell trait with minimal risk for sickling; sickling may occur only under extreme conditions.
- Pathophysiology
    - Sickling of red blood cells occur under conditions of stress: hypoxemia, acidosis, hypothermia, hypovolemia.
    - Precipitation of sickled hemoglobin leads to tactoid formation and conformational change to the red blood cell (sickle cell).
    - Vaso-occlusion (crisis) occurs from thrombus formation and vasospasm.
- Testing
    - Sickledex – screening test for presence of sickle hemoglobin; unable to differentiate type of sickle cell disease.
    - Hemoglobin electrophoresis – detects proportion of different hemoglobin types and can differentiate between sickle cell disease and sickle trait.
    - Isoelectric focusing, high performance liquid chromatography – very sensitive and commonly used for newborn screening.
- Perioperative management
    - Preoperative hydration recommended.

Handbook of Critical Incidents and Essential Topics in Pediatric Anesthesiology, ed. David A. Young and Olutoyin A. Olutoye. Published by Cambridge University Press. © Cambridge University Press 2015.

- Consider pre-procedure transfusion, either exchange or simple, based on surgical procedure and hemoglobin value.
- Maintain normothermia.
- Provide effective perioperative pain control.
- Provide postoperative supplemental oxygen and hydration.

- Transfusion therapy
  - Exchange – replace HbS blood with HbA blood by blood transfusion with a goal of 10 g/dL total hemoglobin and ≤ 30% sickle hemoglobin.
  - Simple – transfuse HbA blood; transfusion goal 10 g/dL total hemoglobin.
  - Choice of transfusion therapy based on patient's condition, starting Hb and procedure.

- Complications
  - Alloimmunization.
  - Transfusion reactions.
  - Hemochromatosis.
  - Hyperviscosity syndrome from over transfusion, >16 g/dL total hemoglobin.
  - Acute chest syndrome.

Von Willebrand disease

- Von Willebrand disease (vWD) is the most common bleeding disorder, prevalence estimated at 1% of population.
- Genetics
  - Mutations of the von Willebrand disease gene.
  - Autosomal dominant inheritance pattern, except for types 2N and 3 which are autosomal recessive.

- Pathophysiology
  - Role of von Willebrand factor (vWF) in coagulation cascade: adherence of platelets to damaged subendothelium and transporting factor VIII in plasma.
  - Coagulopathy related to quantitative (types 1 and 3) and qualitative (type 2) abnormalities.

- Testing and diagnosis
  - Common preoperative symptoms include easy bruising, epistaxis, menorrhagia.
  - Prolonged bleeding time and prolonged PTT (partial thromboplastin time); may have normal values in mild disease.
  - Platelet functional assay (PFA-100) is approximately 90% sensitive for diagnosis.
  - Platelet count is typically normal except in type 2B.

- Perioperative management
  - Consult hematologist; determine type of vWD.
  - Administer DDAVP if patient has responsive type (types 2 ineffective, subtype 2B contraindicated).

- DDAVP administration associated with tachyphylaxis and free water retention.
- Administer factor concentrates: factor VIII and vWF, if unresponsive to DDAVP.
- Administer cryoprecipitate if vWF concentrate unavailable.
- Strong consideration for avoidance of procedures associated with increased bleeding risk (e.g., intramuscular injections, nasogastric tubes).
- Decision to perform regional anesthesia must consider risk: benefit ratio.

Hemophilia

- Types: Factor VIII deficiency (hemophilia A) and factor IX deficiency (hemophilia B or Christmas disease), factor XI (hemophilia C, mild form with infrequent need for therapy).
- Prevalence of hemophilia A is 10.5:100,000 male births.
- Prevalence of hemophilia B is 2.9:100,000 male births.
- Associated with frequent nosebleeds, abnormal intraoperative bleeding.
- Genetics
  - X-linked recessive inheritance for hemophilia A and B.
  - Daughter of affected father is obligate carrier; 50% chance of inheritance by son.
  - *De novo* mutations relatively common.
  - Autosomal recessive form, hemophilia C, affects primarily Ashkenazi Jews.
- Pathophysiology
  - Coagulation cascade interrupted by lack of factor IX and XI.
  - Reduced or absent factor IX and VIII results in decreased to absent conversion of prothrombin to thrombin.
  - This results in reduced or absent conversion of fibrinogen to fibrin.
- Testing
  - Female carriers average 50% of normal factor concentrations; this typically results in no extraordinary bleeding during most surgical procedures.
  - aPTT prolonged in proportion to concentration of factor.
  - Measure specific factor concentrations to confirm diagnosis.
- Perioperative management
  - Replace deficient factor based on procedure and target concentration.
  - DDAVP effective for mild cases of hemophilia A by releasing endogenous factor VIII.
  - Tachyphylaxis is possible with repeated use of DDAVP.
  - Recombinant forms of factors are available.
  - Hemophilia C patients should receive recombinant factor XI or FFP.
  - Children with inhibitors to factor concentrates may benefit from recombinant factor VIIa (rFVIIa).
  - Partially activated prothrombin complex concentrates are effective against inhibitors.
  - Regional anesthesia is relatively contraindicated.

- Maintain factor levels per hematologist recommendations, continue replacement therapy from preoperative period through postoperative period as directed.

Further reading

Coté CJ, Lerman J, Anderson BJ. *Coté and Lerman's A Practice of Anesthesia for Infants and Children*, 5th edition. Philadelphia, PA: Elsevier, 2013; 183–7, 189–92.

Davis PJ, Cladis FP, Motoyama EK. *Smith's Anesthesia for Infants and Children*, 8th edition. Philadelphia: Elsevier Mosby, 2011; 1130–7, 1150–3.

Part C Clinical-based areas in pediatric anesthesiology

Chapter 131

Cardiac surgery
General considerations
Erin A. Gottlieb

Preoperative assessment
- History including anatomy, symptoms, prior intervention, planned repair or palliation.
- Physical examination including cyanosis, venous congestion, edema, signs of poor systemic perfusion.
- Laboratory information including hematocrit.
- Electrocardiogram.
- Imaging
  - Chest X-ray.
  - Echocardiogram.
  - MRI/CT.
- Cardiac catheterization data
  - Pulmonary vascular resistance.
  - Gradients across valves.
  - Ratio of pulmonary to systemic blood flow ($Q_p:Q_s$).
- Anatomy
  - Sources of pulmonary and systemic blood flow.
  - Presence and degree of valvular stenosis and insufficiency.
  - Myocardial function.
  - Presence of pulmonary hypertension or pulmonary vascular disease.

Considerations for planned surgical procedure
- Line placement
  - For most cases, arterial and central venous access are required.
  - Site considerations
    - Venous (see Table 131.1)
      - Femoral venous placement for patients < 5 kg.
      - Internal jugular vein placement for patients > 5 kg.

Handbook of Critical Incidents and Essential Topics in Pediatric Anesthesiology, ed. David A. Young and Olutoyin A. Olutoye. Published by Cambridge University Press. © Cambridge University Press 2015.

Table 131.1 Recommended double lumen central venous catheter sizes and lengths.

Patient weight (kg)	Internal jugular vein	Femoral vein
< 10	4 Fr, 8 cm	4 Fr, 12 cm
10–30	4 Fr, 12 cm	4 Fr, 12–15 cm
30–50	5 Fr, 12–15 cm	5 Fr, 15 cm
50–70	7 Fr, 15 cm	7 Fr, 20 cm
> 70	8 Fr, 16 cm	8 Fr, 20 cm

Source: Andropoulos DB. Vascular access and monitoring. In *Anesthesia for Congenital Heart Disease*, 2nd edition. Edited by DB Andropoulos, SA Stayer, IA Russell and EB Mossad, Chichester, UK: Wiley-Blackwell, 2010.

- Arterial
  - For patients with a right Blalock-Taussig (BT) shunt or who will have a right BT shunt at the end of the procedure, a right radial arterial line is generally NOT recommended, as it will have a lower pressure than other sites due to pulmonary artery steal from the shunt.
  - For repair of an aortic coarctation, an arterial line placed in a vessel whose takeoff is proximal to the coarctation is recommended (right radial). Other blood pressure sites will be unreliable during the period of aortic cross-clamp.
  - Aberrant right subclavian artery with a left aortic arch is more common in patients with congenital heart disease (CHD) and most common in those with conotruncal anomalies; the arterial line should be placed in an alternate extremity so that the arterial line tracing will not be affected by placement of a transesophageal echocardiography probe.
- Consider need for pre/post bypass vasoactive and inotropic infusions.
  - Depressed function may occur following a long aortic cross-clamp time and in patients with depressed preoperative function.
    - Milrinone.
    - Epinephrine.
    - Dopamine.
    - Calcium chloride (for neonates).
  - Decreased systemic vascular resistance may be encountered
    - Phenylephrine.
    - Vasopressin.
    - Norepinephrine.
  - Postoperative hypertension should be anticipated in cases where left or right heart obstruction is relieved (subaortic membrane resection, aortic coarctation repair, replacement of a stenotic right ventricle to pulmonary artery conduit).
    - Esmolol.
    - Sodium nitroprusside.
    - Nicardipine.
- Risk of post-bypass pulmonary hypertension
  - Inhaled nitric oxide should be readily available, especially for patients at high risk for pulmonary hypertension (e.g., after repair of overcirculated AV canal, truncus arteriosus, obstructed total anomalous pulmonary venous return).

- Milrinone infusion to decrease pulmonary vascular resistance and augment right ventricular function.
  - Maneuvers to decrease pulmonary vascular resistance (see below).
- Blood product transfusion
  - Packed red blood cells (transfuse cyanotic patients to a hematocrit of approximately 45% to maximize oxygen carrying capacity).
  - Platelets and cryoprecipitate may be required post-bypass to correct thrombocytopenia, platelet dysfunction, and hypofibrinogenemia.
  - Factor VIIa may be required for continued bleeding if platelets and clotting factor replacement are ineffective.

Managing the ratio of pulmonary to systemic blood flow ($Q_p:Q_s$)

- In patients who have mixing lesions, pulmonary and systemic blood flow should be balanced to avoid excessive pulmonary blood flow (Q_p) and maximize systemic cardiac output (Q_s).
- Most commonly accomplished by manipulating pulmonary vascular resistance (PVR) to decrease pulmonary blood flow (↑ PVR) or increase pulmonary blood flow (↓ PVR).
- Maneuvers to increase PVR
  - Hypoventilation: allow $PaCO_2$ to increase.
  - Avoidance of hyperoxia: decrease FiO_2 to as low as room air.
  - Mechanical snaring of the pulmonary artery by surgeon.
- Maneuvers to decrease PVR
  - Hyperventilation.
  - Delivery of high FiO_2.
  - Avoidance of acidosis; systemic alkalization.
  - Inhaled nitric oxide.
  - Avoidance of hypothermia.
  - Deep sedation/opioid administration.

Ductal-dependent blood flow

- In patients that have near or complete aortic or pulmonary atresia, blood flow through the ductus arteriosus is critical for systemic or pulmonary blood flow.
- Ductal-dependent systemic blood flow
  - Blood flow from the pulmonary artery to the aorta via the ductus arteriosus is responsible for significant degrees of systemic perfusion.
  - Narrowing or closure of the ductus arteriosus will result in hypotension, systemic and gut hypoperfusion, shock, and cardiac arrest.
- Ductal-dependent pulmonary blood flow
  - Blood flow from the aorta to the pulmonary artery via the ductus arteriosus is required for pulmonary blood flow.

- ○ Narrowing or closure of the duct will result in severe hypoxemia, cyanosis, and hypoxemia-related organ dysfunction and cardiac arrest.
- Prostaglandin E_1 infusion is typically initiated to maintain ductal patency after birth until cardiac lesion can be repaired or palliated.
- Important to maintain PVR to avoid the combination of excessive pulmonary blood flow and decreased systemic blood flow.

Choice of anesthetics
- No specific recommendations.
- Care should be taken with medications that can decrease preload, afterload and contractility such as propofol, high concentrations of volatile agents, or ketamine in catecholamine-depleted patients.

Further reading

Andropoulos DB. Hemodynamic management. In *Anesthesia for Congenital Heart Disease*, 2nd edition. DB Andropoulos, SA Stayer, IA Russell, EB Mossad, eds. Chichester, UK: Wiley-Blackwell, 2010.

Andropoulos DB. Vascular access and monitoring. In *Anesthesia for Congenital Heart Disease*, 2nd edition. DB Andropoulos, SA Stayer, IA Russell, EB Mossad, eds. Chichester, UK: Wiley-Blackwell, 2010.

Part C Clinical-based areas in pediatric anesthesiology

Chapter 132

Cardiac surgery
Acyanotic lesions

Premal M. Trivedi and Pablo Motta

Left-to-right shunts represent the most common type of acyanotic lesion, accounting for ~ 50% of all congenital heart disease (CHD).

Pathophysiology of left-to-right shunts

- Anatomical communication between the systemic and pulmonary circulations results in an increase of pulmonary blood flow and pulmonary pressures
- Communication or shunting may occur at different levels:
  - Atrium = atrial septal defect (ASD).
  - Ventricle = ventricular septal defect (VSD).
  - Atrium and ventricle = complete atrioventricular canal (CAVC).
  - Great arteries = patent ductus arteriosus (PDA) and aortopulmonary window.
- Excessive pulmonary blood flow or overcirculation (pulmonary blood flow (Qp)/systemic blood flow (Qs) > 2:1) results in:
  - Failure to thrive.
  - Congestive heart failure: tachypnea, tachycardia and increased work of breathing
    - Cardiac output increases to maintain systemic blood flow.
  - Recurrent respiratory infections.
  - Pulmonary hypertension and Eisenmenger syndrome (suprasystemic pulmonary artery pressures leading to reversal of shunt) if uncorrected.
- Extent of overcirculation depends on:
  - Size of the defect.
  - Ratio of pulmonary vascular resistance (PVR) to systemic vascular resistance (SVR).
- Cardiac remodeling:
  - Atrial shunting causes right atrial and right ventricular dilation.
  - Ventricular and aorto-pulmonary shunting cause left heart dilation.

Handbook of Critical Incidents and Essential Topics in Pediatric Anesthesiology, ed. David A. Young and Olutoyin A. Olutoye. Published by Cambridge University Press. © Cambridge University Press 2015.

Anesthetic considerations

- Pre-repair
    - Manipulate PVR/SVR to minimize left-to-right shunting
        - Avoid significant decreases in PVR and increases in SVR.
    - Avoid air bubbles in intravenous lines to prevent paradoxical emboli.
- Post-repair
    - Support right ventricular function as needed:
        - Inotropes.
        - Avoid increases in PVR.

Atrial septal defect

- Incidence: 5–10% of CHD.
- Anatomy: five subtypes based on level of defect
    - Secundum: defect at fossa ovalis (most common ~80%).
    - Primum: defect at septum primum (associated with AV canal defects).
    - Sinus venosus: defect at superior or inferior vena cava (associated with partial anomalous pulmonary venous return).
    - Patent foramen ovale (PFO): occurs due to failed fusion between the septum primum and septum secundum (probe patent foramen ovale detectable in 30% of adults).
    - Coronary sinus: occurs as a result of an unroofed coronary sinus (allowing blood to flow from the left atrium to the right atrium).
- Manifestations
    - Low pressure left-to-right shunting.
    - Transient ischemic attacks or cerebrovascular accidents due to paradoxical emboli.
    - Supraventricular arrhythmias due to right atrial dilation.
    - May be asymptomatic until 2nd to 3rd decade of life when congestive heart failure develops.
- Management
    - Close monitoring with serial echocardiograms.
    - Diuretic therapy if symptomatic.
    - Surgical closure indicated when Qp:Qs > 2:1.
- Surgical repair
    - Recommended between ages 3–5 years.
    - Only secundum ASD and PFO are amenable to device closure in the cardiac catheterization laboratory.
    - Large defects with insufficient rims may be unsuitable for device closure.

Ventricular septal defect

- Incidence: ventricular septal defect (VSD) is the most common CHD, can occur in isolation or as part of complex CHD.

- Anatomy
    - Type I – subarterial: located in the outlet septum.
    - Type II – perimembranous: situated in the membranous septum (most common type).
    - Type III – inlet or canal type: detected in the posterior region of the septum under the septal leaflet of the tricuspid valve.
    - Type IV – muscular: discovered at any level of the muscular septum.
- Manifestations
    - Depends on defect size and associated anomalies.
    - Restrictive VSDs are small, usually asymptomatic defects, that limit flow and induce high-pressure gradients across the defect.
    - Non-restrictive VSDs are commonly symptomatic, large defects and do not restrict flow into the right ventricle (RV). The RV and pulmonary artery (PA) are therefore exposed to systemic pressures.
- Management
    - Diuretic therapy if symptomatic.
    - Symptoms, when present, generally worsen after 3 months of life when PVR drops.
    - Surgery is indicated for Qp:Qs > 2:1.
- Surgical repair
    - Muscular VSDs may be closed using a percutaneous device.
    - Patch closure or primary closure (small defects) require cardiopulmonary bypass.

Atrioventricular canal

- Incidence of atrioventricular canal (AVC): 4–5% of CHD.
- Develops due to a failure in fusion of the endocardial cushions.
    - Associated with trisomy 21.
- Three subtypes
    - Partial AVC
        - Ostium primum ASD.
        - Cleft mitral valve (MV).
    - Transitional AVC
        - Ostium primum ASD.
        - Cleft MV.
        - Restrictive inlet VSD.
    - Complete AVC
        - Ostium primum ASD.
        - Non-restrictive inlet VSD.
        - Common atrioventricular valve (AV).
- Surgical repair
    - Septation of the heart with ASD and VSD closure.
    - AV repair adds surgical complexity.

Patent ductus arteriosus
- Incidence: 1 in 2500–5000 live births, common in premature patients.
- Anatomy: communication between the descending aorta and pulmonary artery; may occur in isolation or with complex CHD.
- Management
  - Pharmacologic
    - Indomethacin to decrease prostaglandin levels resulting in closure of ductus.
  - Percutaneous device closure
    - Following unsuccessful indomethacin trial and persistence of symptoms.
  - Surgical repair
    - Performed via left thoracotomy, commonly bedside procedure in the intensive care unit (micro-preemies) or in the operating room (older children).

Aortopulmonary window
- Incidence: rare (0.1–0.6% of CHD).
- Anatomy: communication between the aorta and the pulmonary artery.
- Pulmonary hypertension develops early.
- Surgical repair
  - Performed early in the neonatal period.
  - Postoperative period may be complicated by pulmonary hypertension.

Further reading

Andropoulos DB. *Anesthesia for Congenital Heart Disease*, 2nd edition. Hoboken: Wiley-Blackwell, 2010; 266–9.

Coté CJ, Lerman J, Anderson BJ. *Coté and Lerman's A Practice of Anesthesia for Infants and Children*, 5th edition. Philadelphia, PA: Elsevier, 2013; 339–40.

Gregory GA, Andropoulos DB. *Gregory's Pediatric Anesthesia*, 5th edition. Hoboken: Wiley-Blackwell, 2012; 642–5.

Part C Clinical-based areas in pediatric anesthesiology

Cardiac surgery
Cyanotic lesions

Premal M. Trivedi and Pablo Motta

Mechanisms of cyanosis

- Right-to-left shunts
    - Tetralogy of Fallot.
    - Tricuspid atresia.
    - Pulmonary atresia.
    - Ebstein's anomaly.
- Admixture of systemic and pulmonary venous return
    - Hypoplastic left heart syndrome (HLHS).
    - Truncus arteriosus.
    - Total anomalous pulmonary venous return (TAPVR).
    - Pre-Fontan single ventricle.

Tetralogy of Fallot

- Most common cyanotic lesion (accounts for 6–11% of congenital heart disease).
- Anatomy
    - Non-restrictive ventricular septal defect (VSD).
    - Right ventricular outflow tract obstruction (RVOTO).
        - Fixed component due to subvalvar, valvar, or supravalvar stenosis.
        - Dynamic component due to infundibular spasm.
    - Right ventricular (RV) hypertrophy.
    - Aorta overriding the RV.
- Pathophysiology
    - Severity of cyanosis depends on the relationship between RVOTO and systemic vascular resistance (SVR).
    - If the gradient across the RVOTO > SVR, right-to-left shunting ensues.
    - Similarly, shunting occurs if SVR decreases in relation to a fixed RV afterload.
    - Patients with minimal RVOTO may have normal oxygen saturations.

Handbook of Critical Incidents and Essential Topics in Pediatric Anesthesiology, ed. David A. Young and Olutoyin A. Olutoye. Published by Cambridge University Press. © Cambridge University Press 2015.

- Hypercyanotic or Tet "spells"
  ○ Acute right-to-left shunting due to a sudden increase in RV afterload or decrease in SVR.
  ○ Hypoxemia, hypercapnia, and acidosis exacerbate an increase to PVR and further increase the degree of shunting.
  ○ Triggers: sympathetic stimulation
    . Under anesthesia: spells may occur with surgical stimulation or anesthetic-induced decreases in SVR.
  ○ Management
    . Increase inspired concentration of oxygen (FiO_2).
    . Increase SVR with phenylephrine.
    . Increase preload (administer volume) to diminish RVOTO.
    . Deepen anesthesia with opioids or inhalational agent to decrease infundibular spasm.
    . Consider β-blocker therapy (e.g., esmolol) to decrease spasm and increase diastolic filling.
    . Squatting in the awake child may increase preload and SVR.
- Surgical repair
  ○ Occurs early in life with either a modified Blalock-Taussig shunt followed by complete repair, or complete repair as the first procedure.

Transposition of the great arteries

- Anatomy
  ○ Aorta arises from the right ventricle (RV) while the pulmonary artery arises from the left ventricle (LV).
    . Blood is circulated in parallel rather than in series, and cyanosis results.
  ○ 10–25% will have an associated VSD.
- Mixing
  ○ Can occur at the level of the atrium, ventricle, and ductus arteriosus.
  ○ Mixing at the atrial level is the most important determinant of oxyhemoglobin saturation.
  ○ Balloon atrial septostomy.
    . Performed to improve mixing and decrease pulmonary venous congestion.
- Surgical repair
  ○ Occurs in the first few weeks of life.
    . Arterial switch operation (ASO).
    . Following surgery, left ventricular failure may occur in the presence of increased pressure load.

Total anomalous pulmonary venous return

- Anatomy
  - Pulmonary veins drain to other areas rather than the left atrium.
    - Superior vena cava (SVC) or innominate vein via a vertical vein (supracardiac).
    - Coronary sinus (cardiac).
    - Inferior vena cava (IVC) via a common vein (infracardiac).
- Pathophysiology
  - Systemic and pulmonary venous return are mixed.
  - A right-to-left atrial shunt is obligatory in order to allow left heart filling.
  - Pulmonary venous return can be obstructed.
  - If obstruction is present, saturations decrease, RV afterload increases, and RV dysfunction develops – resulting in worsening cyanosis, acidosis, and ultimately death.
- Surgical repair
  - Performed emergently in the case of obstructed veins.

Truncus arteriosus

- Anatomy
  - Common arterial trunk for the RV and LV.
  - VSD.
  - Types distinguished by origin of the pulmonary arteries from the trunk.
- Pathophysiology
  - Mixing occurs at the arterial level.
  - Pulmonary to systemic blood flow ratio, (Q_p:Q_s) is determined by the relationship between SVR and PVR.
    - Decreases in PVR may compromise systemic and coronary perfusion.
- Surgical repair
  - Occurs during neonatal period.
  - Entails separation of the pulmonary and systemic circulations, repair of the common truncal valve, VSD closure, and creation of a RV to pulmonary artery (PA) conduit.

Hypoplastic left heart syndrome

- Anatomy
  - Hypoplastic LV.
  - Mitral and aortic stenosis or atresia.
  - Hypoplastic aortic arch.
  - Ductal-dependent systemic circulation.

- Pathophysiology
    - Mixing occurs through an obligate atrial level shunt and the ductus arteriosus.
    - $Q_p:Q_s$ is determined by relationship between SVR and PVR.
- Surgical repair
    - Stage 1: Norwood procedure
        - Performed in the neonatal period.
    - Stage 2: Bidirectional Glenn, or superior cavopulmonary anastomosis
        - Performed at 3–6 months.
    - Stage 3: Fontan
        - Performed at 2–4 years.
        - Systemic venous return is now fully directed to the pulmonary artery and the single ventricle receives only pulmonary venous blood.

Consequences of cyanosis

- Polycythemia
    - Erythropoietin levels increase in response to hypoxia.
    - Increased blood viscosity
        - Hematocrit > 65% is associated with impaired microvascular perfusion.
    - Both PVR and SVR increase, but the increase in PVR >> SVR.
    - Predisposes to thrombosis, therefore patients need to be adequately hydrated.
- Increased bleeding tendency due to possible:
    - Thrombocytopenia.
    - Abnormal coagulation due to factor deficiencies.
- Ventilatory response to hypoxia is significantly decreased.

Further reading

Andropoulos DB. *Anesthesia for Congenital Heart Disease*, 2nd edition. Hoboken: Wiley-Blackwell, 2010; 267–77.

Coté CJ, Lerman J, Anderson BJ. *Coté and Lerman's A Practice of Anesthesia for Infants and Children*, 5th edition. Philadelphia, PA: Elsevier, 2013; 342–50.

Gregory GA, Andropoulos DB. *Gregory's Pediatric Anesthesia*, 5th edition. Hoboken: Wiley-Blackwell, 2012; 633–5.

Part C Clinical-based areas in pediatric anesthesiology

Cardiac surgery
Non-cardiac surgery
Erin A. Gottlieb

Risks/Outcomes

- Patients with the following conditions have the highest risk for perioperative complications:
    - Functional single ventricle lesions.
    - Suprasystemic pulmonary hypertension.
    - Left ventricular outflow tract obstruction.
    - Dilated cardiomyopathy.
- Single ventricle (SV) groups with higher perioperative risk include:
    - SV patients who are pre-stage II palliation (pre-superior cavo-pulmonary anastomosis), especially shunt-dependent patients.
    - SV patients with depresssed function and/or significant atrioventricular valve regurgitation.
    - Patients undergoing extensive surgical procedures.
    - Patients on preoperative inotropes, angiotensin-converting enzyme inhibitors, or digoxin.
- Highest risk for mortality after cardiac arrest (POCA registry)
    - Cardiomyopathy (50%).
    - Aortic stenosis (62%).
    - Pre-superior cavo-pulmonary anastomosis (35%).
- Minimizing risk
    - Recognizing patients at increased risk.
    - Appropriate preoperative multidisciplinary discussion and planning.
    - Discussion with family and informed consent should include increased anesthetic risk.
    - Extensive preoperative planning is critical.

Handbook of Critical Incidents and Essential Topics in Pediatric Anesthesiology, ed. David A. Young and Olutoyin A. Olutoye. Published by Cambridge University Press. © Cambridge University Press 2015.

Preoperative planning

- Selection of setting (e.g., outpatient surgery center vs. tertiary care center) based on patient's disease; availability of consult services including intensive care and cardiology; ability to analyze arterial blood gases; blood bank/blood transfusion availability.
- Avoid hypovolemia by minimizing pre-surgery fasting duration period (should be first case of the day) and/or starting intravenous fluid preoperatively.
- Appropriate monitoring for patient disease and planned operative procedure.
- Ensure availability of emergency drugs, defibrillator, inhaled nitric oxide.
- Anticipate need for postoperative intensive care and mechanical ventilation.
- Anesthesia provider with experience caring for patients with congenital heart disease should be assigned to the case.
- Blood should be available; hematocrit should be optimized for patient's condition (e.g., a hematocrit of approximately 45% is recommended for cyanotic patients).
- Inotropes and vasoactive infusions should be prepared in advance of procedure.
- The appropriateness and availability of extracorporeal membrane oxygenation (ECMO) and candidacy for cardiac transplantation should be discussed in advance of procedure.

Stages of single ventricle palliation and non-cardiac surgery

- Preoperative single ventricle with ductal-dependent pulmonary or systemic blood flow
    - Delicate balance between pulmonary and systemic blood flow exists.
    - Manage balance by predominantly manipulating pulmonary vascular resistance (PVR).
    - At substantial risk for decreasing systemic blood flow resulting in coronary, cerebral, mesenteric and renal hypoperfusion.
- Shunted single ventricle
    - Delicate balance between pulmonary and systemic blood flow exists.
    - Important to maintain PVR to avoid excessive runoff into the pulmonary circulation leading to systemic hypoperfusion and myocardial ischemia.
    - Avoid hyperoxygenation and hyperventilation.
    - Aim for SpO_2 80–90%.
- Single ventricle with pulmonary artery band
    - Maintain ventricular function.
    - Adjust ventilation and oxygenation to maintain SpO_2 80–90%.
- Single ventricle s/p superior cavo-pulmonary anastomosis (Glenn)
    - Recognize that pulmonary blood flow is dependent on cerebral blood flow, especially in infants.
    - Avoid hyperventilation, as it decreases cerebral blood flow and thus pulmonary blood flow.
    - Aim for SpO_2 80–90%.

- Considered the most stable stage of single ventricle palliation for non-cardiac surgery (HIGHLY CONSIDER SCHEDULING ELECTIVE PROCEDURES DURING THIS PHASE).
- Single ventricle s/p total cavo-pulmonary anastomosis (Fontan)
  - In the absence of a fenestration, patients should have a baseline oxygen saturation > 95%.
  - Pulmonary blood flow is passive.
  - Minimize positive pressure ventilation (PPV); PPV decreases venous return, pulmonary blood flow, and cardiac output.
  - Maintain volume status, sinus rhythm, and ventricular function.
  - Be prepared to administer volume and vasoconstrictors that increase systemic vascular resistance (phenylephrine or vasopressin).
  - Special care should be taken with Fontan patients that have poor ventricular function, significant atrioventricular valve regurgitation, or high PVR.

Endocarditis prophylaxis

- The most recent 2007 American Heart Association Infectious Endocarditis (IE) Guidelines limit the cardiac conditions requiring prophylaxis and the procedures for which IE prophylaxis is recommended.
- IE prophylaxis for dental procedures is recommended with the following coexisting conditions:
  - Prosthetic cardiac valve or prosthetic material used for valve repair.
  - Previous infectious endocarditis.
  - Unrepaired cyanotic congenital heart disease, including shunts and conduits.
  - Completely repaired CHD (via surgery or catheter) with prosthetic material or device during the first 6 months after repair.
  - Repaired CHD with a residual defect at the site or adjacent to the site of prosthetic patch or device.
  - Heart transplant patients who develop a cardiac valvulopathy in the transplanted organ.
- IE prophylaxis with gastrointestinal or genitourinary procedures is no longer recommended; this includes esophagogastroduodenoscopy and colonoscopy.
- IE prophylaxis is recommended for patients undergoing invasive respiratory tract surgery such as tonsillectomy and adenoidectomy, but it is not recommended for bronchoscopy unless an incision is involved.
- IE prophylaxis with dental procedures in pediatric patients:
  - Amoxicillin 50 mg/kg PO; or ampicillin, cefazolin, or ceftriaxone 50 mg/kg IM or IV.
  - For penicillin- or ampicillin-allergic patients taking oral medication, cephalexin 50 mg/kg, clindamycin 20 mg/kg, or azithromycin/clarithromycin 15 mg/kg PO.
  - For penicillin- or ampicillin-allergic patients not taking oral medication, cefazolin or ceftriaxone 50 mg/kg or clindamycin 20 mg/kg IM or IV.

Further reading

Gottlieb EA, Andropoulos DB: Anesthesia for the patient with congenital heart disease presenting for noncardiac surgery. *Curr Opin Anaesthesiol.* 2013; 26(3):318–26.

Ramamoorthy C, Haberkern CM, Bhananker SM, et al. Anesthesia-related cardiac arrest in children with heart disease: data from the Pediatric Perioperative Cardiac Arrest (POCA) registry. *Anesth Analg.* 2010; 110:1376–82.

Watkins SC, McNew BS, Donahue BS. Risks of noncardiac operations and other procedures in children with complex congenital heart disease. *Ann Thorac Surg.* 2013; 95:204–11.

Wilson W, Taubert KA, Gewitz M, et al. Prevention of infective endocarditis: a guideline from the American Heart Association Rheumatic Fever, Endocarditis, and Kawasaki Disease Committee, Council on Cardiovascular Disease in the Young, and the Council on Clinical Cardiology, Council on Cardiovascular Surgery and Anesthesia, and the Quality of Care and Outcomes Research Interdisciplinary Working Group, *Circulation.* 2007; 116:1736–54.

Part C Clinical-based areas in pediatric anesthesiology

Chapter 135
Cardiac surgery
Pacemaker/ICD management
Erin A. Gottlieb

Indications for pacemaker placement in pediatric patients
- Symptomatic sinus bradycardia.
- Recurrent bradycardia-tachycardia syndromes.
- Congenital complete atrioventricular (AV) block.
- Advanced second- or third-degree AV block.

Indications for implantable cardioverter defibrillator (ICD) placement in pediatric patients
- Arrhythmogenic right ventricular cardiomyopathy.
- Long QT syndrome.
- Brugada syndrome.
- Hypertrophic cardiomyopathy.
- History of near sudden death events.

Pacemaker codes
See Table 135.1 and Table 135.2.

Table 135.1 NASPE (North American Society of Pacing and Electrophysiology)/BPEG (British Pacing and Electrophysiology group) generic pacemaker code.

Position	I	II	III	IV	V
Category	Chamber(s) Paced	Chamber(s) Sensed	Response to Sensing	Rate Modulation	Multisite Pacing
	O = None A = Atrium V = Ventricle D = Dual (A+V)	O = None A = Atrium V = Ventricle D = Dual (A+V)	I = Inhibited T = Triggered D = Dual (I+T) Response restricted to dual-chamber devices	O = None R = Rate Modulating	O = None A = Atrium V = Ventricle D = Dual (A+V)

Modified from Bernstein AD, Daubert JC, Fletcher RD, et al. The revised NASPE/BPEG generic code for antibradycardia, adaptive-rate, and multi-site pacing. *Pacing Clin Electrophysiol* 2002; 25:260–264.

Handbook of Critical Incidents and Essential Topics in Pediatric Anesthesiology, ed. David A. Young and Olutoyin A. Olutoye. Published by Cambridge University Press. © Cambridge University Press 2015.

Table 135.2 Most common pacing modes.

Single-Chamber Pacing
- AAI: Atrial pacing and sensing, inhibited on sensed beat
- VVI: Ventricular pacing and sensing, inhibited on sensed beat

Asynchronous Pacing
- AOO: fixed rate atrial pacing, no sensing
- VOO: fixed rate ventricular pacing, no sensing
- DOO: fixed rate AV pacing, no sensing

Dual-Chamber Pacing
- DDD: paces and senses both chambers

Modified from Table 14-5 in Gertler R, Miller-Hance WC. Essentials of cardiology. In A Practice of Anesthesia for Infants and Children, 5th edition. Edited by CJ Coté, J Lerman and BJ Anderson. Philadephia: Elsevier, 2013.

Preoperative management

- Critical information to obtain includes type of device, generator location, indication for device placement, coexisting cardiac disease, and verification of adequate remaining battery life.
- Determine underlying rhythm, settings, and whether patient is pacemaker dependent.
- Have cardiovascular implantable electronic device (CIED) programmer interrogate and reprogram to an asynchronous mode with a rate greater than patient's intrinsic rate if electromagnetic interference (EMI) is likely; see below.
- Turn off anti-tachycardia function if EMI is likely.

Intraoperative management

- PATIENT MUST BE MONITORED FOR A PERFUSING RHYTHM WITH AN ARTERIAL OR PLETHYSMOGRAPHIC WAVEFORM (PULSE OXIMETRY).
- Monitor EKG and pacemaker activity.
- Temporary pacing/defibrillation equipment must be present; ensure appropriately sized equipment for patient.
- Device capture may change with metabolic derangements including acidosis, alkalosis, and some electrolyte abnormalities; consider treatment and/or temporary pacing.
- It is possible that the device output may need to be changed intraoperatively to optimize hemodynamics.

Postoperative management

- Device must be interrogated and reprogrammed after procedure.
- DO NOT DISCONTINUE WAVEFORM MONITORING UNTIL DEVICE HAS BEEN INTERROGATED AND REPROGRAMMED, AND ANTI-TACHYCARDIA FUNCTION IS REENABLED.

Magnet use

- A magnet (typically 90 gauss) should be readily available.
- Magnet application can have unpredictable consequences including pacing at a rate that does not meet the patient's cardiovascular demands.
- Magnet application is not a substitute for preoperative interrogation and reprogramming.
- Information on magnet mode and the expected magnet response should be determined.
- For pacemakers, magnet application *usually* results in a change to an asynchronous mode (AOO, VOO, DOO) at a fixed rate.
- For ICDs, magnet application usually results in deactivation of the antitachycardia function; it DOES NOT change a coexisting pacemaker to asynchronous mode.
- If a magnet is used to disable the anti-tachycardia function or change the pacemaker mode to asynchronous mode, the patient should still be monitored for a perfusing rhythm.
- If the patient develops ventricular fibrillation or ventricular tachycardia while the magnet is being applied, the magnet should be quickly removed, and the tachyarrhythmia can be treated by the ICD.
- After the procedure, the device must be interrogated and reprogrammed.

Electromagnetic interference

- EMI is caused by radiofrequency waves in the 50–60 Hz range.
- EMI can be generated by electrocautery, transthoracic defibrillation, therapeutic radiation, radiofrequency ablation, and multiple other therapeutic and diagnostic modalities.
- MONOPOLAR ELECTROCAUTERY IS THE MOST COMMON SOURCE OF EMI IN THE OPERATING ROOM.
- EMI can cause inappropriate triggering or inhibition of pacing, reversion to asynchronous mode, inappropriate shock/antitachycardia therapy, and induction of current in leads, resulting in damage to myocardium.
- OVERSENSING IS THE ADVERSE INTERACTION MOST LIKELY TO OCCUR WHEN A CIED IS EXPOSED TO EMI.
- EMI can be reduced by using bipolar instead of monopolar diathermy, the use of short bursts of cutting instead of coagulation current when monopolar is required, and carefully placing the grounding pad far from the site of the CIED.

Further reading

Bernstein AD, Daubert JC, Fletcher RD, et al. The revised NASPE/BPEG generic code for antibradycardia, adaptive-rate, and multi-site pacing. *Pacing Clin Electrophysiol.* 2002; 25:260–4.

Crossley GH, Poole JE, Rozner MA, et al. The Heart Rhythm Society (HRS)/ American Society of Anesthesiologists (ASA) Expert Consensus Statement on the perioperative management of patients with implantable defibrillators, pacemakers and arrhythmia monitors: facilities and patient management. *Heart Rhythm* 2011; 8:114–54.

Gertler R, Miller-Hance WC. Essentials of Cardiology. In *A Practice of Anesthesia for Infants and Children*, 5th edition. CJ Coté, J Lerman, BJ Anderson, eds. Philadelphia, PA: Elsevier, 2013.

Kim JJ, Collins KK, Miller-Hance WC. Arrhythmias: diagnosis and management. In *Anesthesia for Congenital Heart Disease 2010*, 2nd Edition. DB Andropoulos, SA Stayer, IA Russell and EB Mossad, eds. West Sussex, UK: Wiley-Blackwell, 2010.

Navaratnam M, Dubin A. Pediatric pacemakers and ICDs: how to optimize perioperative care. *Pediatric Anesthesia* 2011; 21: 512–521.

Clinical-based areas in pediatric anesthesiology

Cardiac surgery
Cardiac bypass

Premal M. Trivedi and Pablo Motta

Basic circuit set-up

- Pumps provide non-pulsatile flow by two different mechanisms:
    - Non-occlusive roller pump.
    - Centrifugal pump.
- Cannula and tubing: selection is based on body surface area.
- **Membrane oxygenator:** allows oxygen delivery and removal of carbon dioxide (CO_2) across a thin membrane without direct blood gas contact. The membrane contains thousands of bundled microporous hollow fibers (diameters 200–300 μm).
- Heat exchanger: The countercurrent flow of water against the patient's blood is responsible for the cooling and rewarming process during cardiac bypass (CPB). The temperature gradient between the blood and the water is kept under 10°C to avoid changes in gas solubility. The heater temperature is always below 40°C to avoid damaging the blood and causing hyperthermia.
- Arterial filter: removes blood contaminants (e.g., bone, fat, etc.), thus reducing macro/micro-emboli.
- Blood hemoconcentrator: removes excess fluid resulting in an increased hematocrit.
- Monitors
    - Oxygen saturation.
    - Hematocrit.
    - Temperature.
    - Reservoir low volume.
    - Arterial line pressure.
- Priming solution: should be physiologic including crystalloids, packed red blood cells (patients < 18 kg), colloid (e.g., albumin) and/or fresh frozen plasma. Other supplements to the prime are heparin, buffer solution (e.g., sodium bicarbonate), mannitol, and steroids. The levels of electrolytes, calcium, glucose, and lactate should be checked and adjusted to as near normal as possible.
- Miniature CPB circuit: reduces priming volumes (~110 mL) and patient hemodilution, thereby decreasing need to transfuse.

Handbook of Critical Incidents and Essential Topics in Pediatric Anesthesiology, ed. David A. Young and Olutoyin A. Olutoye. Published by Cambridge University Press. © Cambridge University Press 2015.

Patient preparation

- Cannulation
  - Arterial: placed first, most commonly in the ascending aorta, allowing for quick transfusion during venous cannulation. Other sites for arterial cannulation include grafts to the innominate artery that can also be used for selective antegrade cerebral perfusion (SACP).
  - Venous: direct cannulation of the superior vena cava and inferior vena cava is necessary for intracardiac repairs. Single venous cannulation of the right atrial appendage is used for procedures that do not require opening of the right-sided chambers.
- Antifibrinolytics: ε-aminocaproic acid (EACA) and tranexamic acid (TA) are lysine analogs that exert their antifibrinolytic effects by affecting the binding of plasminogen to fibrin. Their administration has been associated with decreased perioperative bleeding.
- Heparinization
  - Target activated clotting time (ACT) is 480 seconds.
  - The infant and pediatric doses to achieve this ACT value are 400 U/kg and 300 U/kg, respectively.

Management of cardiac bypass

- Cardiac bypass (CPB) is initiated by starting the arterial pump slowly and, once forward flow is confirmed, the heart is allowed to drain by gravity to the venous reservoir.
- Venous drainage can be enhanced by increasing the height difference between the reservoir and the patient; increasing the size of the venous cannulas and/or the use of a vacuum.
- The pump flow (Q) is maintained by this formula:

  Q = Wt (kg) × 150 mL/kg/min in patients < 10 kg
  Q = BSA (body surface area) × cardiac index (age dependent) in patients > 10 kg

- The cardiac index decreases with age from 3.0–3.2 mL/min/m^2 for children under 2 years to 2.4 mL/min/m^2 for patients over 10 years.
- Vasodilators can be used to maximize CPB flow in blood prime cases.
- The aorta is cross-clamped once mild hypothermia (~34°C) is achieved and the heart is arrested using cardioplegia.
- The blood gas management is pH stat in cases involving hypothermic CPB. Here, CO_2 is introduced to the oxygenator in order to maintain the pH and arterial partial pressure of carbon dioxide (pCO_2). This method improves tissue oxygenation and cerebral blood flow while cooling.
- The degree of hypothermia instituted depends on the patient's size and type of surgical repair:

- Mild (> 32°C): short CPB cases (< 60 min) without aortic cross-clamping (e.g., bidirectional Glenn shunt placement).
- Moderate (25–32°C): moderate CPB duration (< 120 min) with aortic cross-clamping (e.g., ventricular septal defect repair).
- Deep (< 20°C): long CPB duration (> 120 min) with aortic cross-clamping and extensive aortic reconstruction (e.g., Norwood procedure).

- Deep hypothermic circulatory arrest (DHCA) and SACP is used for brain protection.
- Low flow bypass (LFB): is considered when the CPB flows are under 50 mL/kg/min and is preferred to DHCA due to better neurodevelopmental outcomes.
- Hematocrit: higher hematocrit (~30%) on CPB is associated with better neurodevelopmental outcomes in infants undergoing complex surgeries (e.g., Norwood).
- Neuromonitors: are used during the periods of DHCA, LFB, and SACP. Transcranial Doppler (TCD) and near-infrared spectroscopy (NIRS) allow early detection of cerebral desaturation.
- Steroids downregulate proinflammatory mediators and upregulate anti-inflammatory cytokines but their impact on outcome is still controversial.
- Glucose levels are followed closely on CPB. Hyperglycemia is common but transient and rarely requires treatment.

Weaning off cardiac bypass

- Ultrafiltration: conventional or modified ultrafiltration is used during the rewarming phase of bypass. The goal is to remove excess fluid and decrease inflammatory mediators.
- Rewarming is achieved by progressively increasing CPB temperature to normal (nasopharyngeal temperature 36.5°C or rectal temperature 35.5°C).
- Transesophageal echocardiography (TEE) is used to certify that all air has been removed from the heart chambers.
- Trendelenburg position is used to minimize risk of central nervous system emboli of undetected air.
- The aortic cross-clamp is released and the heart spontaneously restores its sinus rhythm.
- Ventricular fibrillation is treated with lidocaine 1 mg/kg IV and internal defibrillation.
- Ventilation is resumed after suctioning.
- Once acid–base and electrolytes are normalized and a desirable hematocrit is achieved, CPB is gradually weaned off by stopping the venous drainage and allowing the heart to fill and start beating.
- TEE is used to confirm the adequacy of the repair and ventricular function.
- Reversal of heparinization is accomplished with protamine sulfate in a protamine–heparin ratio of 1:1.2 and then cannulas are removed.

Complications

- Equipment failure
    - Pump malfunction.
    - Line disconnection.
    - Negative pressure complication causing air emboli.
    - Electrical failure.
- Surgical cannulation problems
    - Aortic dissection.
    - Preferential perfusion detected by uneven NIRS reading.
    - Superior and/or inferior vena cava obstruction.
    - Massive blood loss.
    - Atrial arrhythmias.
- Long-term complications
    - Poor neurodevelopmental outcomes due to end-organ damage during low flow CPB or DHCA.

Further reading

Andropoulos DB. *Anesthesia for Congenital Heart Disease*, 2nd edition. Chichester: Wiley-Blackwell, 2010; 96–103.

Bissonnette, B. *Pediatric Anesthesia. Basic Principles – State of the Art – Future*. Shelton, CT: People's Medical Publishing House, 2011; 94–5.

Coté CJ, Lerman J, Anderson BJ. *Coté and Lerman's A Practice of Anesthesia for Infants and Children*, 5th edition. Philadelphia, PA: Elsevier, 2013; 393–5.

Gregory GA, Andropoulos DB. *Gregory's Pediatric Anesthesia*, 5th edition. Hoboken: Wiley-Blackwell, 2012; 610–14.

Part C Clinical-based areas in pediatric anesthesiology

Chapter 137

Cardiac surgery
Cardiac transplantation
Primal M. Trivedi and Pablo Motta

Indications
- Unacceptable quality of life in the setting of irreversible heart disease.
- Patients in whom survival beyond 1–2 years without transplantation is unlikely.

Common diagnoses in pediatric heart transplant recipients
- Congenital heart disease
    - Most common cause in infants.
- Cardiomyopathy
    - Most common in older children and adolescents; different types:
        - Dilated.
        - Hypertrophic.
        - Restrictive.
        - Arrhythmogenic.
        - Non-compaction.
- Viral myocarditis.
- Malignancy.
- Coronary disease
    - Anomalous left coronary artery arising from the pulmonary artery.
    - Kawasaki disease.
    - Coronary disease associated with a transplanted heart.

Potential contraindications to transplantation
- Recipient pulmonary hypertension (pHTN)
    - If significant, can induce failure of the newly transplanted heart.
    - Assessment is made whether the pHTN is reactive or fixed.
    - If fixed, the patient may be a candidate for heart–lung transplantation, lung transplantation, or heterotopic heart transplantation.

Handbook of Critical Incidents and Essential Topics in Pediatric Anesthesiology, ed. David A. Young and Olutoyin A. Olutoye. Published by Cambridge University Press. © Cambridge University Press 2015.

- Pulmonary vascular resistance (PVR) > 6–10 Wood units or a fixed transpulmonary gradient > 15 mmHg are concerning for poor outcome following cardiac transplantation.
- Multiple congenital anomalies.
- Marked prematurity.
- Low birth weight.
- Active infection, malignancy, or metabolic disease.

Recipient evaluation

- Liver and kidney function tests.
- Prothrombin time/international normalized ratio (INR)/partial thromboplastin time.
- Complete blood count and differential.
- Serologies for
    - HIV.
    - Hepatitis.
    - Cytomegalovirus.
    - Epstein–Barr virus.
    - *Toxoplasma gondii*.
    - Syphilis.
- Immunization status and purified protein derivative (PPD) skin test.
- Cardiomyopathy workup
    - Thyroid function tests.
    - Blood lactate, pyruvate, ammonia, acylcarnitine.
    - Urine organic acids.
    - Skeletal muscle biopsy.
    - Karyotype.
- Cardiopulmonary workup
    - Cardiac catheterization.
    - Echocardiogram.
    - Radionuclide angiography.
    - Endomyocardial biopsy.
    - Electrocardiogram.
    - Chest radiograph.
    - Pulmonary function tests.
    - Maximal oxygen consumption (VO_{2max}).
- Psychosocial evaluation.
- Panel reactive antibody (PRA) level
    - Measures antibodies to random human leukocyte antigens that may be present in the recipient's blood.
    - The greater the number of antibodies, the greater the risk for graft dysfunction and rejection, both acute and chronic.

- High PRA levels correlate positively with history of blood transfusions, mechanical circulatory support, and use of homografts in prior surgeries.
    - Blood products for potential transplant recipients should therefore be leuko-reduced and irradiated.

Listing status

- Mean time from listing to transplant ~3 months
    - Ranking is dependent on
        - Severity of heart failure.
        - Time on the list.
        - ABO blood type.
        - Size of patient.
        - Geographic proximity to the donor.
- Status 1
    - Patients who are most ill.
    - Further divided into
        - Status 1A: highest priority, life expectancy < 1 month, on mechanical ventilation, high dose inotropes, and/or mechanical circulatory support.
        - Status 1B: on low-dose inotropes.
- Status 2
    - Stable at home but in need of transplantation.
- Status 7
    - Temporarily unsuitable to receive transplantation
        - Infection.

Pre-transplant evaluation

- Patients' level of support at the time of transplantation can vary markedly.
    - Natural airway on minimal or no hemodynamic support.
    - Mechanical ventilation with inotropic support.
    - Extracorporeal membrane oxygenation (ECMO).
        - Antithrombin III levels may be deficient in patients on chronic heparin therapy.
        - More commonly used in infants.
    - Ventricular assist device (VAD)
        - Exposure to aspirin or coumadin.
    - ~25% of transplant patients are bridged to transplant with mechanical support.
- Evaluation of end-organ function.
- History of prior sternotomies.
    - Increased risk of arrhythmias with repeat sternotomies

- Ensure availability of defibrillator pads.
  - Increased risk of bleeding
    - Ensure blood is readily available and checked.
- Review venous lines and any history of venous occlusion.

Anesthetic management

- Induction
  - The end-stage heart is extremely sensitive to changes in preload, afterload, heart rate, contractility, and PVR.
  - Goals for induction are to minimize changes to these variables and optimize oxygenation and ventilation.
  - Pre-induction invasive hemodynamic monitoring may be indicated if feasible.
  - Patients on VAD support have a more stable physiology and generally tolerate induction well.
- Maintenance: Balanced technique using opioids, benzodiazepines, low dose inhalation agents, and neuromuscular blocking agents.
- Weaning off cardiopulmonary bypass
  - Right ventricular failure is common and therapy should be tailored to manage this:
    - Control of PVR with optimal oxygenation and ventilation.
    - Inotropic support with milrinone, epinephrine, and/or isoproterenol.
    - Ensure availability of nitric oxide.

Anesthetic considerations following transplantation

- Denervation of the donor heart
  - Baroreceptor reflex is disrupted such that heart rate (HR) and contractility do not increase acutely in response to hypovolemia or change in position.
  - Minimal effect of anticholinergic agents on HR.
- Ischemia-reperfusion injury
  - May manifest as left ventricular diastolic dysfunction.
    - Inotropy may be required.
  - Sinoatrial node dysfunction and arrhythmias are common.
    - Isoproterenol or epinephrine can maintain HR perioperatively.
- Hyperacute rejection
  - Due to preexisting antibodies to donor antigens.
- Blood product administration
  - Potentially long cardiopulmonary bypass period with preexisting platelet dysfunction or coagulation abnormalities may predispose to significant bleeding.
  - Platelets, cryoprecipitate, and fresh frozen plasma should be available.

Late anesthetic considerations
- Graft function
    - A concern at all times following transplantation.
- Coronary artery vasculopathy
    - Prevalence increases with time.
- At > 3 years from transplantation, graft failure and coronary vasculopathy account for > 50% of deaths.
- Post-transplant comorbidities at 5 years
    - Hypertension (61%).
    - Hyperlipidemia (21%).
    - Renal dysfunction (9%).
    - Diabetes mellitus (5%).
    - Lymphoma.
    - Cerebrovascular accident.

Further reading
Andropoulos DB. *Anesthesia for Congenital Heart Disease*, 2nd edition. Hoboken: Wiley-Blackwell, 2010; 493–500.

Coté CJ, Lerman J, Anderson BJ. *Coté and Lerman's A Practice of Anesthesia for Infants and Children*, 5th edition. Philadelphia, PA: Elsevier, 2013; 612–18.

Kirk R, Dipchand AI, Edwards LB. The Registry of the International Society for Heart and Lung Transplantation: Fifteenth Pediatric Heart Transplantation Report – 2012. *J Heart Lung Transplant*. 2012; 31(10):1065–72.

Part C Clinical-based areas in pediatric anesthesiology

Fetal surgery
General considerations
Kha M. Tran

Indications
- Fetus must be at risk of death or severe morbidity from a process that can be diagnosed and treated *in utero*.
- Hydrops fetalis (accumulation of fluid in one or more fetal body cavities) is a common end point demonstrating severity of disease in the fetus.

Specific fetal conditions requiring intervention or surgery
- Complicated twin or multiple gestations
    - Twin-twin transfusion syndrome: unbalanced flow between twins sharing vascular connections in the placenta with blood transfusion occurring from one twin (donor) to the other (recipient).
    - Donor twin becomes hypovolemic and oliguric while the recipient twin suffers from fluid overload; both twins are at increased risk of morbidity and mortality.
        - Preterm delivery.
        - Heart failure.
        - Neurologic morbidity.
- Twin-reversed arterial perfusion sequence (TRAP) sequence: unbalanced flow between a normal-appearing twin and an acardiac or anencephalic twin.
- Neurologic disease: myelomeningocele – not immediately life-threatening, associated with increased morbidity (impaired ambulation, hydrocephalus) later in life.
- Airway lesions: typically do not require mid-gestation intervention and are addressed near term or at delivery (see Chapter 139, Fetal surgery: EXIT procedure).
    - Extrinsic obstruction by neck masses (e.g., cystic hygromas or cervical teratoma).
    - Intrinsic obstruction (e.g., congenital high airway obstruction syndrome (CHAOS) secondary to internal cysts, webs, or atresia.
    - While the placenta is the organ of respiration, a completely obstructed airway will not allow egress of lung fluid and may cause massive overdistension of the lungs in utero. This eventually compresses the heart, resulting in hydrops fetalis and intrauterine death.

Handbook of Critical Incidents and Essential Topics in Pediatric Anesthesiology, ed. David A. Young and Olutoyin A. Olutoye. Published by Cambridge University Press. © Cambridge University Press 2015.

138: Fetal surgery: general considerations

- Lung lesions
    - Congenital cystic adenomatoid malformation (CCAM) and bronchopulmonary sequestration (BPS): large lung lesions which compress the heart and adjacent normal lung tissue.
    - Congenital diaphragmatic hernia (CDH): herniation of abdominal contents into thorax and compression of the lung on the ipsilateral side resulting in hypoplastic lung development.
- Cardiac lesions: hypoplastic left heart syndrome (HLHS) with intact atrial septum.
- Obstructive uropathy.
- Miscellaneous processes
    - Sacrococcygeal teratoma.
    - Cardiac teratoma.

Types of mid-gestation procedure

- Minimally invasive procedure
    - The uterus is accessed percutaneously with small fetoscopes and laser ablation of abnormal placental vessels is performed.
    - Intrauterine transfusion is performed through the umbilical vessels or into the fetal abdomen.
- Open procedure
    - Involves the following steps: laparotomy, hysterotomy, exposure of fetus, surgery on fetus, uterine closure, and abdominal closure.

Anesthetic considerations

Maternal physiology

- Increased aspiration risk: Consider preoperative ranitidine, metoclopramide, and sodium bicitrate.
- Prone to aortocaval compression leading to supine hypotension: Supine positioning with left uterine tilt is recommended.
- Airway mucosal swelling may result in challenging intubation.
- Other physiologic effects of pregnancy include:
    - Dilutional anemia.
    - Hypercoagulability.
    - Increased blood flow to uterus.
    - Decreased functional residual capacity.
    - Compensated respiratory alkalosis.
    - Increased glomerular filtration rate.

Fetal physiology

- Placenta is organ of respiration.
- Maintenance of uterine blood flow is crucial to fetal well-being.
- Fetal blood volume: 90–100 mL/kg estimated fetal weight (EFW) depending on gestational age.
- Normal fetal heart rate: 120–150 bpm.
- Normal fetal oxygen saturation is 50–70%.
- Coagulation factors are immature.
- Glucose is derived from mother's circulation.
- Drug metabolism is either immature or dependent on mother's metabolism.
- Thermoregulation depends on mother.
- Disease process: Untreated fetal pathology commonly results in hydrops fetalis or fetal cardiac failure.

Anesthetic management

- Minimally invasive procedures
    - Type of anesthesia depends on requirements for procedure and local practice patterns.
- Sedation. Options include:
    - Low dose propofol or remifentanil infusions, or dexmedetomidine infusion +/− intermittent doses of midazolam.
- Depending on the procedure, the fetus may require analgesia and immobilization (administration of IM fetal atropine 20 μg/kg, fentanyl 5–10 μg/kg, and vecuronium 0.2–0.4 mg/kg).
- Neuraxial
    - Level of block dependent on the location of access to the uterine cavity.
- General anesthesia with intubation
    - May be indicated in presence of an anterior placenta which requires a laparascopy-assisted procedure.

Open fetal surgery

- General anesthesia is routinely employed except when contraindications exist.
- Epidural catheter is placed preoperatively for use towards the end of the procedure.
- Large bore intravenous access.
- Rapid sequence induction.
- Uterine relaxation achieved with volatile anesthetics (2–3 times minimal anesthetic concentration) or nitroglycerin (uterine effect not easily titratable).
- Hypotension may occur, requiring vasopressors.
- Pulmonary edema may occur as patients are placed on magnesium tocolysis at end of the procedure.
- Administration of epidural local anesthetic and opioid begins as uterus is being closed; volatile anesthetic concentration is also decreased at this time to facilitate emergence.

- Magnesium tocolysis is started at this point as well: 4–6 g IV bolus and 2 g/hr infusion.
- Supplemental intravenous anesthesia technique: has been described to limit fetal exposure to high-dose volatile anesthetics and decrease risk of myocardial depression:
  - Propofol and remifentanil infusions are started after induction and high-dose volatile agents are only initiated just before uterine incision is made.
- Neuraxial anesthesia as sole anesthetic: has been described for EXIT procedures, with nitroglycerin used for uterine relaxation.

Fetal resuscitation

- Depending on nature of surgery, fetal monitoring is typically via ultrasound.
- Management of fetal compromise
  - Rule out maternal hemorrhage, placental abruption, hypotension, hypoxemia, and confirm left uterine displacement.
  - Rule out umbilical cord compression or hemorrhage.
  - Confirm adequate amniotic fluid volume is present.
- Medications/fluids may be administered to both fetus and mother as required:
  - Epinephrine.
  - Atropine.
  - Calcium.
  - Lactated Ringer's fluid bolus.
  - Packed red blood cells (fetus – type O negative blood; this should be cross matched against the mother's blood sample in case her anitbodies have crossed the placenta; mother – type-specific blood).
- Fetal chest compressions may be required.

Further reading

Boat A. Supplementing desflurane with intravenous anesthesia reduces fetal cardiac dysfunction during open fetal surgery. *Paediatr Anaesth.* 2010; 20(8):748–56.

Davis PJ. *Smith's Anesthesia for Infants and Children*, 8th edition. Philadelphia: Elsevier, 2011; 583–604.

Lin EE, Tran KM. Anesthesia for fetal surgery. *Semin Pediatr Surg.* 2013; 22(1):50–5.

Part C Clinical-based areas in pediatric anesthesiology

Chapter 139

Fetal surgery
EXIT procedure
Kha M. Tran

- EXIT (*ex utero* intrapartum therapy) procedure involves institution of fetal therapy at delivery while the fetus is on uteroplacental bypass.
- It allows time to facilitate the fetus's chance of extrauterine survival following therapy performed under controlled conditions.
- A multidisciplinary team approach is routinely employed. Practitioners involved may vary depending on the institution but include: obstetricians, pediatric surgeons, cardiologists, anesthesiologists, neonatologists and ear, nose & throat specialists.
- Basic premise of an EXIT is different than that of mid-gestational fetal procedures.
    - The goal of a fetal procedure is to palliate or cure a fetal disease process and let the fetus continue to grow and develop to term.
    - The EXIT procedure is performed on fetuses near term with a disease process that will not allow successful transition to extrauterine life.

Indications

- Fetal conditions that pose an immediate threat to survival at delivery.
- Indications determine type of EXIT procedure performed.
    - Airway obstruction: most common indication for EXIT-to-airway procedure.
        - Extrinsic: oral teratoma, cervical hygroma, or cervical teratoma – mass obstructing the airway, precluding spontaneous respiration following delivery.
        - Intrinsic: congenital high airway obstruction syndrome (CHAOS) due to laryngeal cysts, webs or atresia.
    - Large fetal lung mass, e.g., congenital cystic adenomatoid malformation (CCAM) or bronchopulmonary sequestration (BPS), particularly masses associated with *in utero* mediastinal shift or signs of fetal cardiac failure (hydrops fetalis).
        - These masses may compress the contralateral lung and have the propensity to cause cardiovascular collapse upon institution of positive pressure ventilation after delivery.
    - Large sacrococcygeal teratomas causing high output cardiac failure.
        - For both large lung masses and sacrococcygeal teratomas, the mass is resected or exteriorized at delivery while the fetus is on uteroplacental support in the EXIT-to-resection procedure.

Handbook of Critical Incidents and Essential Topics in Pediatric Anesthesiology, ed. David A. Young and Olutoyin A. Olutoye. Published by Cambridge University Press. © Cambridge University Press 2015.

○ Very severe congenital diaphragmatic hernias in isolation or associated with congenital heart disease, may be treated with the EXIT to ECMO (Extracorporeal membrane oxygenation) strategy.

Resources required

- Two operating rooms may be required, particularly if the fetus would require additional surgery upon separation from uteroplacental bypass.
- Primary operating room is dedicated to care of the mother and also contains equipment for initial fetus/baby management:
  ○ Separate pulse oximeter for fetus, sterilized neonatal airway equipment, pediatric intravenous fluid, echocardiogram machine to monitor baby intraoperatively.
  ○ Airway instruments for fetus: bronchoscopy, different sized endotracheal tubes, ECMO machine if indicated.
  ○ Blood for transfusion of baby if required: approximately 60 mL of type O negative blood should be readily available.
  ○ Medications for resuscitation of baby should be prepared and drawn up based on baby's weight:
    - Epinephrine: 1 µg/kg and 10 µg/kg.
    - Atropine: 20 µg/kg.
    - Calcium gluconate: 50–100 mg/kg.
    - Lactated Ringer's: 3 syringes of 10 mL each.
- Second operating room
  ○ Prepared for management of baby in case of fetal decompensation during EXIT (refractory bradycardia, abruption or for complete resection of mass or completion of thoracotomy).
  ○ A second team of surgeons, anesthesiologists, nurses, and technicians should be readily available for this room.

Anesthetic considerations

- Maternal: consider preoperative management of pregnant mother for surgery.
  ○ Aspiration precautions.
  ○ Airway mucosal swelling.
- Fetal
  ○ Obtain estimated weight of baby in order to prepare combination medication for baby (fentanyl 5–10 µg/kg, vecuronium 0.2–0.4 mg/kg, and atropine 20 µg/kg).

Anesthetic management

Management of mother

- Epidural may be placed preoperatively to be activated at the end of surgery; alternatively intrathecal morphine 100–150 µg may be administered preoperatively to provide postoperative analgesia.

- Large bore intravenous access.
- Rapid sequence intubation with propofol 2 mg/kg and succinylcholine 1 mg/kg.
- Uterine relaxation is achieved with volatile anesthetics at 2–3 times minimal anesthetic concentration (MAC).
- Regional anesthesia has been performed in some institutions as the sole anesthetic; intravenous nitroglycerin is used for uterine relaxation in this instance.
- Vasopressor therapy with ephedrine or phenylephrine may be required to treat volatile agent induced hypotension.
- Following management of fetus and delivery, uterine relaxation must be rapidly reversed with uterotonic agents: oxytocin 40 units in 1,000 mL of lactated Ringer's solution.
- Other uterotonic agents must be readily available: (e.g., methylergometrine, carboprost tromethamine).

Management of fetus

- Upon delivery of fetal head and upper extremity, a pulse oximeter is applied to the fetal hand (normal oxygen saturations 50–70%).
- Intramuscular injection of a combination of medications is administered to the fetus (fentanyl 5–10 µg/kg, vecuronium 0.2–0.4 mg/kg, and atropine 20 µg/kg).
- Additional fetal monitoring is by the cardiologist on the surgical field who assesses cardiac function and fluid status. Normal fetal heart rate: 120–150 BPM.
- Intravenous access is secured prior to establishing airway, starting thoracotomy or inserting an ECMO cannulae.
- For thoracotomy procedures with lung mass resection, once the airway is secured with an endotracheal tube, positive pressure ventilation should only be instituted after the lung mass has been exteriorized in order to reduce cardiovascular collapse with positive pressure ventilation.
- Umbilical cord clamping occurs once the fetal therapy has been completed (airway has been secured, lung mass exteriorized, insertion of ECMO cannulae has been completed or the sacrococcygeal teratoma has been resected).

Further reading

Coté CJ, Lerman J, Anderson BJ. *Coté and Lerman's A Practice of Anesthesia for Infants and Children*, 5th edition. Philadelphia, PA: Elsevier, 2013; 784–7.

Garcia PJ. Case scenario: anesthesia for maternal-fetal surgery: the Ex Utero Intrapartum Therapy (EXIT) procedure. *Anesthesiology*. 2011; 114(6):1446–52.

Lin EE, Tran KM. Anesthesia for fetal surgery. *Semin Pediatr Surg*. 2013; 22(1):50–5.

Part C Clinical-based areas in pediatric anesthesiology

Chapter 140

General surgery
General considerations
Mary A. Felberg

- General surgical procedures can be varied in the complexity of procedure (abscess drainage, bowel perforation, vascular access) and medical condition of the patient (healthy, critically ill neonate).
- Surgeries of the abdomen in children range from simple outpatient procedures (e.g., umbilical hernia repair) to complex high-risk procedures such as liver transplantation.
- As with any patient, a thorough preoperative evaluation is the foundation for an effective perioperative plan.

Elective vs. emergent

- Elective cases imply time to optimize medical conditions (transfusion of red blood cells) and adhere to fasting guidelines.
- Full stomach precautions should be considered for all cases with increased potential for pulmonary aspiration of gastric contents.
  - A pre-induction gastric tube with suctioning may be indicated (i.e., pyloromyotomy).

Open vs. minimally invasive surgery

- The surgical technique selected impacts the choice of airway management, anticipated fluid requirements, and perioperative analgesia management.
- Laparoscopic procedures often require endotracheal intubation with controlled ventilation, minimal fluid replacement for insensible losses, less intensive perioperative pain management (local anesthetic infiltration of port sites, moderate opioid/non-steroidal anti-inflammatory medications, nerve blocks, e.g., rectus sheath block).
- Open procedures may also necessitate endotracheal intubation, have increased insensible losses, and may require more intensive pain management (e.g., continuous epidural infusion for open fundoplication).

Fluid status

- Many anesthetic management decisions are based on calculations of estimated blood volume.

Handbook of Critical Incidents and Essential Topics in Pediatric Anesthesiology, ed. David A. Young and Olutoyin A. Olutoye. Published by Cambridge University Press. © Cambridge University Press 2015.

- Significant fluid shifts may occur with obstructed or ischemic bowel, especially during open surgical procedures.
- Assess and estimate the volume status by using the following:
  - Physical examination: vital signs, mucous membranes, skin turgor, size of fontanelles, level of consciousness.
  - History: prolonged nausea/vomiting/diarrhea, recently receiving a bowel preparation, and having an extended fasting time.
  - Laboratory data: increased hematocrit, electrolytes such as an increased blood urea nitrogen (BUN).
  - Current intravenous replacement orders, type of solution, and rate.
- Replace deficits with an isotonic balanced salt solution.
- Remember that hypotension is a late finding of hypovolemic shock.
- Adequate vascular access for complex procedures or children with comorbid conditions may include peripheral, arterial, and perhaps central line placement.

Bowel status

- Vasoactive substances released by ischemic or dead bowel may result in hemodynamic instability and the development of metabolic acidosis.
- Assess the need for additional intravenous access and/or arterial line placement.
- Additional fluid requirements should be expected including the possible need for transfusion of blood products.
- Medications to treat hemodynamic instability should be readily available (e.g., epinephrine, vasopressin).

Perioperative analgesia

- Develop a perioperative pain management plan which may include regional anesthesia, non-opioid medications, as well as traditional opioid therapy.

Further reading

Coté CJ, Lerman J, Anderson BJ. *Coté and Lerman's A Practice of Anesthesia for Infants and Children*, 5th edition. Philadelphia, PA: Elsevier, 2013; 583–94.

Gregory GA, Andropoulos DB. *Gregory's Pediatric Anesthesia*, 5th edition. Hoboken: Wiley-Blackwell, 2012; 720–39.

Part C Clinical-based areas in pediatric anesthesiology

Chapter 141 General surgery
Laparoscopy/abdominal procedures
Mary A. Felberg

- Conventional laparoscopic surgery is the most common type of minimally invasive surgery used in the pediatric population; robotic surgery is evolving.
- Laparoscopic procedures are now commonplace for pediatric patients due to the development of pediatric-sized instrumentation and is the preferred approach by many surgeons.
- The variety of abdominal pediatric procedures done with laparoscopy are numerous and include:
  - Diagnostic examination or tissue biopsy.
  - Appendectomy.
  - Pyloromyotomy.
  - Cholecystectomy.
  - Inguinal hernia repair.
  - Nissen fundoplication.
  - Gastrotomy tube placement.
  - Bowel pull-through.
  - Pyeloplasty.
  - Removal of large organs (e.g., kidney or spleen).
- Not all patients are candidates for laparoscopic procedures; conditions which may preclude this technique include:
  - Severe cardiopulmonary disease.
  - Severe prematurity.
  - Severe abdominal distention.
  - A history of multiple abdominal procedures with severe adhesions.

Pneumoperitoneum
- Visualization of the intraabdominal structures is accomplished by creating a pneumoperitoneum using carbon dioxide.
- A pneumoperitoneum has potential for adverse physiologic consequences.
  - Pediatric insufflation pressures are typically 8–12 mmHg.
    - Higher pressures may compress the inferior vena cava, resulting in decreased venous return and hypotension.

Handbook of Critical Incidents and Essential Topics in Pediatric Anesthesiology, ed. David A. Young and Olutoyin A. Olutoye. Published by Cambridge University Press. © Cambridge University Press 2015.

- High pressures may also compromise blood flow to the liver and kidneys with the potential for organ dysfunction.
- Oliguria or anuria may be seen intraoperatively during insufflation; urine output is typically reestablished after discontinuation of the pneumoperitoneum.
- Carbon dioxide (CO_2) is utilized as the insufflating agent due to its non-flammability, rapid elimination from the abdominal cavity, and having a neutral effect on air-filled spaces.
- Adverse effects from CO_2 insufflation include the development of hypercarbia and the potential for intravascular embolization.
  - CO_2 is rapidly absorbed from the abdominal cavity, the absorption rate is higher in infants than adults.
  - An increase in minute ventilation up to 75% may be necessary to offset the CO_2-induced hypercarbia.
  - Hypercarbia may trigger a sympathetic response including increased heart rate and blood pressure, and the development of ventricular dysrhythmias.
  - Intravascular embolization of CO_2 may result in catastrophic cardiovascular collapse.
- Decompression of both the stomach and the bladder may be indicated prior to the start of the procedure.
- Consider antiemetic medications for prophylaxis of postoperative nausea and vomiting.

Respiratory considerations

- Changes in respiratory parameters that result from insufflation include decreased tidal volume and functional residual capacity, lower closing volumes, and increased CO_2.
- Infants have pliable chest walls and are more dependent on diaphragm excursion for ventilation; hypoxia can ensue after insufflation in the head-down position (due to atelectasis development) or with head-up position (due to ventilation/perfusion mismatch).

Positioning

- Positioning may vary by procedure from steep head-down to steep head-up accompanied by lateral rotation; multiple changes in position may also occur during the same procedure.
- Meticulous padding and securing of the patient is highly recommended.

Physiologic considerations

- Placement of vascular access lines in an upper extremity may optimize resuscitation if cross-clamping of the inferior vena cava or aorta becomes necessary due to severe bleeding during trocar placement.
- Consider the administration of additional isotonic crystalloid to restore intravascular volume prior to insufflation.
- Titrate mechanical ventilator settings to compensate for changes in respiratory mechanics due to insufflation.

- Endotracheal intubation utilizing a cuffed tube will help to minimize airway leak and effectively deliver the increased ventilation commonly required.
- Controlled ventilation modes are most frequently utilized during laparoscopic procedures in order to regulate the associated hypercarbia.
- Consider the addition of positive end-expiratory pressure (PEEP) to minimize atelectasis.

- Mainstem bronchial intubation may occur more often in infants and small children. This may also develop when transitioning to abdominal insufflation or from the supine to the head-down position; assess for bilateral breath sounds after any position change

Complications

- Surgical complications occur in 4–5% of procedures. These include:
    - Inadvertent puncture of a vessel or the bladder with introduction of the trocar (the bladder is an intraperitoneal structure in children under 3 years old).
    - Perforation of a hollow viscus (bowel).
    - Embolization of CO_2 and the possible development of cardiovascular depression.
    - Trauma to solid organs (liver).
- Conversion to an open procedure occurs in 5–10% of complications; uncontrolled bleeding is a leading indication.
- Hypothermia due to prolonged insufflation of cool gases.
- Postoperative complications may include right shoulder pain (referred pain due to residual intraperitoneal gas), nausea, and vomiting.

Further reading

Coté CJ, Lerman J, Anderson BJ. *Coté and Lerman's A Practice of Anesthesia for Infants and Children*, 5th edition. Philadelphia, PA: Elsevier, 2013; 583–94.

Gregory GA. *Gregory's Pediatric Anesthesia*, 5th edition. Hoboken: Wiley-Blackwell, 2012; 730–9, 913–16.

Wedgewood J, Doyle E. Review Article: Anesthesia and laparoscopic surgery in children. *Ped Anes*. 2001; 11(4):391–9.

Part C Clinical-based areas in pediatric anesthesiology

Chapter 142

Neonatal surgery
General considerations
Carlos Rodriguez

- Neonates are probably considered the most challenging group of patients to manage in the perioperative period. Neonates have an overall increased anesthesia risk and are commonly scheduled for urgent or emergent procedures. Furthermore, compared to a few decades ago, the survival rate of premature neonates has increased dramatically despite significant morbidity. Neonates have distinct characteristics that impact their anesthetic management.
- Neonates have a relatively large head and tongue in comparison to older children. This places the head in a relatively flexed position that may contribute to airway obstruction and increased difficulty with tracheal intubation. The cricoid ring is the narrowest part of the airway; it is important to place an appropriately sized tracheal tube that will generate an audible leak and reduce the risk for post-extubation stridor. The epiglottis is large and floppy; a straight laryngoscope blade is the optimal blade to utilize since this blade can be used to directly lift the epiglottis and expose the larynx. Subglottic stenosis may develop in patients who have had prolonged periods of tracheal intubation.
- Respiratory distress syndrome is present in many ex-premature babies; this may progress to chronic lung disease (CLD). Patients with CLD tend to have dysplastic pulmonary vasculature, decrease in number of alveoli, and an increase in alveoli size. This leads to overall inefficient lung function and decreased gas transfer. Many of these patients require long-term mechanical ventilation and chronic treatment with diuretics. Oxygen concentration should be carefully titrated due to the concern for oxygen toxicity and retinopathy of prematurity. The lungs of the neonate are particularly sensitive to hyperinflation such as during aggressive manual ventilation. Permissive hypercapnia, rapid respiratory rates, and smaller tidal volumes are all strategies used to reduce pulmonary-associated morbidity. Many patients with CLD may require relatively increased mechanical ventilatory pressures to maintain acceptable oxygenation and ventilation.
- Apnea (apnea of prematurity and postoperative apnea) is common in this age group and the incidence is inversely proportional to the post-conceptual age of the patient. Many factors contribute to apnea in the premature infant but the main cause is an immature central nervous system. Neonates without preexisting apnea are at increased risk of postoperative apnea until approximately 60 weeks post-conceptual age.

Handbook of Critical Incidents and Essential Topics in Pediatric Anesthesiology, ed. David A. Young and Olutoyin A. Olutoye. Published by Cambridge University Press. © Cambridge University Press 2015.

- Cardiac output is heart rate dependent in the neonate. Decreases in heart rate may lead to dramatic reductions in blood pressure. Volume administration should be carefully titrated in neonates to prevent volume overload. Critically ill neonates may have varying degrees of pulmonary hypertension as well as unrepaired congenital heart disease.
- Neonates may have residual neurologic damage from previous events such as anoxic injuries, intraventricular hemorrhage, and seizures. These defects may require surgical management and could lead to future deficits in cognition and development.
- Hypothermia can be detrimental to neonates; it increases oxygen consumption and can lead to hypoxemia, acidosis, and apnea. Concerted efforts should be taken to keep neonates warm throughout the perioperative period.
- Due to reduced immunity, neonates have an increased risk for infection. Sterility should be maintained during all relevant procedures (e.g., regional anesthesia, medication administration).
- Retinopathy of prematurity (ROP) is uncommon in full-term neonates. Oxygen is a major factor in the development of ROP. Commonly accepted goals for oxygen saturation values are between 85% and 93%.
- Neonates are prone to develop hypoglycemia; therefore these infants should receive glucose-containing maintenance fluid infusions. Ideal serum glucose levels should be maintained at 50–90 mg/dL; glucose levels should be checked as clinically indicated.
- Neonatal renal function is not as developed as in older age groups. There is reduced renal blood flow, glomerular filtration rate, and solute excretion. Neonates are less able to regulate sodium and concentrate urine. Due to limited ability to handle a solute load, relatively hypotonic intravenous solutions (e.g., D10W, D51/4NS, etc.) are commonly administered to neonates.
- Neonatal hepatic function is immature, which leads to inefficient metabolism and synthesis of many proteins. Prolonged duration of action of medications and a decrease in coagulation factors may be observed.

Further reading

Davis PJ, Cladis FP, Motoyama EK. *Smith's Anesthesia for Infants and Children*, 8th edition. Philadelphia: Elsevier Mosby, 2011; 517–43, 554–9.

Gregory GA, Andropoulos DB. *Gregory's Pediatric Anesthesia*, 5th edition. Hoboken: Wiley-Blackwell, 2012; 475–501.

Part C Clinical-based areas in pediatric anesthesiology

Neonatal surgery
PDA ligation/CDH
Carlos Rodriguez

Ligation of patent ductus arteriosus

- Patent ductus arteriosus (PDA) is a persistent communication between the pulmonary artery and the aorta. It occurs more commonly in infants that are delivered prematurely. This communication results in a left-to-right shunt and can lead to overcirculation into the pulmonary arteries with the development of congestive heart failure. The ductus arteriosus plays a vital role in the fetal circulation. After birth, the ductus arteriosus typically closes within 24–72 hours secondary to smooth muscle contraction as a result of increasing oxygen concentration.
- Treatment of PDA initially includes administration of indomethacin. If the PDA does not close with medical treatment, then either surgical ligation in the operating room or at the bedside; closure in the cardiac catheterization laboratory may also be considered.
- Most patients requiring PDA closure are premature. Many of these patients may be on inotropic and mechanical ventilatory support. All anesthetic considerations related to the care of the neonate should be followed. Due to the critically ill nature of the patient, a bedside surgical procedure may be performed; these cases are typically performed by administering a total intravenous anesthesia technique. Blood pressure cuffs and pulse oximeter probes should be ideally placed on preductal (right arm) and postductal locations in the event the surgeon needs to clamp the aorta. Once the PDA is ligated, the left ventricle experiences an increase in afterload; this may be demonstrated by an observed increase in the diastolic blood pressure.
- Complications from PDA ligation include hemorrhage, recurrent laryngeal nerve damage, and inadvertent ligation of other vessels (e.g., aorta).

Congenital diaphragmatic hernia repair

- Congenital diaphragmatic hernia (CDH) occurs with an estimated incidence of 1:3,000. It occurs when there is incomplete diaphragm formation; and this defect leads to herniation of abdominal contents into the thoracic cavity, resulting in an inability of thoracic organs to fully develop *in utero*. The most common defect is located in the left postero-lateral section of the diaphragm.
- Diagnosis of CDH usually occurs in the prenatal period during ultrasound of the fetus. At birth, patients may be found to be in significant respiratory distress. Physical examination may demonstrate a scaphoid-shaped abdomen, bowel sounds heard in

Handbook of Critical Incidents and Essential Topics in Pediatric Anesthesiology, ed. David A. Young and Olutoyin A. Olutoye. Published by Cambridge University Press. © Cambridge University Press 2015.

the chest, and decreased breath sounds in the ipsilateral chest (typically the left chest). Diagnosis can be confirmed with chest X-rays showing loops of bowel within the chest.
- Accompanying pulmonary hypoplasia leads to dysfunction in ventilation and oxygenation. Many patients with develop CDH will develop hypoxemia, hypercarbia, and acidosis; each of the previously mentioned conditions results in further pulmonary vascular constriction. This vicious cycle places these patients at risk for developing pulmonary hypertension. Patients may develop respiratory distress soon after birth and require tracheal intubation.
- Current practice favors medical stabilization prior to surgical repair. Ventilation is ideally achieved using smaller tidal volumes (5–7 mL/kg) despite the potential development of moderate hypercarbia. Some patients may not tolerate conventional mechanical ventilation and may require a transition to high frequency oscillatory ventilation, nitric oxide, and possibly extracorporeal membrane oxygenation (ECMO).
- Surgical intervention may be performed either in the operating room or at the bedside in the neonatal intensive care unit. Intra-arterial monitoring and central venous access may be beneficial and should be determined on an individual basis. Many patients are critically ill and commonly a decision is made to perform the procedure at the bedside; these cases are performed by administering a total intravenous anesthesia technique.
- Intraoperative management should include adequate analgesia in an attempt to prevent increased pulmonary vascular reactivity. Patients may benefit from neuromuscular blockade and high doses of opioids (e.g., 25–50 µg/kg of fentanyl).
- The anesthesiologist should be prepared to transfuse blood products, administer vasoactive medications, and modify mechanical ventilatory support settings during surgery.
- Sudden cardiovascular collapse should immediately suggest the development of either a pulmonary hypertensive crisis or a tension pneumothorax on the contralateral side to the defect (typically the right chest).
- Patients with CDH have an increased risk for significant morbidity and mortality. Long-term disorders are also more likely to occur such as obstructive lung disease, gastroesophageal reflux, and developmental disorders.

Further reading

Davis PJ, Cladis FP, Motoyama EK. *Smith's Anesthesia for Infants and Children*, 8th edition. Philadelphia: Elsevier Mosby, 2011; 567–73, 696–7.

Gregory GA, Andropoulos DB. *Gregory's Pediatric Anesthesia*, 5th edition. Hoboken: Wiley-Blackwell, 2012; 479, 500, 510–12.

Part C Clinical-based areas in pediatric anesthesiology

Chapter 144

Neonatal surgery
Necrotizing enterocolitis/abdominal wall defects

Carlos Rodriguez

Necrotizing enterocolitis

- Necrotizing enterocolitis (NEC) is most prevalent in premature neonates and is associated with significant morbidity and mortality. The risk of NEC is inversely related to birth weight and gestational age.
- The etiology of NEC is considered to be multifactorial. It is a result of gut ischemia, bacterial translocation, and inflammation. An immature immune system may also play a role in reduced protection from inflammation and bacterial insult.
- Many cases of NEC are medically managed using bowel decompression, bowel rest, antibiotics, and parenteral nutrition.
- Surgical management is necessary when bowel perforation is suspected.
- Neonates may present with symptoms of vomiting, increased gastric residuals, and guaiac-positive stools. These symptoms are nonspecific and in the absence of radiologic evidence, patients presenting with only these symptoms are considered to have stage 1 (mild) disease. Stage 2 disease includes a definitive diagnosis of NEC with the appearance of pneumatosis intestinalis on radiographs. These patients are also initially managed medically. Patients considered to have stage 3 disease have more systemic involvement; this includes signs of sepsis with hemodynamic, respiratory, and hematologic instability.
- Supportive therapy such as fluid resuscitation, electrolyte therapy, inotropic support in unstable patients, and correction of coagulopathies may be required. Most patients have preexisting mechanical ventilatory support due to underlying apnea and respiratory distress syndrome; many patients will require additional ventilatory support (i.e., increased peak airway pressures, increased oxygen concentration) with the development of NEC.
- Intraoperative management is dependent on patient stability. All anesthetic considerations related to the care of the neonate should be followed. Many patients are critically ill and as such it is not uncommon for a bedside procedure to be performed; these cases are performed by administering a total intravenous anesthesia technique. Unstable patients on inotropic therapy will likely need arterial blood pressure monitoring and central line access. Blood products (e.g., packed red blood cells, fresh frozen plasma and platelets) should be immediately available, especially in the presence of anemia and coagulopathy. Many patients are hypovolemic due to

---

Handbook of Critical Incidents and Essential Topics in Pediatric Anesthesiology, ed. David A. Young and Olutoyin A. Olutoye. Published by Cambridge University Press. © Cambridge University Press 2015.

significant third space fluid losses. Anticipate administering large amounts of volume (e.g., 100 mL/kg) during surgery. Fluids should ideally be warmed in order to reduce the development of hypothermia.
- Postoperatively these patients should remain sedated and on mechanical ventilation.
- Mortality from NEC is high (10–30%). There is also a long-term complication of short gut syndrome (20–25%). Short gut syndrome results from extensive bowel resection resulting in the patient being permanently dependent on total parenteral nutrition.

Abdominal wall defects: gastroschisis and omphalocele

- Gastroschisis and omphalocele are the two most common abdominal wall defects with an estimated incidence of 1:10,000 and 1:6,000, respectively. They are usually diagnosed in the antenatal period via ultrasound.
- The treatment and anesthetic management for both defects is similar even though their embryologic origins are different.
- In gastroschisis, there is a defect in the abdominal wall allowing for contents of the abdomen to herniate. The defect is usually located to the right of the umbilicus. It is important to note that the abdominal contents in this defect are not enclosed within any sac. The presence of additional congenital anomalies is also rare with this defect.
- The defect of an omphalocele is situated in the midline. The abdominal contents herniate through the umbilical ring. The contents of the abdomen are lined with a sac. It is important to note that many patients born with an omphalocele may have another congenital anomaly and will require additional evaluations (e.g., echocardiogram).
- After birth, for either defect, special care is taken to cover the exposed bowel with sterile dressings. Significant fluid and heat loss can occur through the defect.
- Depending on the size of the defect, patients may either initially go to the operating room for attempted primary closure or temporarily receive a silo cover placed at the bedside. All anesthetic considerations related to the care of the neonate should be followed.
- Closure of large defects can lead to difficulty in ventilation and hemodynamic depression. Anticipate additional fluid requirements due to third space losses. The development of an abdominal compartment syndrome is also possible.
- Patients who do not tolerate complete closure may tolerate partial closure with a silo placed over the remaining abdominal defect.

Further reading

Davis PJ, Cladis FP, Motoyama EK. *Smith's Anesthesia for Infants and Children*, 8th edition. Philadelphia: Elsevier Mosby, 2011; 564–84.

Gregory GA, Andropoulos DB. *Gregory's Pediatric Anesthesia*, 5th edition. Hoboken: Wiley-Blackwell, 2012; 158–9, 503–6.

Part C Clinical-based areas in pediatric anesthesiology

Chapter 145

Neurosurgery

General considerations

Yang Liu

Cranial procedure

- Key goals of anesthesia during craniotomy
    - Protection of the brain from further injury during the perioperative period.
    - Control and normalization of intracranial pressure (ICP), cerebral blood flow (CBF), and cerebral perfusion pressure (CPP).
    - Provide a "relaxed" brain (decreased ICP) to optimize surgical exposure.
    - Anesthesia technique should facilitate neuromonitoring (if required).
    - Facilitate early postoperative neurologic assessment.
- Preoperative assessment
    - A child with major or acute onset cranial pathology is likely to present with increased ICP. The signs of increased ICP include:
        - Irritability.
        - Headache.
        - Vomiting.
        - Full fontanelle.
        - Cranial enlargement.
        - Altered level of consciousness.
        - Ipsilateral pupil dilation.
    - History and physical examination
        - Identify preoperative medications: anticonvulsant therapy may affect anesthetic management.
        - Patients with cardiac shunts are at risk of paradoxical air emboli.
        - Radiology images provide details of the size and site of any lesion, the presence of hydrocephalus, and any cerebral pressure effects.
    - Anxiolytics should be used judiciously under monitored circumstances.
- Induction of anesthesia
    - Avoid increases in ICP during induction of anesthesia.
        - Intravenous induction with propofol, local anesthetics, opioids, and nondepolarizing neuromuscular blocking agents are commonly utilized.

Handbook of Critical Incidents and Essential Topics in Pediatric Anesthesiology, ed. David A. Young and Olutoyin A. Olutoye. Published by Cambridge University Press. © Cambridge University Press 2015.

- Hypercapnia, hypoxemia, variations in mean arterial pressure, and volatile agents may all increase ICP.
- Inhalation induction with sevoflurane may be considered in patients with difficult intravenous access to prevent crying, which further increases ICP.

- Monitoring
  - Standard ASA monitoring.
  - Arterial line placement is important both for blood pressure and arterial carbon dioxide ($PaCO_2$) monitoring.
    - The arterial line transducer should be zeroed at the level of the circle of Willis (external auditory meatus).
  - Urethral catheterization and close monitoring of urine output is mandatory for long surgical procedures.
  - Neurophysiologic monitoring may be required to detect neurologic injury.
  - Precordial Doppler or transesophageal echocardiography (TEE) for detection of venous air embolism (VAE) should be used in sitting position craniotomy procedures.
  - Consider placement of a central venous line for cases with large expected blood loss.
- Patient positioning
  - Protect all vulnerable pressure areas.
  - Prone position
    - Tracheal tube displacement and obstruction from kinking may occur with neck flexion, especially in infants.
  - Sitting position
    - May be utilized for posterior fossa surgery to improve surgical access and reduce bleeding. Posterior fossa procedures are typically performed using the prone or lateral positions.
    - Is associated with a high incidence of VAE, hypotension, and complications related to positioning.
- Maintenance of anesthesia
  - Volatile agents or total intravenous anesthesia in combination with opioids and neuromuscular blocking agents may be used.
  - Volatile agents should be limited to less than 1 minimum alveolar concentration (MAC) to avoid an increase in CBF.
  - Mild hyperventilation with the $PaCO_2$ maintained no less than 30 mmHg will help control increased ICP.
  - Hypotonic intravenous fluids or those containing glucose should not be used.
  - Mannitol may be required to attenuate increases in ICP.
  - Corticosteroids (administered to decrease swelling) may result in hyperglycemia.
  - Fluid warmers, warm air devices, or heated mattresses are required for temperature control.
- Postoperative management
  - A controlled quick emergence is important for early neurologic assessment.

- Coughing, bucking, and retching during emergence can cause dramatic increases in ICP and should be minimized.
- Ensure effective analgesia.

Spine procedure

- Preoperative assessment
  - Common diseases that require surgery include neural tube defects, Arnold Chiari malformations, scoliosis, primary spinal cord tumors, and acute spinal cord injuries.
  - Identify other congenital defects.
  - Evaluate for anatomical abnormalities that may result in a difficult airway.
  - Be aware of the potential for latex allergy.
  - Discuss positioning and the need for neuromonitoring with neurosurgeon.
- Induction of anesthesia
  - Routine ASA monitoring; also consider invasive, arterial line monitoring.
  - Consider fiberoptic intubation for a difficult airway or unstable cervical spine.
- Patient positioning
  - Most pediatric spine operations are performed in the prone position.
    - Properly secure the endotracheal tube.
    - Ensure adequate padding of the patient.
- Maintenance of anesthesia
  - Standard inhalation or total intravenous anesthetic (TIVA) technique can be used for maintenance of anesthesia.
  - Propofol and short-acting opioids (TIVA) should be used to facilitate spinal cord monitoring.
  - Consider blood conservation techniques in procedures with high potential for massive hemorrhage.
- Postoperative management
  - Infiltration of local anesthetic into the wound at the end of surgery will improve pain relief in the immediate postoperative period.

Further reading

Cote CJ. *A Practice of Anesthesia for Infants and Children*, 5th edition. Philadelphia: Elsevier, 2013; 513–20.

Gregory GA, Andropoulos DB. *Gregory's Pediatric Anesthesia*, 5th edition. Hoboken: Wiley-Blackwell, 2012; 540–68.

Soundararajan N, Cunliffe M. Anaesthesia for spinal surgery in children. *Br J Anaesth.* 2007;99:86–94.

Part C **Clinical-based areas in pediatric anesthesiology**

Neurosurgery
Hydrocephalus/VP shunts
Julia Chen

Hydrocephalus
- Etiology
  - Overproduction or impaired drainage of cerebrospinal fluid (CSF) resulting in abnormal accumulation of CSF and increased intracranial CSF volume.
    - Overproduction of CSF. Causes include choroid plexus papilloma.
    - Impaired drainage of CSF (most common category) secondary to internal obstruction of CSF flow or impaired absorption of CSF by the arachnoid villi. Causes include hemorrhage, trauma, infection, tumors, congenital anomalies (aqueductal stenosis, Arnold Chiari malformation)
- Pathophysiology
  - Increased intracranial CSF volume may increase intracranial pressure (ICP). The degree of increase in ICP will depend on intracranial compliance, acuity of increase in CSF volume, and effectiveness of compensatory mechanisms.
    - Infants with open anterior and posterior fontanelles may accommodate gradual increases in CSF volume; these children may present with widened cranial sutures, persistent open fontanelles, failure of fusion of cranial bones, and increases in head circumference.
    - The anterior fontanelle typically closes by age 6–18 months while the posterior fontanelle is typically closed by age 1–2 months.
    - Older children with fused cranial sutures cannot effectively accommodate large increases in CSF volume and are at higher risk of developing clinical signs of increased ICP (see below).
    - Compensatory mechanisms when increased CSF volume is present include shifting a larger proportion of CSF cephalad into the spinal canal and the expansion of ventricles (which results in the development of hydrocephalus).
- Diagnosis
  - Clinical assessment
    - Clinical signs of increased ICP include: headache, vomiting, irritability, decreased level of consciousness, hypertension, bradycardia, focal neurologic signs, unequal pupils, and altered respiratory rate.

Handbook of Critical Incidents and Essential Topics in Pediatric Anesthesiology, ed. David A. Young and Olutoyin A. Olutoye. Published by Cambridge University Press. © Cambridge University Press 2015.

- Neuroimaging
    - Computed tomography (CT) is rapid, reliable, and can typically be accomplished without sedation.
    - Magnetic resonance imaging (MRI) offers detailed neuroanatomy; however, is time consuming and may require pharmacologic agents to obtain imaging.
- Surgical treatment
    - Temporary external ventricular drain (EVD).
    - Ventriculoperitoneal (VP) shunt
        - Transports CSF from the lateral ventricles to the peritoneal cavity.
        - Ventriculopleural and ventriculoatrial shunts are alternative shunt choices if there is difficulty with peritoneal cavity absorption of CSF.
    - Endoscopic third ventriculostomy
        - Effective for certain cases of obstructive hydrocephalus.
        - Formation of a communicating opening from the third ventricle to the subarachnoid space of a basal cranial cistern.

Anesthetic considerations

- Preoperative
    - Patients may present with signs and symptoms of increased ICP.
    - Proximal shunt tapping may be an option in some patients to reduce ICP preoperatively.
    - Patients may have other coexisting conditions (e.g., difficult airway, prematurity) that must be considered and integrated into the anesthetic management plan.
- Intraoperative
    - Consider rapid sequence induction and tracheal intubation for patients with clinical evidence of increased ICP; these patients may be at risk for vomiting and pulmonary aspiration. A standard inhalation or intravenous induction may be considered for children without clinical evidence of increased ICP.
    - Maintenance of anesthesia is typically accomplished with the use of volatile anesthetics, neuromuscular blocking agents, and judicious use of opioids.
    - In patients with increased ICP, avoid acute increases in ICP prior to relief of the hydrocephalus, such as an inadequate depth of anesthesia during airway management.
    - Avoid hypotension as this will decrease cerebral perfusion pressure (CPP) in patients with increased ICP; CPP = mean arterial pressure – ICP.
    - Increasing the anesthetic depth and the use of short-acting opioids may attenuate the hemodynamic response to surgical incision and catheter tunneling.
- Postoperative
    - Frequent neurological observations and vital sign monitoring should be carried out postoperatively to detect new neurologic findings (e.g., postoperative intracranial hemorrhage).
- Special considerations
    - External ventricular drain.

- Care should be taken during transport to avoid dislodgement of the ventricular tubing. Extreme changes in height of the drainage bag in relation to the patient's head should also be avoided, as this can acutely change the rate of CSF drainage and ICP.
  o Third ventriculostomy
    - Surgical complications include damage to basilar artery, neural injury, and need to convert to craniotomy.
  o Ventriculoperitoneal (VP) shunt
    - May require revision or replacement secondary to patient growth, mechanical malfunction, or infection.
  o Ventriculoatrial shunt
    - Venous air embolism may occur during distal placement of shunt.
  o Ventriculopleural shunt
    - CSF accumulation in pleural space may impair respiration, possibly requiring thoracentesis or placement of a chest tube.

Further reading

Barash PG. *Clinical Anesthesia*, 7th edition. Philadelphia: Lippincott Williams & Wilkins, 2013; 1209.

Coté CJ, Lerman J, Anderson BJ. *Coté and Lerman's A Practice of Anesthesia for Infants and Children*, 5th edition. Philadelphia, PA: Elsevier, 2013; 527–5.

Gregory GA, Andropoulos DB. *Gregory's Pediatric Anesthesia*, 5th edition. Hoboken: Wiley-Blackwell, 2012; 549–51, 976.

Part C Clinical-based areas in pediatric anesthesiology

Chapter 147
Neurosurgery
Brain tumors/neural tube defects
Yang Liu

Brain tumors

- General considerations
  - Approximately 4,000 children per year in the United States are diagnosed with a brain tumor; 70% of these children are < 15 years of age.
  - Brain tumors comprise the second most common childhood cancer (after leukemia).
  - Two-thirds of childhood brain tumors are located in the posterior fossa.
  - Children with brain tumors frequently require sedation or general anesthesia for neuro-imaging and diagnostic procedures.
  - Most common symptoms are headaches and vomiting.
  - Brain tumors may result in:
    - Increased intracranial pressure (ICP) and decreased cerebral perfusion pressure (CPP).
    - Cerebral herniation.

- Preoperative assessment
  - Recognize signs of increased intracranial pressure.
  - Examine patient for signs of major neurologic deficits.
  - Review computed tomography scan and/or magnetic resonance images for the location of the brain tumor and determine whether obstruction of cerebrospinal fluid flow is present.
  - Review preoperative medications, with a particular focus on antiepileptic drugs and steroids.
  - Evaluate laboratory values – electrolytes, hemoglobin, coagulation status; obtain crossmatched packed red blood cells.
  - Communicate with neurosurgeon about planned surgery: patient position, duration of procedure, potential for blood loss, and the need for specific monitoring.

- Induction and maintenance of anesthesia
  - Opioids, local anesthetics, and nondepolarizing muscle relaxants are recommended for induction of anesthesia.
  - Carefully pad all pressure points.

Handbook of Critical Incidents and Essential Topics in Pediatric Anesthesiology, ed. David A. Young and Olutoyin A. Olutoye. Published by Cambridge University Press. © Cambridge University Press 2015.

- If increased ICP is present, keep arterial carbon dioxide ($PaCO_2$) around 30 mmHg with appropriate mechanical ventilation.
- Avoid hypoventilation, which can further increase ICP.
- Avoid excessive hyperventilation, which may lead to excessive cerebral vasoconstriction and cerebral ischemia.
- Avoid hypotension, which decreases CPP, especially in patients with increased ICP.
- Consider combination of inhalational anesthesia with intravenous anesthesia techniques and tailor to the clinical situation.
- Maintain adequate fluid balance.
- Maintain normothermia.
- Consider initiation of prophylactic antiepileptic treatment during surgery.

- Emergence and postoperative management
    - Most patients require overnight intensive care unit monitoring.
    - A preliminary decision to either extubate the patient or keep the patient sedated and intubated postoperatively should be made before surgery. This decision may be modified based on the intraoperative events.
    - Analgesics should be carefully titrated to allow for proper neurologic assessment after surgery.

- Special consideration for supratentorial tumors
    - Patient usually is positioned supine with the head slightly elevated and turned to one side to facilitate surgical exposure.
    - Avoid extreme flexion, extension, or rotation of the neck.

- Special consideration for infratentorial tumors
    - Medulloblastoma, astrocytoma, and ependymoma are the most common infratentorial tumors.
    - Posterior fossa tumors are often associated with acute obstruction of the aqueduct and obstructive hydrocephalus.
    - Prone positioning is typically utilized for infratentorial tumor surgery.
    - Consider the use of precordial Doppler or echocardiography for detection of air embolism if surgery is performed in the sitting position.
    - Somatosensory evoked potentials may be indicated for intramedullary or brainstem lesions.
    - The patient's face must be carefully padded if a horseshoe headrest is used.
    - The multipin head holder provides better fixation for patients older than 3 years of age.

- Special consideration for midline supratentorial tumors
    - Craniopharyngiomas are benign neuroepithelial intracranial tumors predominately observed in children 5–10 years of age.
    - Craniopharyngiomas commonly cause important endocrine dysfunction and neurologic deficits.
    - Perioperative administration of steroids should be considered.
    - Diabetes insipidus is common and can be successfully managed with desmopressin (DDAVP) or vasopressin.

- The patient's electrolyte status and urine output should determine fluid replacement requirements.
- Location of the tumor and complications of curative therapy can result in significant morbidity.

Neural tube defects

- General considerations
  - Neural tube defects are congenital defects of the brain, spine, or spinal cord; the etiology is unknown.
  - Spina bifida and anencephaly are the two most common neural tube defects.
  - Folate deficiency has been associated with the development of spina bifida (myelomeningocele).
  - The most common forms of spinal bifida are spina bifida occulta, meningocele, myelomeningocele, and tethered cord.
  - Myelomeningocele is the most severe form of caudal neural tube defect. About 70–80% of patients also have Arnold Chiari type II malformation and hydrocephalus.
  - In anencephaly, most of the brain and skull do not develop; affected babies are either stillborn or die shortly after birth.
- Special consideration for myelomeningocele
  - Prophylaxis with broad-spectrum antibiotics is recommended until surgical closure of the lesion.
  - Surgical repair should be performed within the first 24 hours of life to prevent infection of the nervous system and possible progressive neural damage.
  - Avoid any pressure on the open neural plate. Induction should be performed in either the lateral position or supine with the sac positioned within a cushioned ring.
  - Latex precautions should be utilized.

Further reading

Coté CJ, Lerman J, Anderson BJ. *Coté and Lerman's A Practice of Anesthesia for Infants and Children*, 5th edition. Philadelphia, PA: Elsevier, 2013; 479.

Gregory GA, Andropoulos DB. *Gregory's Pediatric Anesthesia*, 5th edition. Hoboken: Wiley-Blackwell, 2012; 540–68.

Part C Clinical-based areas in pediatric anesthesiology

Chapter 148

Ophthalmologic surgery
General considerations
Mary A. Felberg

- Infants and children are commonly unable to cooperate for a full ophthalmologic examination.
- General anesthesia is often required even for diagnostic examinations of the eye if absolute immobility is required.
- Many surgical procedures may be brief, but involve airway avoidance (turning the table 90°); the airway is often secured with a supraglottic airway device or endotracheal tube.

Ophthalmologic physiology

Intraocular pressure
- Intraocular pressure (IOP) is the internal pressure of the eye exerted on the sclera and conjunctiva.
- Normal IOP for neonates averages 9.5 mmHg.
- After age 5, IOP reaches adult values in the range 10–20 mmHg.
- IOP greater than 25 mmHg is considered elevated.
- In general (excluding ketamine), anesthetic medications (e.g., inhalational agents, induction agents, opioids) decrease IOP.
- Succinylcholine has been shown to increase IOP transiently by as much as 7–9 mmHg. The use of succinylcholine in patients with open globes or known increased IOP is controversial.
- Ketamine has been shown in several studies to both increase and decrease IOP; there is no consensus for using ketamine when there is a concern for increased IOP.
- Coughing, crying, vomiting, laryngoscopy, hypertension, acidosis, and hypercarbia have all been implicated in significantly increasing IOP, perhaps greater than the increase from succinylcholine.
- Suggested strategies to prevent increases in IOP include:
  - Premedication of the anxious patient.
  - Prior to laryngoscopy:
    - Administer lidocaine 1–2 mg/kg IV.
    - Ensure a deep level of anesthesia prior to airway management.

Handbook of Critical Incidents and Essential Topics in Pediatric Anesthesiology, ed. David A. Young and Olutoyin A. Olutoye. Published by Cambridge University Press. © Cambridge University Press 2015.

- Consider airway management with a supraglottic airway device if appropriate.
- Consider deep extubation.
- Preemptive antiemetics to reduce postoperative vomiting.

Aqueous humor production and drainage

- Aqueous humor is produced by the ciliary body in the posterior chamber of the eye and flows into the anterior chamber. Drainage from the anterior chamber is via the canal of Schlemm where absorption occurs in the episcleral veins.
- Glaucoma may develop in patients with ineffective drainage of aqueous humor.

Oculocardiac reflex

- The incidence of the oculocardiac reflex (OCR) in pediatric ophthalmic surgery is as high as 80%.
- Traction on the extraocular muscles is the most common trigger for OCR although it can occur with intraorbital or retrobulbar injections, enucleation, and endoscopic sinus surgery.
- The afferent limb of the OCR is the ophthalmic division of the trigeminal nerve (cranial nerve V) and the efferent limb is the vagus nerve (cranial nerve X) with resultant parasympathetic response.
- Bradycardia is the most common response from the OCR; junctional rhythm, premature ventricular contractions, atrioventricular block, and asystole have all been reported.
- Administration of an anticholinergic medication, such as atropine or glycopyrrolate, with induction of anesthesia may reduce but not reliably prevent the OCR from occurring.
- Termination of the noxious stimuli (i.e., stopping surgery) typically eliminates the parasympathetic response within 10–20 seconds.
- The OCR fatigues over time.

Implications of ophthalmic medications

- Topically applied ophthalmic medications may be systemically absorbed and can have undesirable physiologic effects (see Table 148.1).

Preoperative assessment

- Ocular disorders requiring anesthesia for intervention may be congenital (e.g., congenital cataracts, strabismus, retinoblastoma) or acquired (e.g., retinopathy of prematurity, open globe injury); they may be isolated occurrences or associated with systemic disorders.
- Associated systemic disorders include:
  - Trisomy 21 – cataracts, strabismus, nasolacrimal duct stenosis, glaucoma.
  - Marfan syndrome – retinal detachment, lens displacement, cataracts, glaucoma.
  - Mucopolysaccharidoses – glaucoma, corneal opacities.
  - Prematurity – retinopathy of prematurity (ROP).

Table 148.1 Common opthalmic medications, indications, and undesirable effects.

Medication	Ophthalmic indication	Undesired effects
Atropine (1%)	Mydriasis, cycloplegia	Tachycardia, flushing, dry mouth, photosensitivity
Cyclopentolate (1%)	Mydriasis, cycloplegia	Tachycardia, flushing, dry mouth, photosensitivity
Echothiophate (0.25%)	Glaucoma	Possible prolongation of succinylcholine and medications metabolized by plasma cholinesterase
Phenylephrine (1–2.5%)	Mydriasis, cycloplegia, decongestion	Hypertension, bradycardia
Timolol (0.25%)	Glaucoma	Decreased heart rate, blood pressure; bronchospasm

Postoperative nausea and vomiting

- Postoperative nausea and vomiting (PONV) is the most common anesthesia-related adverse event from ophthalmic surgery, with an incidence of 50–80%.
- PONV accounts for > 50% of unanticipated overnight hospital admissions.
- A multimodal approach for decreasing PONV includes:
  - Preoperative anxiolysis if indicated.
  - IV fluid hydration, up to 30 ml/kg of an isotonic crystalloid.
  - Avoidance of nitrous oxide.
  - Consider placement of gastric a decompression tube.
  - Preemptive administration of antiemetics from two different drug classes:
    - 5-HT3 receptor antagonists (e.g., ondansetron).
    - Cortiosteroids (e.g., dexamethasone).
    - Antidopaminergic agents (e.g., metoclopramide).
  - Minimizing the use of opioids by utilizing adjuvant agents such as acetaminophen and/or ketorolac.

Anesthesia, open globe, and the full stomach

- The risk of increasing IOP resulting in extrusion of ocular contents must be weighed against the benefit of using a rapid sequence technique for minimizing pulmonary aspiration.
- Rocuronium 1.2 mg/kg is an acceptable alternative to succinylcholine.
- Major priority includes producing a deep plane of anesthesia prior to airway management.

Further reading

Coté CJ, Lerman J, Anderson BJ. *Coté and Lerman's A Practice of Anesthesia for Infants and Children*, 5th edition. Philadelphia, PA: Elsevier, 2013; 685–98.

Gregory GA, Andropoulos DB. *Gregory's Pediatric Anesthesia*, 5th edition. Hoboken: Wiley-Blackwell, 2012; 800–6.

Part C Clinical-based areas in pediatric anesthesiology

Chapter 149

Ophthalmologic surgery
Retinopathy of prematurity/ strabismus surgery

Mary A. Felberg

Retinopathy of prematurity

- Definition: Retinopathy of prematurity (ROP) is a vasoproliferative disease of the retinal blood vessels that can result in permanent visual impairment or blindness.
- More than 50% of premature infants with birthweights < 1,000 grams develop ROP; however, many of these patients have spontaneous regression of these retinal changes.

Risk factors

- Prematurity, low birth weight, and high concentrations of supplemental oxygen.
- The younger the gestational age and the lower the birth weight, the higher the risk for ROP.

Pathophysiology

- The definitive etiology of ROP and the exact role supplemental oxygen plays in the development of ROP is not completely understood. Studies have shown that limiting oxygen concentrations has decreased the incidence of ROP. Some infants will develop ROP despite minimizing oxygen supplementation, implying that the development of ROP is multifactorial.
- Retinal blood vessel development begins during the 16th week of gestation; complete retinal vascularization occurs by 42 weeks.
- Unlike normal vessel branching patterns, the neovasculature is chaotic or "tangled", fragile and bleeds easily. Post hemorrhage, fibrin threads attach to vitreous strands causing the vitreous to contract, resulting in retinal detachment.
- Untreated retinal detachment leads to visual impairment or blindness.
- ROP may spontaneously regress without visual impairment.

Treatment

- Treatment is linked to classification. ROP is classified in five stages according to progression of disease.
- Stage 1 and 2 require serial retinal examinations, usually performed at the bedside with or without minimal sedation.

Handbook of Critical Incidents and Essential Topics in Pediatric Anesthesiology, ed. David A. Young and Olutoyin A. Olutoye. Published by Cambridge University Press. © Cambridge University Press 2015.

- There are four surgical treatments for ROP stages 3–5, guided by the stage of the disease:
  - Laser photocoagulation – used to treat stage 3 disease. Can be performed at the bedside.
  - Cryotherapy – used to treat stage 3 disease. Commonly performed in the operating room under general anesthesia.
  - Scleral buckling – used to treat stage 4 disease (partial retinal detachment); performed in the operating room under general anesthesia.
  - Vitrectomy – used to treat stage 5 disease (complete retinal detachment); performed under general anesthesia.
- Rapidly progressing ROP can become a surgical emergency; there is a limited time period to reduce permanent visual loss.

Anesthetic management

- Comorbidities of the premature infant will influence the anesthetic management (e.g., temperature management, minimal intravenous fluid administration, presence of chronic lung disease).
- Target levels of oxygenation for the patient can be obtained with an oxygen saturation of 90–95%.
- General anesthesia with an endotracheal tube is commonly used for airway management; many of these patients will have a preexisting tracheal tube.
- Postoperative ventilation may be required due to the increased risk for apnea of prematurity or the need for increased ventilatory requirements due to preexisting pulmonary disease.

Strabismus surgery

- Strabismus is misalignment of the visual axes; it can be congenital or acquired.
- It is one of the most commonly performed ophthalmologic surgeries in children.
- Primary anesthetic considerations:
  - Identifying associated conditions.
  - Cardiovascular effects of topical eye medications.
  - Oculocardiac reflex (OCR).
  - Postoperative nausea and vomiting (PONV).

Associated conditions

- Strabismus surgery does not involve major fluid shifts or blood loss; the anesthetic implications of associated conditions influence the choice of induction, airway management, and management of OCR.
- Associated conditions include:
  - Cerebral palsy.
  - Noonan syndrome.
  - Retinopathy of prematurity.

- Retinoblastoma.
- Traumatic brain injury.
- Trisomy 21.
- Studies have disproven the notion that patients with congenital strabismus are at an increased risk for malignant hyperthermia.

Effects of topical eye medications
- Topically applied ophthalmic medications are systemically absorbed and can have undesirable physiologic effects.
- Phenylephrine (1–2.5%), cyclopentolate (0.5%), and tropicamide (0.5%) are used to achieve mydriasis and hemostasis.
- Phenylephrine may cause severe vasoconstriction and hypertension.

Oculocardiac reflex
- The incidence of the OCR during strabismus surgery is as high as 80%.
- Triggered by traction on the extraocular muscles, OCR can also occur with intraorbital or retrobulbar injections, enucleation, and endoscopic sinus surgery.
- The afferent limb of the OCR is the ophthalmic division of the trigeminal nerve (cranial nerve V) and the efferent limb is the vagus nerve (cranial nerve X) with resultant parasympathetic response.
- Bradycardia is the most common response; junctional rhythm, premature ventricular contractions, atrioventricular block, and asystole have all been reported.
- Administration of an anticholinergic medication such as atropine or glycopyrrolate during induction of anesthesia may attenuate the OCR.
- Termination of muscle traction by the surgeon should eliminate the parasympathetic response of the OCR within 10–20 seconds.
- Consider the administration of an anticholinergic if the OCR persists.
- OCR fatigues over time.

Postoperative nausea and vomiting
- Postoperative nausea and vomiting (PONV) is the most common adverse event for ophthalmic surgery with a reported incidence of 50–80%.
- PONV accounts for >50% of unanticipated overnight hospital admissions after strabismus repair.
- A multimodal approach to decreasing PONV includes:
    - Preoperative anxiolysis if indicated (e.g., midazolam).
    - IV fluid hydration, up to 30 ml/kg of an isotonic crystalloid.
    - Avoidance of nitrous oxide.
    - Preemptive administration of antiemetics from two different drug classes
        - 5-HT3 receptor antagonists (e.g., ondansetron).
        - Cortiosteroids (e.g., dexamethasone).

- Antidopaminergic agents (e.g., metoclopramide).
- Droperidol is no longer a first-line antiemetic due to concerns for QT prolongation.
  ○ Minimizing opioids by utilizing adjuvant medications such as acetaminophen and ketorolac.

Further reading

Coté CJ, Lerman J, Anderson BJ. *Coté and Lerman's A Practice of Anesthesia for Infants and Children*, 5th edition. Philadelphia, PA: Elsevier, 2013; 693–6.

Davis PJ, Cladis FP, Motoyama EK. *Smith's Anesthesia for Infants and Children*, 8th edition. Philadelphia: Elsevier Mosby, 2011; 883–5.

Gregory GA, Andropoulos DB. *Gregory's Pediatric Anesthesia*, 5th edition. Hoboken: Wiley-Blackwell, 2012; 482–83, 806.

Orthopedic surgery
General considerations
Andrew J. Costandi and Senthilkumar Sadhasivam

Introduction
- The majority of children presenting for orthopedic procedures require repeated admissions and surgeries. This should be taken into consideration for the administration of preoperative anxiolytic agents.
- In many instances the anesthetic plan depends on the child's age, operative site, and emergent nature of surgery; in other instances, the patient's medical condition and associated anomalies determine the perioperative anesthetic plan.
- Children with cerebral palsy, neuromuscular or metabolic disorders present frequently for orthopedic surgeries, mandating careful review of their medical history in order to anticipate respective anesthetic challenges.
- Proper positioning with padding of the pressure points is extremely important, especially among children with neuromuscular disorders undergoing prolonged procedures.
- Blood loss may be significant in many orthopedic surgeries, requiring adequate vascular access and preparation for transfusion of blood products.
- Conservation of body temperature can be challenging, especially in procedures involving the back in the prone position or other procedures with large exposure areas.
- Major orthopedic surgery, such as spine fusion for scoliosis, is covered in Chapter 151.

Use of a tourniquet
- A tourniquet is mainly used to minimize blood loss and provide optimal operating conditions.
- Physiologic changes and complications:
  - Cellular ischemia leading to tissue hypoxia and acidosis. These changes are usually reversible if tourniquet inflation time is < 2 hours and the inflation pressure is ≤ 100 mmHg above the systolic blood pressure.
  - Metabolic changes: Occurs with cuff deflation and reperfusion resulting in an increase in lactic acid, creatine phosphokinase (CPK), potassium (peak increase 0.32 mEq/L), and carbon dioxide (peak increase 8–18 mmHg). Values return to baseline typically within 30 minutes.

Handbook of Critical Incidents and Essential Topics in Pediatric Anesthesiology, ed. David A. Young and Olutoyin A. Olutoye. Published by Cambridge University Press. © Cambridge University Press 2015.

- Muscle damage: "Post–tourniquet syndrome"; edema, stiffness, pallor, weakness, and numbness. Myoglobinuria from muscle injury can cause renal failure; recovery usually occurs within 7 days.
- Nerve damage: Due to direct nerve compression rather than nerve ischemia. Incidence is greater in upper compared to lower limbs, frequently affecting the radial nerve.
- Pain: starts approximately 45 minutes after tourniquet inflation and is associated with increased heart rate and blood pressure despite adequate regional/general anesthesia. Pain often subsides with tourniquet deflation.

- Recommendations
  - Tourniquet time should be limited to a maximum of 2 hours; allow at least a 30-minute deflation period prior to reinflation of the tourniquet.
  - Avoid tourniquet use in patients with sickle cell disease to avoid sickling and ischemic injuries.

Fat embolism
- Characterized by the triad of hypoxemia, neurologic abnormalities, and petechial rash.
- Develops to some extent in nearly all patients with long bone fractures or during orthopedic procedures but is usually asymptomatic.
- Significant cardiovascular collapse can occur in severe cases; initial presentation may include hypotension, bronchospasm, and decreased end tidal carbon dioxide ($ETCO_2$).
- High index of suspicion is needed to make the diagnosis intraoperatively.
- Treatment is mainly supportive and may require cardiopulmonary resuscitation.

Pain control
- Postoperative pain is usually moderate to severe after most orthopedic procedures; the use of regional analgesia is encouraged when feasible, especially among cognitively impaired patients.
- Regimens utilizing multimodal approaches for pain control with the use of opioid and non-opioid adjuvants in addition to regional anesthesia are often effective.
- There is a concern that regional anesthesia may mask compartment syndrome which may complicate orthopedic trauma injuries. Discussion with the surgeon and increased postoperative vigilance is strongly encouraged.

Cerebral palsy
Cerebral palsy is a static encephalopathy that is defined as a non-progressive disorder.
- Aspiration pneumonia, recurrent respiratory infections, obstructive sleep apnea, gastric reflux, seizures, and neurologic impairment including bulbar dysfunction are all very likely to be present and may influence anesthetic management.
- Higher overall incidence of latex allergy; latex precautions should be strongly considered.

- Patients should continue their seizure management medications into the pre-operative period.
- Medications such as etomidate and ketamine should be used with caution in children with seizure disorders.
- Affected patients appear to have a lower MAC than unaffected children.
- Patients may be unable to communicate their postoperative pain, making pain assessment challenging.
- Muscle spasms are very common and are treated effectively with skeletal muscle relaxants such as baclofen, methocarbamol, and diazepam.

Arthrogryposis multiplex congenita

Arthrogryposis multiplex congenital (AMC) is a group of disorders characterized by non-progressive congenital joint contractures due to fetal akinesia.
- Surgical management is directed at correcting the extremity deformities.
- Anesthetic management is complicated because of associated congenital abnormalities such as congenital heart disease, pulmonary hypertension, abnormal upper airway, difficulty in intubation and positioning difficulties.
- Patients with AMC are not considered to be at an increased risk of malignant hyperthermia.

Osteogenesis imperfecta

Osteogenesis imperfect (OI) is a disorder of collagen production with four subtypes, all characterized with fragile bones.
- Management is mainly surgical and rehabilitative; these patients frequently present for surgery due to multiple fractures after little or no apparent trauma.
- Anesthetic management is focused on handling these patients gently especially during transport, positioning, and airway management.
- Warming the patient intraoperatively and the use of antimuscarinic agents should be limited as these patients may develop a hypermetabolic state and develop hyperthermia.

Further reading

Coté CJ, Lerman J, Anderson BJ. *Coté and Lerman's A Practice of Anesthesia for Infants and Children*, 5th edition. Philadelphia, PA: Elsevier, 2013; 866–9.

Davis PJ, Cladis FP, Motoyama EK. *Smith's Anesthesia for Infants and Children*, 8th edition. Philadelphia: Elsevier Mosby, 2011; 640–51.

Part C Clinical-based areas in pediatric anesthesiology

Chapter 151

Orthopedic surgery
Scoliosis surgery
Luigi Viola and Senthilkumar Sadhasivam

Introduction
- Scoliosis: lateral curvature of any part of the spine resulting in rotation of the vertebral bodies; prevalence approximately 1%.
- Classification: idiopathic (70% of cases); congenital (bone or spinal cord anomalies); neuromuscular (neuropathic or myopathic); miscellaneous (neurofibromatosis, connective tissue disorders, trauma, infections, tumors).
- Common technique involves posterior spinal fusion with or without instrumentation to achieve stabilization of the curve. The fusion extends from the vertebra above the curve to the second vertebra below; this may incorporate many vertebral levels.
- Instrumentation devices (Harrington Rod, pedicle screws) are inserted to hold the spine in the best possible position. Anterior release and instrumentation of the spine is occasionally required in complex cases.

Preoperative evaluation
- Initial evaluation should determine location and length of deformity, Cobb angle, presence of cardiopulmonary symptoms, and any comorbid conditions.
- Assessment of the severity of cardiorespiratory dysfunction correlates with the angle of spinal curvature (Cobb angle). Cobb angles > 65° are associated with restrictive lung disease, > 100° with dyspnea on exertion and decreased exercise tolerance.
- The Cobb angle helps predict the likelihood of post-surgical mechanical ventilation requirement (increased likelihood if angle > 65°).
- Recommended preoperative testing: chest radiography, echocardiography, pulmonary function tests, complete blood count, coagulation profile, electrolytes, blood crossmatch, and renal panel.
- Pulmonary function tests: useful in establishing the risk for postoperative pulmonary complications. FVC (forced vital capacity) < 30 mL/kg (< 50% of predicted) or FEV_1 (forced expiratory volume in 1 second) less than 50% of predicted correlates with post-surgical respiratory insufficiency and the increased potential for postoperative mechanical ventilation. Blood gas analysis may also be helpful in cases of severe deformity or neuromuscular patients, to evaluate for chronic hypoxemia.
- EKG and cardiac echocardiography should be obtained when scoliosis or the primary neuromuscular disorder causes cardiac dysfunction (cardiomyopathies, rhythm

Handbook of Critical Incidents and Essential Topics in Pediatric Anesthesiology, ed. David A. Young and Olutoyin A. Olutoye. Published by Cambridge University Press. © Cambridge University Press 2015.

disorder, cor pulmonale, pulmonary hypertension). Early onset scoliosis should be assessed for pulmonary hypertension.

Positioning

- Prone positioning is necessary for posterior fusion.
- Recommendations for the management of the prone patient for spine surgery may include:
  - Use of a wire-reinforced endotracheal tube (ETT) to avoid kinking.
  - Verify that the ETT is properly and reliably secured.
  - Use of dental guards and soft bite blocks to prevent tongue injuries from intraoperative neurophysiologic monitoring.
  - Pad all pressure points to avoid abrasions and contusions (face, eyes, chest, hips, knees).
  - Avoid brachial plexus stretching by positioning the arms at no more than 90° to the body.
  - Ensure that the abdomen is free in order to reduce respiratory resistance and blood shunting to the paravertebral veins.
  - Consideration for presurgical placement of external defibrillation pads in patients at higher risk.

Anesthetic management

- Most procedures will require standard monitors and an arterial line; patients at increased risk may benefit from monitoring the trend of central venous pressure values.
- Patients should have generous vascular access in order to effectively manage the potential for sudden and significant blood loss.
- Processed EEG monitoring may also be considered, particularly in older children or adolescents without neurologic disorders.
- Combined somatosensory evoked potentials (SSEP) and motor evoked potentials (MEP) are commonly utilized to detect intraoperative spinal cord injuries.
- Many anesthetic agents, particularly inhaled anesthetic gases, and neuromuscular blocking agents significantly interfere with SSEP and MEP monitors.
- Total intravenous anesthesia (TIVA) allows for effective neurophysiologic intraoperative monitoring (IOM) compared to use of volatile anesthetics since inhaled anesthetic agents depress MEP and SSEP amplitudes in a dose-dependent manner.
  - Propofol is usually a central component of TIVA: a major side effect can be hypotension, which can depress MEP amplitude secondary to spinal cord hypoperfusion. Therefore, it is crucial to maintain a constant level of anesthetic depth and blood pressure (i.e., avoid boluses of propofol).
  - Opioids: another key component of TIVA since they minimally affect the SSEP and MEP.
  - An alternative to consider or in addition to propofol: dexmedetomidine.
  - Midazolam can depress the SSEP amplitude.

- In the event of intraoperative acute loss or significant reduction of SSEP or MEP amplitude or increased latency:
    - Increase mean arterial blood pressure to ≥ 90 mmHg (reduce anesthetic depth, administer fluid bolus, and/or a vasoactive agent).
    - Optimize: hematocrit, temperature, oxygen and CO_2 tensions, acid–base balance.
    - Discuss with surgeon the "spinal cord injury protocol" (methylprednisolone 30 mg/kg IV followed by 5.4 mg/kg/hr for the next 23 hours).
    - Perform a "wake-up" test if loss persists despite therapy.

Intraoperative blood loss

- The degree of blood loss is significantly associated with type of scoliosis (patients with neuromuscular scoliosis typically have more blood loss than a patient with idiopathic scoliosis), body weight, number of the spinal levels involved, duration of surgical instrumentation, type of bone graft, and blood pressure.
- Strategies to reduce blood loss:
    - Moderate hypotension (systolic blood pressure lowered 20 mmHg from baseline).
    - Antifibrinolytic agents (tranexamic acid, TXA; aminocaproic acid).
    - Modification of patient position (ensuring that the abdomen is not compressed).
- Alternatives to homologous blood products:
    - Intraoperative blood salvage (cell saver).
    - Preoperative autologous blood donation.
    - Normovolemic hemodilution.

Other intraoperative complications

- Paralysis.
- Peripheral nerve injuries.
- Tongue laceration, soft tissue positional injuries.
- Vision loss (ischemic optic neuropathy, corneal abrasion).
- Intraoperative awareness.
- Pulmonary embolism.
- Deep venous thrombosis.
- Rhabdomyolysis.
- Coagulopathy.

Postoperative care

- Pain control
    - Postoperative pain can be severe following spine surgery.
    - Patient-controlled analgesia (PCA) is a common technique. Possible adjuncts are intravenous acetaminophen, ketorolac, and diazepam.
    - Epidural catheters can be placed under direct vision by the surgeon for postoperative pain management.

- Intensive care unit admission should be considered for the following patients:
  - Neuromuscular scoliosis.
  - Comorbidity conditions.
  - Combined anterior and posterior spinal fusions.
  - Intraoperative complications (major blood loss, loss of SSEP/MEP, cardiorespiratory insufficiency).
  - Significant fluid shifts/massive transfusion.

Further reading

Abu-Kishk I, Kozer E, et al. Pediatric scoliosis surgery – is postoperative intensive care unit admission really necessary? *Pediatr Anesth.* 2013; 23:271–7.

Bissonnette B. *Pediatric Anesthesia*. Shelton, CT: People's Medical Publishing House, 2011; 91:1527–50.

Davis PJ, Cladis FP, Motoyama EK. *Smith's Anesthesia for Infants and Children*, 8th edition. Philadelphia: Elsevier Mosby, 2011; 844–57.

Sethna NF, Zurakowski D, et al. Tranexamic acid reduces intraoperative blood loss in pediatric patients undergoing scoliosis surgery. *Anesthesiology.* 2005; 102(4):727–32.

Soundararajan N, Cunliffe M. Anaesthesia for spinal surgery in children. *Br J Anaesth.* 2007; 99:86–94.

Part C Clinical-based areas in pediatric anesthesiology

Chapter 152

Otolaryngology
General considerations
John E. Fiadjoe

- Surgery of the ear, nose and throat (ENT) is very common among children.
- Pressure equalizing tube (PET) placement and adenotonsillectomy are the most common performed surgeries in this category.
- The surgeon and anesthesiologist both share the airway. The table is often rotated 90° away from the anesthesiologist.
- Communication and cooperation between both teams is critical for a safe perioperative course.
- Upper respiratory tract infection (URI) is common in children presenting for surgery:
  ○ Surgery on children with fever and/or other signs of lower respiratory tract infection should be postponed. Surgery may proceed with mild URI symptoms.
  ○ Children with URI have increased airway reactivity during anesthesia (e.g., bronchospasm, laryngospasm, stridor, oxygen desaturation).
  ○ Parental input with regard to change in feeding habits or decreased activity level can be valuable in helping to make a decision to proceed or reschedule surgery.
  ○ Risk factors for adverse respiratory events in children with URI include copious secretions, nasal congestion, tracheal intubation, history of prematurity, history of reactive airway disease, parental smoking, and airway surgery.
- Laryngospasm occurs more frequently in children with URIs; management includes:
  ○ Positive pressure with 100% oxygen, jaw thrust.
  ○ Removal of laryngeal stimulus such as secretions and blood.
  ○ Deepening of anesthetic (e.g., inhaled agents, propofol).
  ○ Succinylcholine and atropine may be necessary to treat refractory laryngospasm.
- Obstructive sleep apnea is an indication for adenotonsillectomy. It may be obstructive, central or mixed:
  ○ Central apnea: absent airflow with no respiratory effort.
  ○ Obstructive: more than 90% reduction in airflow with respiratory efforts.
  ○ Airway features of patients with OSA include: long oval face, high palate, small triangular chin.
  ○ Patients with severe OSA need to be monitored in the ICU post procedure.

Handbook of Critical Incidents and Essential Topics in Pediatric Anesthesiology, ed. David A. Young and Olutoyin A. Olutoye. Published by Cambridge University Press. © Cambridge University Press 2015.

- Emergence agitation commonly occurs following ENT surgery:
  - Characterized by disorientation, screaming, kicking, incoherence.
  - Unclear etiology; hypotheses include rapid emergence from anesthesia, variable central nervous system recovery, pain.
  - Risk factors: Usually occurs in children < 5 years of age, parental anxiety, rapid emergence or use of sevoflurane.
  - May result in self-injury, bleeding, removal of surgical dressings, and dislodgement of intravenous catheters.
  - Severity can be assessed using the Pediatric Anesthesia Emergence Delirium Scale (PAEDS).
  - Five criteria: eye contact, purposeful movement, awareness of environment, restlessness, inconsolability.
- Nausea and vomiting is another common complication of ENT surgery.
  - Is common cause of delayed discharge from post-anesthesia care unit (PACU).
  - Prophylaxis includes administration of dexamethasone (0.2–0.5 mg/kg) at beginning of surgery and ondansetron 0.1–0.15 mg/kg towards end of surgery.
  - Side effects of ondansetron include headaches, dizziness, and (with high doses) prolonged QT.

Further reading

Coté CJ, Lerman J, Anderson BJ. *Coté and Lerman's A Practice of Anesthesia for Infants and Children*, 5th edition. Philadelphia, PA: Elsevier, 2013; 390–2.

Levine A, Govindaraj S, DeMaria S. *Anesthesiology and Otolaryngology*. New York: Springer, 2013; 333–62.

Part C Clinical-based areas in pediatric anesthesiology

Chapter 153

Otolaryngology
Adenotonsillectomy/otologic procedures

John E. Fiadjoe and Senthilkumar Sadhasivam

Adenotonsillectomy

- Each year, approximately 500,000 adenotonsillectomies are performed in the United States.
- Obstructive sleep apnea (OSA) and recurrent tonsillitis are the two most common indications for adenotonsillectomy.
- OSA is a major public health concern as its incidence and severity are increasing in direct correlation to the obesity epidemic.
- Approximately one in eight American children will undergo tonsillectomy; adenotonsillar hypertrophy is the major contributing factor to OSA and adenotonsillectomy is the curative surgical treatment.
- With an increasing prevalence of obesity and OSA in childhood, more children are expected to receive anesthesia in the future for adenotonsillectomy. In children, OSA is often associated with substantial perioperative morbidity and even mortality.

Peri-operative anesthetic management

- Preoperative assessment and optimization of OSA in a child presenting for adenotonsillectomy is valuable.
- If the child has been diagnosed with OSA, it is important to inquire about the severity and current management such as home monitoring, respiratory support, supplemental oxygen administration, and preferred sleep position.
- The diagnosis of OSA is commonly made based on the clinical symptoms preoperatively without a traditional sleep study.
- If preoperative polysomnography was performed, important information to evaluate includes number of apneic/bradycardia episodes, the nadir and duration of oxygen saturation, as well as the peak $ETCO_2$ measurements.
- Patients with nadir episodes of oxygen desaturation reaching 70% during sleep may develop chronic hypercarbia and subsequently increased pulmonary pressures resulting in cor pulmonale.
- These patients require an electrocardiogram, echocardiogram, and evaluation by a cardiologist before elective surgery.

Handbook of Critical Incidents and Essential Topics in Pediatric Anesthesiology, ed. David A. Young and Olutoyin A. Olutoye. Published by Cambridge University Press. © Cambridge University Press 2015.

Premedication
- Anesthesiologists must be cautious with sedating premedication in children with severe OSA in the setting of inadequate monitoring as significant airway obstruction and severe oxygen desaturation may occur.
- Continuous pulse oximetry and clinical observation are strongly recommended.
- Residual effects from the premedication may persist, especially after a relatively short tonsillectomy procedure, and may exacerbate postoperative respiratory complications.

Induction of anesthesia
- Inhalation induction of children with significant OSA can often lead to significant airway obstruction: inhalational anesthetic agents reduce pharyngeal muscular tone, resulting in a subsequent upper airway obstruction.
- Upper airway obstruction during induction of general anesthesia should be expected; continuous positive airway pressure (CPAP) may significantly reduce upper airway obstruction.
- On the contrary, airway collapsibility and respiratory depression seem to be relatively less after the administration of ketamine and dexmedetomidine.
- Increased sensitivity to intraoperative and postoperative opioids in children with OSA should be expected due to an upregulation of μ opioid receptors from recurrent episodes of hypoxia.
- Co-administration of non-opioid analgesics (e.g., dexmedetomidine, acetaminophen, ketamine, and dexamethasone) often reduces opioid requirements and subsequent opioid-related respiratory depression.

Post-anesthetic emergence
Post-anesthetic emergence in children with severe OSA can be a challenge; awake extubation with full recovery of strength and minimal residual anesthetic drug concentrations may reduce postoperative respiratory conditions.

Postoperative pain management
- Postoperative pain management follows the same principles as described above.
- The use of non-opioid analgesics and techniques must be strongly considered to decrease the doses of opioid administration.
- Children older than 3 years of age with OSA may benefit from overnight postoperative observation; it is common practice to require postoperative observation for children less than 3 years of age.
- Largest reports of mortality following tonsillectomy revealed that events not related to post-tonsillectomy bleeding, such as use of opioids, account for a significant number of deaths and anoxic brain injury.
- A major limitation of opioids in children with OSA undergoing tonsillectomy is life-threatening respiratory depression, especially in unmonitored home settings.
- Ultrarapid metabolizers of codeine are especially at higher risk for postoperative respiratory depression and death. Following multiple deaths and respiratory

complications from the use of codeine, the US Food and Drug Administration recently added a black box warning against the use of codeine in children following adenotonsillectomy to manage postoperative pain.
- Planned administration of opioid-sparing analgesics such as acetaminophen, ibuprofen, and dexamethasone, avoiding automatic use of potent opioids (especially opioids dependent on the CYP2D6 pathway such as codeine and tramadol), and use of the lowest effective doses of non-CYP2D6 opioids on an as-needed basis are expected to increase safety and efficacy of post-tonsillectomy pain management.

Further reading

Brown KA, Laferriere A, Lakheeram I, Moss IR. Recurrent hypoxemia in children is associated with increased analgesic sensitivity to opiates. *Anesthesiology* 2006; 105:665–9.

Cote CJ, Posner KL, Domino KB. Death or Neurologic Injury after Tonsillectomy in Children with a focus on Obstructive Sleep Apnea: Houston, We Have a Problem! *Anesthesia & Analgesia* 2014; 118: 1276–83.

Davis PJ, Cladis FP, Motoyama EK. *Smith's Anesthesia for Infants and Children*, 8th edition. Philadelphia: Elsevier Mosby, 2011; 794–9.

Food and Drug Administration. Safety review update of codeine use in children; new Boxed Warning and Contraindication on use after tonsillectomy and/or adenoidectomy. *FDA Drug Safety Communication:* 2013: www.fda.gov/Drugs/DrugSafety/ucm339112.htm

Patino M, Sadhasivam S, Mahmoud M. Obstructive sleep apnoea in children. *British Journal of Anaesthesia* December 2013 PGA Special Issue.

Subramanyam R, Varughese A, Willging JP, Sadhasivam S. Future of pediatric tonsillectomy and perioperative outcomes. *Int J Pediatr Otorhinolaryngol.* 2013; 77:194–9.

Part C Clinical-based areas in pediatric anesthesiology

Chapter 154

Otolaryngology
Airway surgery/airway foreign body
John E. Fiadjoe

Laser surgery

- Laser is an acronym for light amplification by stimulated emission of radiation.
- Laser surgery is useful for supraglottoplasty in patients with laryngomalacia, laryngeal papilloma excision, and treatment of hemangiomas.
- Laryngomalacia, laryngeal collapse during inspiration secondary to immature cartilage, is a common cause of stridor in infants.
- Carbon dioxide (CO_2) and KTP (potassium titanyl phosphate) lasers are most commonly used for airway surgery.
- The CO_2 laser has a long wavelength in the infrared spectrum, is absorbed by water, and does not penetrate beyond the first few layers of cells; regular glasses provide protection.
- The KTP laser produces a beam which is visible as a green dot; special eye protection is required.
- Maintain FiO_2 less than 30% during laser use, avoid nitrous oxide, and protect the patient's eyes with shields.
- Most anesthesia techniques utilize maintenance of spontaneous ventilation; total intravenous anesthesia (TIVA) and inhaled agents are both acceptable.
- Complications of surgery include airway fire, eye injury, and vaporized infectious or mutagenic material.
- Airway fire management: remove burning material, stop oxidizer flow, extinguish fire, and evaluate the airway.

Tracheostomy

- Indications: airway obstruction, prolonged mechanical ventilation, pulmonary toilet
    - Airway obstruction: craniofacial abnormalities, congenital or acquired subglottic stenosis, severe tracheomalacia, vocal cord paralysis.
    - Prolonged mechanical ventilation: bronchopulmonary dysplasia, central hypoventilation.
    - Pulmonary toilet: children with severe neurologic or pulmonary disease.
- Good communication between surgery and anesthesia teams is mandatory.
- Avoid neuromuscular blockade if unobstructed airway cannot be maintained.

Handbook of Critical Incidents and Essential Topics in Pediatric Anesthesiology, ed. David A. Young and Olutoyin A. Olutoye. Published by Cambridge University Press. © Cambridge University Press 2015.

- Elective tracheostomies are performed in children requiring prolonged mechanical ventilation.
- The patient is positioned supine with a shoulder roll, neck extended, the incision is made, and stay sutures placed to allow identification of stoma if tracheostomy is dislodged.
- Stay sutures should be marked right and left so that pulling on the sutures in the proper direction results in the opening of the tracheostomy site.
- Decreased inspired concentration of oxygen (FiO_2) is required when electrocautery is in use; the use of electrocautery to enter the trachea should be avoided.
- Prior to making tracheal incision:
  - The anesthesia team should be notified by the otolaryngologist.
  - If a cuffed endotracheal tube is present, the cuff should be deflated.
  - The existing endotracheal tube should be withdrawn prior to insertion of the tracheostomy.
- Upon tracheostomy insertion, end-tidal carbon dioxide should be confirmed prior to complete removal of endotracheal tube from the pharynx.
- Complications: hemorrhage, subcutaneous emphysema, pneumomediastinum, pneumothorax, airway fire, creation of a false passage, recurrent laryngeal nerve injury.
- Patients should recover in the intensive care unit (ICU); a backup tracheostomy tube should be available at the patient's bedside.

Subglottic stenosis

- Defined as diameter < 4 mm at the level of the cricoid in full-term infant, and < 3.5 mm in premature infant. Common in premature babies.
- May be congenital or secondary to intubation trauma, infection, caustic smoke inhalation, blunt trauma, and neoplasms.
- Subglottis is a complete circular cartilage lined by respiratory epithelium.
- High incidence of gastro-esophageal reflux in these patients.
- Evaluation is with rigid bronchoscopy under anesthesia.
- Anesthetic management and goals:
  - Mask induction, application of topical lidocaine under deep anesthesia.
  - Total intravenous anesthesia (TIVA) and/or inhaled anesthetic agents can be used.
  - Ventilation/oxygenation occurs through side port of ventilating bronchoscope.
  - Maintain spontaneous ventilation.
  - Minimize secretions.
  - Decrease airway reflexes.
- Surgical correction is by cricoid split, single or double stage laryngotracheal reconstruction (LTR).
  - Cricoid split – Incision is made through the cricoid ring, first two tracheal rings and lower one-third of thyroid cartilage. Neck is closed with an endotracheal tube (ETT) in place to act as stent.

- LTR can be single stage (cartilage grafts supported by ETT kept in place for prolonged period 2–10 days) or double stage (permanent stent maintains the airway while graft heals). Rib grafts often used.
- Cricotracheal resection (CTR) removes narrowed section and reconnects trachea, performed for severe disease.

Choanal atresia

- No connection between the nasal cavity and aerodigestive tract.
- Signs: cyanosis while feeding, unilateral nasal drainage, respiratory distress.
- Associated syndromes: Apert, Di-George, Trisomy 18, Treacher Collins, CHARGE association.
- May be unilateral or bilateral.
- Oral airway, McGovern nipple (large nipple with cross-cuts in the end) may help, bilateral cases may need tracheostomy.
- Rule of tens for surgery: 10 weeks, 10 pounds, and hemoglobin of 10 g/dL.
- Intravenous induction commonly used, oral RAE tube.
- Intranasal repair involves opening atretic area with dilators and placing stent.
- Transpalatal repair involves removal of part of hard palate and posterior septum.
- Postoperative monitoring in the ICU for bilateral cases.
- Restenosis is a common problem.

Foreign body

- Food is the most commonly aspirated material.
- Children are at highest risk (1–3 years), signs include coughing, wheezing, shortness of breath.
- Preoperative workup includes physical examination, chest X-ray (lateral and supine expiratory film), few foreign bodies (FBs) are radio-opaque but air trapping, atelectasis, hyperinflation, pneumonia, localized emphysema, and asymmetric breath sounds can suggest location of FB.
- Lateral chest film: hyperinflation of affected side due to FB.
- Battery aspiration is an emergency as corrosive chemicals can rapidly erode mucosa.
- Symptoms vary with FB location:
  - Supraglottic: inspiratory stridor, dyspnea and cough.
  - Glottic or subglottic: biphasic stridor, cough and hoarseness.
  - Intrathoracic: expiratory stridor.
- Inhalation or intravenous induction acceptable.
- Avoid nitrous oxide because of hyperinflation and air trapping.
- Some providers prefer TIVA technique instead of inhalational agents due to less operating room pollution and interruption of ventilation. Propofol and remifentanil are commonly used agents.
- Spontaneous vs. controlled ventilation controversial but critically important is endoscopist's preparation, equipment, and skill.

- Topical anesthesia of the vocal cords is necessary if spontaneous ventilation is maintained.
- Spontaneous ventilation typically maintains oxygenation throughout procedure.
- Controlled ventilation may dislodge FB and worsen obstruction.
- Problems encountered include increased work of breathing with spontaneously ventilating patients, leak around the bronchoscope, laryngospasm, bronchospasm, hypoxemia, pneumothorax, pneumomediastinum, obstruction by FB, and cardiac arrest.
- Management of dislodged/obstructing FB:
    - Object in the trachea that cannot be removed promptly should be advanced into a bronchus to allow reestablishment of ventilation.
    - Foreign body that dislodges into unaffected bronchus should be advanced back into original bronchus in order to avoid occluding a "good" bronchus (bronchus that FBs are originally aspirated into tend to be edematous).
- Dexamethasone 0.5 mg/kg helps reduce edema after removal of FB.
- Postoperative disposition depends on preoperative respiratory status, type of FB, duration of impaction, and difficulty of extraction.
    - Uncomplicated cases may go home; patients with respiratory compromise should be observed in the intensive care unit.

Further reading

Coté CJ, Lerman J, Anderson BJ. *Coté and Lerman's A Practice of Anesthesia for Infants and Children*, 5th edition. Philadelphia, PA: Elsevier, 2013; 1068–8.

Gregory GA, Andropoulos DB. *Gregory's Pediatric Anesthesia*, 5th edition. Hoboken: Wiley-Blackwell, 2012; 401–8.

Levine A, Govindaraj S, DeMaria S *Anesthesiology and Otolaryngology*. New York: Springer, 2013; 333–62.

Part C Clinical-based areas in pediatric anesthesiology

Chapter 155

Pain medicine
General considerations
Andrew J. Costandi and Senthilkumar Sadhasivam

Introduction

- Pain is a subjective experience described as "an unpleasant sensory and emotional experience associated with actual or potential tissue damage."
- Pain remains undertreated in children due to difficulty in assessment of pain among this population, lack of pediatric pain management services in many hospitals, lack of in-depth knowledge about inter-individual variability, and misconceptions about opioid safety and addiction.
- Improved understanding of developmental neurobiology, pediatric analgesic pharmacokinetics, and utilizing more effective pain assessment tools should facilitate improved pain management to children.

Pain assessment

- There is evidence that children experience short- and long-term physical, physiological, and psychological effects due to untreated pain.
- Selection of appropriate pain assessment tools should consider age, cognitive level, and the presence of disability, type of pain, and the situation in which pain is occurring.
- Optimal assessment scores provide accurate data about pain location, its intensity, and the effectiveness of the measures used to alleviate or abolish it.
  - Older children and adolescents can be assessed with the standard adult self-report scales such as visual analog scales (VAS) and numerical rating scales (NRS) (0 = no pain and 10 = worst pain).
  - In children 3–6 years old, pain can be assessed using word descriptors or pictures like the "Six-Face Pain Scale."
  - In infants, newborns, and sedated or cognitively impaired patients, the level of pain is assessed by physiologic, observational, and behavioral indices. Physiologic indices of pain include: tachycardia, tachypnea, and hypertension. Observational and behavioral indices include facial expressions, cry characteristics, and body movement. For infants, the revised Face, Legs, Activity, Cry, and Consolability (FLACC) score is commonly used. On the other hand, the COMFORT scale is used more often for neonates and sedated patients.

Handbook of Critical Incidents and Essential Topics in Pediatric Anesthesiology, ed. David A. Young and Olutoyin A. Olutoye. Published by Cambridge University Press. © Cambridge University Press 2015.

Pain neurophysiology

- Besides developmental differences when compared to adults, children exhibit exaggerated emotional and behavioral components of pain including higher anxiety and altered coping mechanisms.
- With the rapid growth of knowledge in infant neurobiology, long-held concepts about the lack of pain perception in the fetus and newborn have been challenged. Fetal stress in response to painful stimuli has been shown. The obliteration of this response by the administration of opioids to the fetus suggests an analgesic effect.
- Thalamocortical connections underpinning the neuroanatomy of pain appear at 20–30 weeks gestational age, and the physiologic mechanisms for pain perception become established by early second trimester.
- Nociceptors are sensory receptors responsible for the detection of noxious stimuli distributed throughout the body (skin, viscera, muscles, joints, and meninges) and can be stimulated by mechanical, thermal, or chemical stimuli.
- Inflammatory mediators (e.g., bradykinin, serotonin, prostaglandins, cytokines, and H^+) are released from damaged tissue and can stimulate nociceptors directly.
- A-delta fibers transmit "first pain," which is rapid, sharp, localized pain that lasts as long as the original stimulus.
- C fibers transmit the "second pain," which is slow, diffuse, dull pain that lasts beyond the termination of the stimulus.
- A-delta and C fibers synapse with secondary afferent neurons in the dorsal horn of the spinal cord that ascend via the spinothalamic tract and the spinoreticular tract to the thalamus and the somatosensory cortex in the brain.
- In newborns and infants, since specific connections in the pain pathway are immature, the receptive field areas in the dorsal horn of the spinal cord that respond to stimulation are relatively large. Moreover, inhibiting descending input from the brain is nonfunctional in the first few weeks of life, leading to exaggerated reflex responses to pain in this age group.

Preemptive analgesia and multimodal approach

- Preemptive analgesia is a treatment that proactively prevents establishment of the altered sensory processing that amplifies postoperative pain. The treatment should cover the entire duration of high-intensity noxious stimulation that can lead to establishment of central and peripheral sensitization caused by incisional or inflammatory injuries.
- The multimodal approach utilizes the concept of preemptive analgesia and aims at targeting multiple sites along the pain pathway to prevent central sensitization and rewiring, avoiding increased pain perception for future painful insults, and maximizing pain control, while minimizing drug-induced adverse side effects. This approach includes both pharmacologic and non-pharmacologic therapies.
- Pharmacologic therapies include: opioid, non-opioid analgesics, and adjuvants.
  - Opioid analgesics are the corner stone in acute pain control. They should be used in a multimodal balanced analgesia approach that minimizes opioid requirements and the degree of their side effects.

- The non-opioid analgesics (acetaminophen, nonsteroidal anti-inflammatory drugs; NSAIDs) are useful alone for mild to moderate pain and provide additive analgesia when combined with opioid drugs.
- Adjuvant analgesics are drugs that have a primary indication other than pain (i.e., NMDA antagonists and alpha-2 adrenergic agonists, corticosteroids, and benzodiazepines). They produce analgesia as a secondary effect and decrease opioid dosing, but display a "ceiling effect" on analgesia, irrespective of the dose administered. Local anesthetics may be utilized in neuraxial and peripheral nerve blocks to ameliorate pain reception.

- Non-pharmacologic therapies include behavioral methods such as distraction, coping mechanisms, and relaxation techniques. It also includes the use of TENS units and acupuncture.

Further reading

Chiaretti A, Pierri F, Valentini P et al. Current practice and recent advances in pediatric pain management. *Eur Rev Med Pharmacol Sci.* 2013; 17(1 Suppl):112–26.

Coté CJ, Lerman J, Anderson BJ. *Coté and Lerman's A Practice of Anesthesia for Infants and Children*, 5th edition. Philadelphia, PA: Elsevier, 2013; 909–15.

Davis PJ, Cladis FP, Motoyama EK. *Smith's Anesthesia for Infants and Children*, 8th edition. Philadelphia: Elsevier Mosby, 2011; 418–24.

Part C Clinical-based areas in pediatric anesthesiology

Chapter 156

Pain medicine
Acute pain management
Vidya Chidambaran and Senthilkumar Sadhasivam

Introduction

- The practice of pediatric pain management has made great progress in the recent past with development of pain assessment tools specific to children, dedicated pain services in major pediatric hospitals, and evidence from pediatric clinical trials.
- However, acute pain remains under-recognized and under-treated even among hospitalized children. Parental behavior and misconceptions regarding pain medications, including fear of opioid addiction and fear of serious adverse drug effects, constitute reasons for suboptimal analgesia.

Preoperative history and pain assessment

- While self-reporting of pain is the gold standard of pain assessment in adults, it is difficult to obtain in non-verbal or developmentally delayed children.
- Special attention to the biopsychosocial nature of pain is essential as this population presents developmental differences in their experience of pain and response to analgesics.
- Pain perception and coping are affected by
  - Fear.
  - Anxiety.
  - Non-comprehension of the situation.
  - Societal or family support.
- Preoperative assessment includes
  - A comprehensive history.
  - Exaggerating and alleviating factors.
  - Pain medications (basal requirements and side effects).
  - Renal, hepatic or respiratory issues.
  - Contraindications for regional techniques.
  - Physical examination.
- Importantly, the goals are
  - To adjust or continue medications whose sudden cessation may provoke withdrawal.
  - Preoperative treatment of pain and anxiety.

Handbook of Critical Incidents and Essential Topics in Pediatric Anesthesiology, ed. David A. Young and Olutoyin A. Olutoye. Published by Cambridge University Press. © Cambridge University Press 2015.

- Patient/family education and informed discussion about the plan for postoperative analgesia.

Pharmacologic interventions

- Opioids are the mainstay of perioperative analgesia. It is advisable to titrate opioids due to their narrow therapeutic indices and inter-individual variability in responses.
- Side effects of opioids include
    - Pruritus.
    - Vomiting/nausea.
    - Constipation.
    - Sedation.
    - Respiratory depression.
- The risk of potentially fatal respiratory depression with opioids is high in the presence of risk factors such as
    - Sleep apnea.
    - Extremes of age.
    - Concomitant administration of sedatives.
- Morphine, fentanyl, and hydromorphone are the most commonly used parenteral opioids.
- Patient/proxy controlled analgesia (PCA)
    - PCA is an effective way of achieving optimal analgesia in children.
    - There are concerns that proxy control bypasses the safety feature of the PCA, wherein an oversedated patient cannot push the button. However, in children < 6 years of age, proxy-controlled PCA is commonly and effectively used.
    - Written and verbal instructions to parents regarding proper use of the PCA, emphasizing the dangers of pressing the button when the child is not in pain, and use of strict sedation and respiratory monitoring, are essential
- Oral opioids
    - Oxycodone commonly used to treat postoperative pain.
    - When used in combination with acetaminophen, the dosage is often restricted by the maximum allowed daily dose of acetaminophen.
    - FDA has recently issued warnings regarding use of codeine as it is metabolized by *CYP2D6* cytochromes in the liver. Ultrarapid metabolizers of *CYP2D6* convert codeine to the active drug morphine at a faster pace, causing serious respiratory depression and even death.
    - Similar to codeine, to some extent other oral opioids such as tramadol, hydrocodone, and oxycodone are also metabolized by the CYP2D6 pathway
- Managing opioid adverse effects
    - Opioid agonist-antagonists (butorphanol, nalbuphine) can be administered to patients sensitive to opioid-induced respiratory depression, pruritus, vomiting, and ileus.
    - Naloxone infusions can be employed to treat pruritus.
    - Hypoventilation is often treated with stimulation and naloxone (in incremental 1µg/kg doses).

- Life-threatening apnea may require controlled ventilation.
- Constipation, a common opioid side effect, slows recovery and remains difficult to treat. The use of stool softeners (docusate sodium), stimulants (senna, bisacodyl) and osmotic (lactulose) laxatives are the mainstay of therapy and prevention.
- Opioid adjuncts are commonly used along with opioids
    - Benzodiazepines such as diazepam (0.05–0.1 mg/kg) and lorazepam (0.05 mg/kg) for muscle relaxation and anxiety.
    - Methocarbamol (10–15 mg/kg), a less sedating skeletal muscle relaxant, is a useful adjunct.
    - Especially useful after major scoliosis, pectus, bladder, and hip surgeries.
- Non-opioid analgesics
    - Intravenous acetaminophen was approved by the FDA in 2010 for use in children > 2 years old.
        - A centrally acting cyclooxygenase inhibitor
        - Intravenous use produces a higher peak serum concentration than oral administration.
        - Recommended pediatric dose (> 2 years) 10–15 mg/kg IV 6-hourly, with a maximum daily dose of 75 mg/kg/day.
    - NSAIDs (e.g., ketorolac) produce analgesia and decrease opioid requirements.
        - Mechanism of action involves inhibition of cyclooxygenases and prostaglandin synthesis, which also produces side effects including impaired renal function, gastric mucosal irritation, decreased platelet activity, and possible delayed bone healing.

Regional analgesia

- In children, use of regional techniques is generally in conjunction with general anesthesia.
- Importantly, infants are more susceptible to toxicity from local anesthetics because of decreased metabolism and protein binding leading to increased free concentrations of local anesthetic.
- Neuraxial techniques
    - Compared to adults, the dural sac and spinal cord in the neonate both terminate lower at levels S3 and L3 respectively.
    - Neuraxial blocks in children have minimal hemodynamic effects compared to adults due to minimal sympathetic blockade.
    - Caudal blocks are the most commonly used regional technique.
    - Doses of 0.5 mL/kg of 0.2% ropivacaine are sufficient for incisions below T12 and 0.75 mL/kg for incisions below T10.
    - Preservative free morphine 50 µg/kg may be added to the local anesthetic mixture for longer acting analgesia; hospitalization for at least 24 hours to have respiratory monitoring is strongly recommended.
    - Intrathecal opioids such as morphine (4–5 µg/kg) can also be used to prolong analgesia.
    - Neuraxial opioids often cause pruritus but rarely produce significant respiratory depression.

- Epidural catheters can be advanced via the caudal route up to thoracic segments in infants.
- To reduce risk of contamination of catheters and colonization with bacteria, subcutaneous tunneling of the catheter to a higher position and use of bio-occlusive barriers has been recommended.
- Use of fluoroscopy, stimulating catheters, and ultrasound can guide accurate placement of the catheters.
- Maximum recommended dose for 0.1% bupivacaine is 0.4 mg/kg/hr for infants > 6 months old. Adjuncts such as opioids and clonidine can be added to the epidural solutions.

- Peripheral nerve blocks
  - Use of ultrasound has led to increased use of peripheral nerve blocks and continuous catheters for orthopedic procedures in anesthetized children.
  - Femoral and sciatic nerve blocks are commonly placed for knee surgeries.
  - Interscalene nerve blocks with a continuous catheter can be utilized in shoulder surgeries to extend analgesia for 2–3 days.
  - Education regarding symptoms and signs of local anesthetic toxicity as well as close follow-up after discharge is essential to maintain safety and efficacy.
  - Use of dilute local anesthetic solutions generally does not mask the development of compartment syndrome.
  - The incidence of peroneal nerve palsy after knee surgery with sciatic nerve blocks is < 1% among the general population but increases in the presence of underlying medical conditions affecting nerves such as rheumatoid arthritis, diabetes mellitus and malignancy (i.e., use of neurotoxic chemotherapy).
  - Use of transversus abdominis plane (TAP) blocks for abdominal surgeries has also been gaining popularity as it is beneficial in reducing opioid requirements without the inherent risks of traditional neuraxial techniques.

Further reading

Chidambaran V, Sadhasivam S. Pediatric acute and surgical pain management: recent advances and future perspectives. *Int Anesthesiol Clin.* 2012; 50(4):66–82. Epub 2012/10/11.

Coté CJ, Lerman J, Anderson BJ. *Coté and Lerman's A Practice of Anesthesia for Infants and Children*, 5th edition. Philadelphia, PA: Elsevier, 2013; 917–33.

Practice guidelines for acute pain management in the perioperative setting: an updated report by the American Society of Anesthesiologists Task Force on Acute Pain Management. *Anesthesiology.* 2012; 116(2):248–73. Epub 2012/01/10.

Sadhasivam S, Chidambaran V. Pharmacogenomics of opioids and perioperative pain management. *Pharmacogenomics.* 2012; 13(15):1719–40. Epub 2012/11/23.

Verghese ST, Hannallah RS. Acute pain management in children. *J Pain Res.* 2010; 3:105–23. Epub 2011/01/05.

Willschke H, Marhofer P, Machata AM, Lonnqvist PA. Current trends in paediatric regional anaesthesia. *Anaesthesia.* 2010; 65 Suppl 1:97–104. Epub 2010/04/14.

Part C — Clinical-based areas in pediatric anesthesiology

Chapter 157

Pain medicine
Chronic pain management
Alexandra Szabova and Kenneth Goldschneider

Patient on long-term opioid analgesics

Perioperative implications

- Significant prolongation of gastrointestinal transit time as a result of opioid use.
    - Potential for increased gastric volumes and perioperative aspiration despite fasting.
- Tolerance to opioid analgesics (increasing doses required to achieve the same analgesic effect). Abrupt cessation of opioids may result in a withdrawal syndrome.
    - Mechanisms for tolerance are complex and involve several CNS receptor and mediator pathways.
- Tolerance raises perioperative opioid requirements.

Management strategies

- Preoperative
    - Have patient take morning dose of opioid with a sip of water.
    - If unable to take enteral opioids, provide intravenous equivalent of baseline opioid.
- Intraoperative
    - Consider managing induction and emergence as for a patient with a full stomach.
    - Be prepared for higher than expected opioid requirements.
    - Consider regional anesthesia/analgesia whenever possible.
    - Consider use of opioid adjuncts: ketamine, acetaminophen, ketorolac (and methadone as an alternative opioid).
- Postoperative
    - Continue the equivalent of the preoperative opioid regimen in addition to any planned analgesia.
    - May need to aggressively titrate opioids to gain effective pain control.
    - Utilize epidural/nerve catheter techniques for postoperative analgesia as much as possible.

Handbook of Critical Incidents and Essential Topics in Pediatric Anesthesiology, ed. David A. Young and Olutoyin A. Olutoye. Published by Cambridge University Press. © Cambridge University Press 2015.

- Consult with primary pain physician before altering home pain regimen or sending prescriptions home with patient.

Patient with complex regional pain syndrome

Perioperative implications

- Complex regional pain syndrome (CRPS) is a prototypical neuropathic pain characterized by persistent severe pain (with or without specific nerve injury) and sensory, vasomotor, trophic, and motor signs.
- Perioperative goal: prevent flare-up of ongoing or resolved CRPS.
- Emotional stress and surgical trauma can trigger increased symptoms.
- Reassure the patient about perioperative pain care, continue outpatient therapies, and provide acute anxiolysis when needed.

Management strategies

- Preoperative
    - Consider vitamin C supplementation, 1 gram daily PO, 3–7 days prior to surgery.
    - Start anticonvulsant (e.g., gabapentin 5 mg/kg at bedtime for 3 nights, then increase to 10 mg/kg at bedtime) or tricyclic antidepressant (e.g., amitriptyline 0.5 mg/kg at bedtime).
    - Consider starting dextromethorphan for its NMDA-antagonist effects.
- Intraoperative
    - Use regional anesthesia/analgesia whenever possible.
    - Ketamine and methadone may also be useful.
- Postoperative
    - Consider nerve catheter techniques for analgesia.
    - Titrate opioids to effect.
    - Continue vitamin C and neuropathic medications. Wean when symptoms are stable or after approximately 2 months, if asymptomatic.

Preparing for phantom limb pain

Perioperative implications

- Phantom limb pain (PLP) affects 42–78% of patients.
- Can occur any time after 1 week postoperatively.
- Risk factors: females, preexisting pain in amputated extremity, stump pain (pain in remaining portion of the limb), upper extremity amputation.
- PLP results from loss of normal interactions among peripheral, spinal and brain efferent, afferent and integrative pathways.
- PLP is difficult to treat; emphasis is on prevention.

Management strategies

- Preoperative
  - Educate patient about differences between PLP, phantom limb sensation (non-painful feelings of the amputated extremity still being present), and stump pain.
  - Strongly consider administering gabapentin, vitamin C, or dextromethorphan.
  - Ideally, start conduction blockade 24 hours prior to amputation.
- Intraoperative
  - Neuraxial or peripheral nerve block via catheter techniques to achieve dense block.
  - Consider ketamine and methadone.
- Postoperative
  - Continue nerve conduction blockade for 3–7 days.
  - Continue gabapentin, vitamin C, dextromethorphan for 1–2 months.
  - Consider methadone when transitioning to oral analgesia.

Chronic pain medications in the perioperative period

Perioperative implications

- Most chronic pain medications have associated withdrawal syndromes if stopped abruptly.
- Baclofen has no IV form and withdrawal can be life-threatening.
- NSAIDs: hold or continue per surgical preference.
- Methadone can prolong QT interval; use caution when administering other perioperative medications that can prolong the QT interval (e.g., ondansetron).

Management strategies

- Patients should take their home medications with a sip of water preoperatively when possible.
- Oral medications should be converted to intravenous or transdermal forms while the patient is fasting.
- Medications that are only available in enteral forms may be managed by:
  - Holding for a dose or two, and restart as soon as possible.
  - If prolonged fasting is anticipated, wean off ahead of time.
  - Finding an acceptable alternative that can be given by the intravenous route.

Chronic pain patient in the post-anesthesia care unit

Perioperative implications

- Tolerance, prior sensitization, anxiety, and often maladaptive coping all account for increased analgesic requirements.
- In patient with high baseline pain levels, reports of high pain levels postoperatively should be expected and may be misinterpreted as poor pain control.

- Do not treat pain scale numbers in isolation. Use a combination of numeric, subjective and observational reports.

Management strategies
- Assess preexisting and situational anxiety.
- Consider use of anxiolytics. Delay often results in administering large amounts of opioid followed by benzodiazepines which may then lead to respiratory depression.
- Consider utilizing non-pharmacologic treatments such as child life specialists, psychologists, and specialists in integrative medicine.

Further reading

Abraham BR, Marouani N, Kollender Y, Meller I, Weinbroum AA. Dextromethorphan for phantom pain attenuation in cancer amputees: a double-blind crossover trial involving three patients. *Clin J Pain*. 2002; 18(5):282–5.

Cote CJ, Lerman J, Anderson BJ. *A Practice of Anesthesia for Infants and Children*, 5th edition. Philadelphia: Churchill Livingstone Elsevier, 2013; 951–61.

Dworkin RH et al. Recommendations for the pharmacological management of neuropathic pain: an overview and literature update. *Mayo Clin Proc*. 2010; 85(3 Suppl): S3–S14.

Geary T, Negus A, Anderson BJ, Zernikow B. Perioperative management of the child on long-term opioids. *Paediatr Anaesth*. 2012; 22(3):189–202.

Zollinger PE, Kreis RW, van der Meulen HG, Maarten van der Elst, Breederveld RS, Tuinebreijer WE. No higher risk of CRPS after external fixation of distal radial fractures – subgroup analysis under randomised vitamin C prophylaxis. *Open Orthop J*. 2010; 4:71–7.

Part C Clinical-based areas in pediatric anesthesiology

Plastic surgery
General considerations
Rajeev Subramanyam and Senthilkumar Sadhasivam

General concepts

- Plastic surgery is performed in children of all ages with the majority between 1 and 9 years of age.
- A thorough preoperative assessment of the existing defects, associated comorbidities, and a multidisciplinary approach will contribute to a successful outcome.
- The most common anesthetic considerations are a suspected difficult airway and substantial intraoperative bleeding.
- Some common surgeries are discussed below. Craniofacial reconstruction (Chapter 159) and cleft surgery (Chapter 160) are discussed separately.

Hemifacial microsomia

- Hemifacial microsomia (HM) is the second most common facial defect after cleft lip/palate. The embryologic defect of HM involves the first and second branchial arch.
- Difficult airway, cardiac anomalies, renal defects, neurologic defects, and presence of sleep apnea are significant anesthetic considerations.
- Difficult airway management plans should be developed and equipment should be immediately available to manage any unanticipated difficulty in ventilation and/or intubation.
- Appropriate eye protection is necessary in order to reduce orbital compression and possible vision loss.
- Cardiac anomalies may require appropriate infective endocarditis prophylaxis.
- Frequent positioning changes to the head are sometimes required during surgery; care should be taken to prevent tracheal tube displacement.

Midface procedures

- A midface procedure is performed for maxillary hypoplasia which can be present in some congenital syndromes.
- Associated choanal atresia may make mask ventilation difficult even after insertion of an oral airway.
- Intubation is usually uncomplicated. Tongue-lip adhesion release and mandibular distractions typically require nasal intubation.

Handbook of Critical Incidents and Essential Topics in Pediatric Anesthesiology, ed. David A. Young and Olutoyin A. Olutoye. Published by Cambridge University Press. © Cambridge University Press 2015.

- Surgeons may request the intraoperative change from an oral to a nasal tracheal tube.
- Although blood loss can occur, it is not as significant as for craniofacial reconstruction. Generous vascular access should be secured and cross-matched red blood cells should be available.
- A nasogastric tube is usually placed for gastric decompression.
- If intermaxillary fixation is performed, a wire cutter should be immediately available at the bedside postoperatively.

Orthognathic surgery

- Indications are malocclusion due to facial hypoplasia and any other disorder affecting the face or jaw.
- Surgery is performed after completion of maxillary and mandibular growth; these patients tend to be adolescents.
- Anesthetic considerations include possible difficult airway and increased intraoperative bleeding.

Orbital hypertelorism

- Orbital hypertelorism comprises abnormally separated orbits.
- May be a part of other congenital abnormalities.
- Repair is usually performed at 5 years of age and the child may have undergone previous reconstructive surgeries.
- Either a subcranial or an intracranial approach is employed.
- Anesthetic considerations include presence of a difficult airway, significant blood loss and transfusion requirements, and oculocardiac reflex resulting in bradycardia. Oculocardiac reflex is reduced by atropine or glycopyrrolate and discontinuation of surgical stimulus.
- Awake extubation and postoperative monitoring for airway obstruction are both strongly encouraged.

Cystic hygromas

- Cystic hygroma is a rare lymphatic malformation of the head and neck occurring in 1:16,000 births.
- Associated with Noonan and Turner syndromes.
- Requires thorough airway evaluation and assessment for underlying syndromes.
- Increased vigilance for postoperative complications such as laryngeal edema, airway obstruction, pneumonia, and facial palsy is necessary.

Hemangiomas

- Hemangiomas may require surgical excision. Laser therapy under general anesthesia is more commonly utilized than excision.
- Oral propranolol reduces the need for surgical intervention and children may be on this medication preoperatively.
- Nitrous oxide is safe for induction, but may pose a fire hazard for lesions close to the face if continued during surgery.

- Airway malformations can cause respiratory obstruction. Laser therapy may initially cause swelling and can worsen preexisting respiratory obstruction.

Tissue expanders

- Expanders consist of silicone shell. They are used to treat congenital nevi, hemangiomas, abdominal wall defects, myelomeningocele, and burn scar reconstructions.
- Require a minimum of two surgeries: one to insert and the other to remove the silicone when expansion is complete.

Hand surgery

- Most hand anomalies are managed after the first year of life.
- Syndactyly may require correction during infancy.
- Superficial extra digits are commonly removed during the neonatal or infancy period.
- Constriction bands may require urgent surgical intervention.

Brachial plexus surgery

- Brachial plexus injury is believed to result from birth trauma. Erb's palsy involves nerve roots C5–7 and Klumpke's palsy C8 and T1.
- Small proportion of patients may also have clinically significant diaphragmatic involvement.
- Anesthetic considerations include the long duration of surgery, use of neuromonitoring, and maintenance of normotherma.
- Total intravenous anesthesia techniques without neuromuscular blocking agents are commonly selected when neuromonitoring is required.
- Typically the only site for intravenous access is the contralateral arm. Both legs are commonly prepared sterile for sural nerve harvesting.
- Indwelling urinary catheter, vigilance for over-infusing crystalloids, proper pressure padding, and multiple warming devices are other important intraoperative considerations.
- Postoperative analgesic requirements are usually minimal. Acetaminophen and NSAIDs may provide adequate analgesia without the requirement for opioids.

Cosmetic procedures

- Patients are generally healthy and routine general anesthesia is used.
- Postoperative nausea and vomiting and postoperative pain may be more common.
- Liposuction involves use of high dose of lidocaine. Possibilities of lidocaine toxicity and fluid accumulation should be anticipated.

Further reading

Coté CJ, Lerman J, Anderson BJ. *Coté and Lerman's A Practice of Anesthesia for Infants and Children*, 5th edition. Philadelphia, PA: Elsevier, 2013; 697–711.

Davis PJ. *Smith's Anesthesia for Infants and Children*, 8th edition. Philadelphia: Elsevier, 2013; 821–41.

Part C Clinical-based areas in pediatric anesthesiology

Chapter 159

Plastic surgery

Craniofacial reconstruction

Rajeev Subramanyam and Senthilkumar Sadhasivam

General concepts

- Craniosynostosis is a condition in which one or more of the cranial sutures have closed prematurely.
- This premature closure may lead to restricted brain growth and increased intracranial pressure.
- The most common variant (about 80%) is simple or non-syndromic involving only one suture. The less common variant (about 20%) is complex or syndromic involving multiple sutures.
- Presence of syndromes requires evaluation for involvement of other organs particularly the heart; this may necessitate obtaining a preoperative echocardiogram.
- Repair involves cranial vault reconstruction typically performed in infancy. Less invasive techniques include extended strip craniectomy, endoscopic strip craniectomy, and spring-assisted cranioplasty.
- Indications for cranial vault reconstruction include increased intracranial pressure, severe exophthalmos, sleep apnea, craniofacial deformity, and psychosocial reasons.

Preoperative assessment

- The main focus of the preoperative assessment should focus on the airway evaluation and the presence of comorbid conditions.
- Obstructive sleep apnea may be present in children with syndromic craniosynostosis and may necessitate preoperative tonsillectomy or midfacial advancement.

Anesthetic considerations

- Anesthetic considerations should focus on airway management, eye protection, perioperative bleeding/transfusion, possible intracranial pressure, venous air embolism, prolonged surgery, and safety of pressure points.

Handbook of Critical Incidents and Essential Topics in Pediatric Anesthesiology, ed. David A. Young and Olutoyin A. Olutoye. Published by Cambridge University Press. © Cambridge University Press 2015.

Airway management

- The main focus of the preoperative assessment should focus on the evaluation of the airway. Airway management is complicated by presence of a syndrome associated with difficult airway and/or presence of sleep apnea.
- Awake intubation is not practical in young children and hence the anesthesiologist must be familiar with various airway securement techniques.
- Clear communication with the surgeon regarding the specific plan for securing the airway should be performed to reduce inadvertent tracheal tube dislodgment.

Bleeding and transfusion

- Blood loss is a significant contributor to morbidity and mortality. Blood loss can be sudden and significant.
- Various blood conservation strategies can be used. These include preoperative recombinant erythropoietin, use of cell saver, controlled hypotension, meticulous surgical technique, adrenaline infiltration, acute normovolemic hemodilution, and hypervolemic hemodilution.
- Consideration for use of arterial pressure monitoring and obtaining serial blood gas analysis, hematocrit, coagulation profile [prothrombin time (PT), international normalized ratio (INR), activated partial thromboplastin time (aPTT), and fibrinogen] should occur if the bleeding is sudden or involves more than half of the estimated total blood volume.
- Placement of multiple large-bore intravenous lines and the availability of blood in the operating room are imperative. Routine use of central venous cannula for craniosynostosis should be considered on an individual basis.
- Albumin is a widely used colloid that may also be part of the fluid management plan.

Metabolic disturbances

- This occurs due to significant blood loss and transfusion of blood products.
- Infusion of citrated blood products may result in hypocalcemia and hyperkalemia.
- Significant correlation exists between volume of crystalloid administered (e.g., normal saline, lactated Ringer's solution) and development of intraoperative metabolic acidosis.

Air embolism

- Air embolism is a result of osteotomies and open dural venous sinuses.
- Early signs are decreased oxygen saturation and end-tidal carbon dioxide; in contrast, the arterial carbon dioxide value would be expected to increase. Severe cardiac compromise may also occur. Precordial Doppler is sensitive to detect air, albeit rarely used in routine clinical practice.
- Prevention is via judicious use of bone wax, considering the risks and benefits of head-up position and possibly decreased bleeding, and positive end-expiratory pressure.
- Treatment for air embolism is supportive. Initial management should include flooding the surgical field with saline, administering intravenous fluids and vasopressors, placement in the head-down position, and aspiration of air from the right side of the heart if a central line is present. Resuscitation may be required including performing chest compressions and the administration of epinephrine.

Prolonged surgery

- Nerve palsies, skin pressure necrosis, eye complications, hypothermia, acidosis, and bleeding can all occur.
- Preventing pressure complications is crucial by utilizing appropriate padding of all potential pressure points.
- Eyes can be shielded with a corneal button.
- Hypothermia should be prevented by warming the operating room, forced air warmers, and fluid/blood warmers.

Postoperative care

- Most patients are extubated at the end of surgery or in the immediate postoperative period.
- Severe or syndromic craniosynostosis may require mechanical ventilation in the intensive care unit.
- Postoperative complications include hemorrhage, pain, stridor, apnea, periorbital swelling, electrolyte imbalances, seizures, infections, and altered consciousness.
- Children are at a particularly high risk for hyponatremia related to increased antidiuretic hormone secretion.

Pain management

- Intraoperative pain management is typically with opioids and intravenous acetaminophen.
- Emphasis on titration of intraoperative opioids and vigilance for postoperative airway obstruction should occur.
- Postoperative pain is managed with acetaminophen, non-steroidal anti-inflammatory drugs, and opioids.

Outcome and prognosis

- Following intracranial procedures, major morbidity and mortality are estimated at 0.1%. Hypovolemia due to blood loss was the most frequent cause of death.
- Persistent defects may require a mesh closure and multiple future procedures.

Further reading

Burokas L. Craniosynostosis: caring for infants and their families. *Crit Care Nurse*. 2013; 33(4):39–50.

Coté CJ, Lerman J, Anderson BJ. *Coté and Lerman's A Practice of Anesthesia for Infants and Children*, 5th edition. Philadelphia, PA: Elsevier, 2013; 700–705.

Czerwinski M, Hopper RA, Gruss J, Fearon JA. Major morbidity and mortality rates in craniofacial surgery: an analysis of 8101 major procedures. *Plast Reconstr Surg*. 2010; 126(1):181–6.

Davis PJ. *Smith's Anesthesia for Infants and Children*, 8th edition. Philadelphia: Elsevier, 2013; 821–41.

Hughes C, Thomas K, Johnson D, Das S. Anesthesia for surgery related to craniosynostosis: a review. Part 2. *Paediatr Anaesth*. 2013; 23(1):22–7.

Part C Clinical-based areas in pediatric anesthesiology

Chapter 160

Plastic surgery
Cleft lip and palate surgery
Smokey Clay and Jacquelyn Morillo-Delerme

Overview

- The left and right sides of the hard and soft palates come together between 4 and 12 weeks of gestational age.
- Failure of this process may result in a cleft palate.
- Orofacial clefts are one of the most common birth defects in the United States.
- Risk factors include:
  - Environmental and genetic factors.
  - Intrauterine exposure to phenytoin and cigarette smoke.
- Cleft lip is more common than cleft palate.
- Over 4,000 babies per year are born with a cleft lip and/or cleft palate in the United States.
- Over 2,000 babies are born with an isolated cleft palate each year in the United States.
- Cleft palate alone is more common in females.
- Cleft lip and the combination of cleft lip and cleft palate are more common in males.
- The most common form of cleft palate involves a bifid uvula.

Surgical repair

- Goal of surgical repair is to develop or create a functional seal between the nasal cavity and the oral cavity, thereby allowing normal speech development.
- Timing of surgical repair is variable and attempts to balance earlier correction for speech development and later closure for surgical ease.
- Surgical technique varies between centers.
- Local anesthetic with a vasoconstrictor, normally epinephrine, is used for hemostasis as well as providing analgesia.
- Up to 10μg/kg of epinephrine may be safely infiltrated in children without preexisting congenital heart disease.
- Flaps of tissue are created, mobilized, or advanced, and closed in separate nasal and oral layers.
- More extensive repairs involving bone may be required for more extensive defects.

Handbook of Critical Incidents and Essential Topics in Pediatric Anesthesiology, ed. David A. Young and Olutoyin A. Olutoye. Published by Cambridge University Press. © Cambridge University Press 2015.

Anesthetic considerations

- Consider anxiolytic techniques – parental presence, behavior modification, or medication – for children presenting for repeat surgery.
- Patients require a very thorough and extensive examination of the airway, oral cavity, and craniofacial structures.
- Induction with inhalational agent or intravenous agent.
- Mask ventilation may be difficult due to inability to obtain adequate mask seal.
- Seating of a supraglottic airway device may also be difficult and risks injury to the structures within the cleft.
- Tracheal intubation may be more difficult but is readily achieved in the vast majority of cases.
- Additional anatomic abnormalities, specifically retrognathia, may complicate mask ventilation and/or intubation.
  - Additional airway anomalies may require advanced airway management techniques.
  - Consider maintaining spontaneous ventilation if difficult intubation is anticipated.
- An oral RAE tube may be preferred for adequate surgical exposure and allows fixation of endotracheal tube on the chin.
- Anesthesia is maintained with either intravenous or inhalational agents in combination with opioids.
- The administration of opioid-sparing medications such as intravenous acetaminophen and intravenous steroids should be considered.
- Dosing of opioids should be titrated to effect.
- Surgical retractors and head positioning may result in unanticipated extubation or endotracheal tube occlusion.

Emergence and extubation

- Adequate hemostasis and suctioning should be achieved by the surgeon prior to emergence.
- An orogastric tube should be inserted under direct visualization by the surgeon prior to end of the procedure to adequately empty any stomach contents such as blood.
- Extreme caution should be used if further suction is necessary.
  - Disruption of the palatal closure may occur.
  - Injury to the soft tissue, resulting in more bleeding, may also occur.
- Routine placement of an oral or nasal airway should be avoided as disruption of the palatal closure may occur.
- Consider a tongue stitch in patients with significant anatomic abnormalities or noted tongue edema in order to reduce airway obstruction following extubation.
- Awake extubation with minimal agitation causes little bleeding at the end of the procedure.
  - Reduces risk for laryngospasm that may necessitate maneuvers that would risk injuries as listed above.
  - Allows for handling of secretions by intact airway reflexes.

Postoperative care and considerations

- Airway adjuncts, nasal or oral, may disrupt the cleft repair.
- Humidified oxygen may help prevent drying of secretions.
- Slight trendelenburg position or lateral decubitus position may assist with drainage of secretions and reduce airway obstruction.
- Intravenous or oral acetaminophen are good supplemental analgesics.
- Emergency situations may require re-intubation.
    - Swollen structures may result in a difficult intubation.
    - Release of wound sutures may be required.
- Future preparations for airway management should involve obtaining the history of cleft lip and/or palate repair, any associated airway complications, and should alert the provider to:
    - Potential for airway anomalies.
    - Avoid insertion of equipment through the nares.
    - Avoid trauma to a previously repaired palate.
- Multiple surgical procedures may be required in the process of a complete cleft lip and/or palate repair.

Further reading

Coté CJ, Lerman J, Anderson BJ. *Coté and Lerman's A Practice of Anesthesia for Infants and Children*, 5th edition. Philadelphia, PA: Elsevier, 2013; 697–8.

Davis PJ. *Smith's Anesthesia for Infants and Children*, 8th edition. Philadelphia: Mosby, Inc., 2011; 834–7.

Parker SE, Mai CT, Canfield MA, Rickard R, Wang Y, Meyer RE, et al. for the National Birth Defects Prevention Network. Updated national birth prevalence estimates for selected birth defects in the United States, 2004–2006. *Birth Defects Res A Clin Mol Teratol*. 2010; 88(12):1008–16.

Part C Clinical-based areas in pediatric anesthesiology

Chapter 161

Providing anesthesia in remote locations

General considerations

David Moore and Senthilkumar Sadhasivam

Remote anesthesia locations and specific procedures

- Pediatric anesthesiologists are providing anesthesia services outside of the operating room (OR) boundaries in rising numbers. Frequently, there are patients who need anesthesia outside the routine environment of the OR.
- This may occur due to unique equipment needed (i.e., MRI, CT, radiation therapy) or for procedures not requiring all of the OR capabilities (i.e., renal biopsies, liver biopsies, endoscopies, dental clinic procedures, bronchoscopies, bone marrow biopsies).
- The standards for off-site locations must be the same as found in the OR.
- This would apply to policies, staffing models, fasting requirements, etc.
- The anesthetic preoperative evaluation and preparations of the patient are the same as they are in the OR.
- All anesthesia providers have learned an essential preinduction setup checklist. One such list is "MS MAIDS"– Machine, Stethoscope, Mask, Monitor, Airway, IV, Drugs, and Suction.
- It is essential that the providers performing anesthesia in a remote location outside the OR confirm that appropriate setup has occurred prior to induction of anesthesia.
- Remote locations may not have the same equipment and ancillary assistance that providers typically would have in the OR. The anesthesia machine, airway equipment, and anesthetic medication choices may be limited in remote locations. Many remote locations do not have an anesthesia machine available.

Limitations of remote anesthesia locations

- Consideration for performing procedures in the OR or perhaps postponing the procedure should be given for patients identified as having increased anesthesia risk.
- Examples of risk factors for off-site procedures include
  - higher ASA physical status (ASA 3 and above).
  - active respiratory symptoms.
  - extremes of age and weight.
  - suspected difficult airways.

Handbook of Critical Incidents and Essential Topics in Pediatric Anesthesiology, ed. David A. Young and Olutoyin A. Olutoye. Published by Cambridge University Press. © Cambridge University Press 2015.

- In some cases, such as a suspected or known difficult airway, the patient may have induction and airway management performed in the OR followed by transfer to the off-site procedure area followed by return to the OR for a controlled extubation.

Anesthetic management in remote locations

- Must have distinct areas for preoperative, intraoperative, and postoperative phases of care.
- Must have direct access to a code cart with defibrillator and emergency medications; a malignant hyperthermia cart and difficult airway equipment should also be immediately available.
- Preoperative evaluations should include vital signs, fasting times, history and physical examination, obtaining informed consent, and determining the need for premedication such as anxiolysis.
- Intraoperative procedures include anesthetic induction, establishing vascular access (if needed), securing a definitive airway, anesthesia maintenance, and possible needs for transport (emergency drugs, self-inflating bag/mask/oxygen).
- Postoperative considerations include postoperative pain control and recovery in a post-anesthesia care unit. Standard post-anesthesia discharge criteria should apply such as being awake, hemodynamically stable, and without discomfort.

Examples of common off-site procedures and their anesthetic implications

- Computed tomography (CT)
    - Many CT scans can be performed without requiring pharmacologic support due to the short overall duration of the scan (typically 1–5 minutes).
    - Many patients may have recently (within 1–2 hours) received oral contrast. The best approach for this situation is controversial, due to the potential increased risk for pulmonary aspiration; however, many anesthesiologists will provide anesthesia after the patient has received oral contrast greater than 1 hour previously.
    - Evidence is lacking in the best approach to effectively manage this scenario.
- Radiation therapy
    - Patients receiving radiation therapy (XRT) typically will be scheduled for numerous procedures within a short time period (e.g., once per day for the next 20 days).
    - In addition, the XRT procedure is typically short in duration (10–30 minutes) as well as the requirement for complete immobility.
    - Anesthesia providers are not allowed to be physically present in the room during delivery of radiation.
    - Many anesthesia providers select techniques (e.g., propofol infusion, supraglottic airway device) that avoid tracheal intubation, because of the repetition of procedures.

- Magnetic resonance imaging (MRI)
    - MRI studies may take on average 30–180 minutes.
    - Patients typically are required to restrict their movement to the minimum during the MRI in order to reduce the development of motion artifacts.
    - MRI-compatible equipment is required (non-ferrous); the equipment includes anesthesia-related items (e.g., anesthesia machine, stethoscope, laryngoscope) as well as all ancillary objects (e.g., bed, intravenous line poles). Many anesthetic techniques are acceptable for MRI (i.e., propofol infusion, tracheal intubation, supraglottic airway device).

Further reading

Committee of Origin: Ambulatory Surgical Care. Guidelines for Office-Based Anesthesia. (Approved by the ASA House of Delegates on October 13, 1999, and last affirmed on October 21, 2009.)

Committee of Origin: Standards and Practice Parameters. Statement on Nonoperating Room Anesthetizing Locations. (Approved by the ASA House of Delegates on October 15, 2003 and amended on October 22, 2008.)

Coté CJ, Lerman J, Anderson BJ. *Coté and Lerman's A Practice of Anesthesia for Infants and Children*, 5th edition. Philadelphia, PA: Elsevier, 2013; 963–79.

Lee HH, Milgrom P, Starks H, Burke W. Trends in death associated with pediatric dental sedation and general anesthesia. *Pediatr Anesth*. 2013; 23:741–6.

Urman RD, Punwani N, Shapiro FE. Office-based surgical and medical procedures: educational gaps. *Ochsner J*. 2012 Winter; 12(4):383–8.

Part C Clinical-based areas in pediatric anesthesiology

Chapter 162

Thoracic surgery
General considerations/lung isolation techniques

Kha M. Tran

Preoperative considerations

- Alveoli increase in number after birth until the age of 8 years and increase in size until growth of the chest wall ceases.
- Functional residual capacity is lower in infants, this combined with increased metabolic rate contributes to rapid development of hypoxemia.
- Lungs of infants are more prone to alveolar collapse and atelectasis.
- Ventilation/perfusion (V/Q) mismatch occurs more readily due to higher oxygen demand.

Indications for thoracic surgery

- Congenital
  - Cystic adenomatoid malformation.
  - Bronchopulmonary sequestration.
  - Lobar emphysema.
  - Tracheo-esophageal fistula.
  - Duplication cysts.
  - Congenital diaphragmatic hernia.
  - Patent ductus arteriosus.
- Infectious
  - Empyema.
  - Abscess.
- Neoplastic
  - Primary.
  - Metastatic.
- Trauma.
- Chest wall anomalies
  - Pectus excavatum.
  - Pectus carinatum, "sliding ribs."

Handbook of Critical Incidents and Essential Topics in Pediatric Anesthesiology, ed. David A. Young and Olutoyin A. Olutoye. Published by Cambridge University Press. © Cambridge University Press 2015.

- Other
  - Sympathectomy.
  - Thymectomy.
  - Anterior spinal fusion.

Pathophysiology

- Depending on condition, the diseased lung is either poorly functional or non-functional.
- Non-diseased lung may be hypoplastic or compressed by the diseased lung.
- Increased risk of V/Q mismatch.
- Possibility of cardiovascular compression with expanding intrathoracic masses.
- Air trapping may occur.
- Poor lung compliance may predispose patients to pneumothorax.

Preoperative preparation

- Required laboratory work and further studies will be directed by the history and physical examination, disease process, and the planned procedure.
- Optimization of medical conditions may include:
  - Bronchodilator therapy.
  - Vasoactive medications.
  - Nitric oxide therapy.
  - Drainage of effusions.
  - Extracorporeal membrane oxygenation.
- Risk of disease progression and time required for optimization must be balanced.

Intraoperative considerations

- Inhalation or intravenous induction may be employed.
- Intravenous (IV) access:
  - Upper extremity is the preferred location.
  - Consider lower extremity placement of peripheral IV in presence of superior vena cava syndrome due to compression by intrathoracic mass.
- Consider invasive monitoring such as arterial line and central venous pressure for intrathoracic procedures and procedures with potential for massive blood loss, respectively.
- Consider utilization of two pulse oximeters to help exclude artifact and to assess pre- and post-ductal saturations (in presence of patent ductus arteriosus).
- Endotracheal intubation
  - If lung isolation is not required, use of a low pressure micro-cuffed endotracheal tube (ETT) is sufficient for neonates.
  - A low pressure cuff adequately eliminates circuit leak and reduces mucosal injury when intubation is prolonged.

- Depending on size of lung mass, surgeon may be able to perform the procedure without lung isolation; however, decreased tidal volumes may be required and increased respiratory rate will decrease hypercarbia and may be necessary.
- Positioning
  - Lateral decubitus position with use of an axillary roll, ensure access to hands, face and confirm ETT is free of compression.
- Maintenance of anesthesia
  - Isoflurane may preserve hypoxic pulmonary vasoconstriction better than other volatile agents.
  - Consider 100% inspired oxygen, wean as tolerated.
  - Consider opioids or neuraxial block for intraoperative analgesia.
- Surgery
  - Know steps of surgical procedure and follow progress.
  - Observe closely for compression, retraction on lung tissue or airways and for compression/kinking of ETT.
  - Have blood readily available in operating room.

Lung isolation

- The age and size of child, along with familiarity and availability of equipment, dictate method of isolation.
- Main stem intubation.
- This is an option for neonatal/infant lung isolation.
- Slightly smaller tube size than expected may be required to adequately fit into the main stem.
- Use of ETT without a Murphy eye may minimize chances of inadvertent ventilation of the operative lung.
- Right mainstem intubation
  - Intentionally position ETT into right mainstem, confirm with auscultation, unilateral chest rise, and consider fiberoptic bronchoscopy (FOB) confirmation.
- Left mainstem intubation: more complicated
  - Position head to right, turn ETT with bevel facing the right, advance tube, and confirm with auscultation.
  - Confirm placement in left main bronchus with the fiberoptic scope or fluoroscopy.
- Other options for lung isolation
  - Bronchial blockers: single tube with the blocker positioned in the tracheal lumen, but outside of ETT lumen. Major drawbacks include inability to suction or provide continuous positive pressure.
  - Fogarty catheter: tip of stylet is directed toward bronchus on the operative side with the aid of fiberoptic scope or fluoroscopy.
  - Arndt endobronchial blocker: blocker is passed through special adaptor that is placed at proximal end of ETT.

- Available in two pediatric sizes 5F (fits ETT sizes 4.5–5.5) & 7F (fits ETT sizes 6.0–7.0).
- The special adapters allow visualization, ventilation and manipulation of blocker.
- Positioning is best accomplished with fiberoptic scope and fluoroscopy.
  - Univent tube
    - Has a channel for the blocker, which can be bent for guidance with aid of FOB.
    - Available in sizes adequate for children 6 years and older.
    - Less risk of blocker migration.
    - Smaller tubes have high resistance to airway flow.
    - Possible to provide continuous positive airway pressure (CPAP); suction is possible, but only in larger sized tubes.
  - Double lumen endotracheal tube
    - Size is limiting factor as the smallest size is 26F, no sizes available for neonates, infants or young children.
    - Most suitable method due to ease of placement, and ability to isolate lungs.
    - Have capability for suctioning and provision of CPAP.

Management of single lung ventilation

- 100% oxygen is recommended; may be weaned as tolerated.
- Permissive hypercarbia may be tolerated, depending on patient, surgeon and duration of procedure.
- Hypoxemia during one lung ventilation:
- Confirm there is no compression of ETT.
  - Check for appropriate lung isolation.
  - Suction ETT.
  - Operative lung: optimize ventilation, increase inspired concentration of oxygen, lung volumes, and apply CPAP.
  - Non-operative lung: apply positive end-expiratory pressure (PEEP).
  - Convert back to two-lung ventilation if above measures are ineffective.
- Consider clamping of the pulmonary artery if all other measures are ineffective.

Pain management

- Depending on amount of opioids administered, postoperative extubation is usually possible.
- Consider admission to step-down or intensive care unit.
- Neuraxial blockade
  - Facilitates postoperative extubation.
  - Postoperative pain may cause splinting and hypoxemia in patients extubated at the end of surgery.
  - Epidural catheters:

- - May be placed directly at the thoracic levels.
  - May be threaded from the caudal space up to thoracic levels.
- Threaded catheters are prone to fecal soiling and also become more technically challenging as children grow older.
  - Epidural catheters with in-situ stylets have decreased chance of kinking.
  - Position can be confirmed with radiocontrast media, Tsui stimulating technique, ultrasound or fluoroscopy.
  - Radiopaque catheter placement can be guided in real time with fluoroscopy.

Further reading

Coté CJ, Lerman J, Anderson BJ. *Coté and Lerman's A Practice of Anesthesia for Infants and Children*, 5th edition. Philadelphia, PA: Elsevier, 2013; 279–84.

Davis PJ. *Smith's Anesthesia for Infants and Children*, 8th edition. Philadelphia: Elsevier, 2011; 767–70.

Part C Clinical-based areas in pediatric anesthesiology

Chapter 163

Thoracic surgery
Mediastinal masses
Andrew J. Costandi and Senthilkumar Sadhasivam

Mediastinal masses

Anatomy
- The mediastinum is an anatomic space bound by the sternum anteriorly, the ribs and spine posterolaterally, the thoracic inlet cranially, and the diaphragm caudally.
- Functionally, the mediastinum is subdivided into anterior, middle, and posterior mediastinal spaces.

Etiology
- Neoplastic masses – primary tumors that arise from the adjacent structures: lung, pleura, and other mediastinal organs or may be of metastatic origin.
- Non-neoplastic masses – vascular malformations, granulomas, cysts, and cystic hygromas.

Classification
- Anterior mediastinal masses (AMM): usually from a hematologic source (lymphoblastic lymphomas and Hodgkin's disease). Less frequently: teratomas, lymphangiomas, thymomas, neurogenic, and mesenchymal tumors. Large AMM are associated with increased perioperative morbidity and mortality. Patients with these lesions may present with varying degrees of cardiopulmonary distress.
- Middle mediastinal masses: bronchogenic cysts and granulomas. Patients with these lesions may initially be asymptomatic but may subsequently present with signs of lower airway obstruction not responding to medical therapy.
- Posterior mediastinal masses: usually enteric cysts and tumors of neurogenic origin. Patients with these lesions have less threatening anesthetic implications. Enteric cysts are lined with secretory epithelium and can cause dysphagia, ulceration, and bleeding. Neurogenic tumors are usually asymptomatic, but may cause tracheobronchial compression leading to atelectasis and recurrent pneumonias.
- The remaining portion of this chapter will concentrate on the AMM.

Handbook of Critical Incidents and Essential Topics in Pediatric Anesthesiology, ed. David A. Young and Olutoyin A. Olutoye. Published by Cambridge University Press. © Cambridge University Press 2015.

Anterior mediastinal mass

Presentation
- The presentation of an AMM varies greatly depending on its location and size.
- Constitutional manifestations: fever, malaise, and weight loss.
- Signs and symptoms suggestive of airway and vascular compression: chest tightness, dyspnea, orthopnea, stridor, coughing, superior vena cava (SVC) syndrome (recurrent headaches, swelling of the upper arm, face and neck), and pleural effusion.
- Patients with AMM may prefer sitting up or lying on a particular side.

Pathophysiology
Induction of general anesthesia in children with AMM may lead to catastrophic respiratory and cardiovascular complications. This may occur in apparently asymptomatic children due to cessation of spontaneous ventilation and the reduction of the overall airway and oropharyngeal tone.

Preoperative evaluation
- Physical examination: Evaluate the severity of signs and symptoms by listening to breath sounds (stridor, wheezing), vital signs (respiratory rate, oxygen saturation), examining for signs of SVC syndrome (upper torso swelling, cyanosis), and noting the position(s) most comfortable for the patient in regard to breathing (sitting, prone, lateral).
- Imaging such as computed tomography scans delineates the extent of the mass and detects tracheobronchial and vascular compression. There is increased anesthetic risk if the tracheal area is < 50% of normal.
- Flow volume loops: These tests detect the dynamic qualities of the airway including the severity of intrathoracic airway obstruction. A supine peak expiratory flow rate (PEFR) less than 50% of predicted normal is an indicator of a compressed airway.
- Echocardiography: In upright and supine positions evaluates for cardiac, superior vena cava, and pulmonary outflow tract compression/obstruction.

Perioperative considerations
- Every effort should be made to complete the procedure under local anesthesia and/or minimal sedation if feasible. This can occasionally be performed by obtaining biopsies from superficial nodes.
- In patients with life-threatening mass compression, administering a 24-hour steroid burst, initiating chemotherapy, and/or radiotherapy will likely decrease the size of the tumor and may relieve the compression before obtaining a tissue diagnosis.
- Discussion with the surgeon and oncologist should take place to determine the contingency plans if the biopsy is unable to be obtained with sedation and, more importantly, if severe cardiopulmonary compromise occurs.
- Discussion of and preparation for emergency resuscitation therapies such as rigid bronchoscopy and cardiopulmonary bypass should occur prior to induction of anesthesia.

Preinduction
- Avoid or minimize the use of sedatives.
- Large-bore lower extremity vascular access should be placed in patients with SVC syndrome to ensure delivery of fluids and medications.
- Preload with fluids prior to induction to minimize hemodynamic instability.
- Consider arterial line placement under local anesthesia.
- Nebulized lidocaine may help to minimize airway reactivity during intubation.
- All backup equipment and personnel should be immediately available.

Induction
- A skilled bronchoscopist should be in the room during induction as a rigid bronchoscope may facilitate re-establishment of ventilation and oxygenation in cases of airway collapse.
- Median sternotomy and cardiopulmonary bypass may be impractical unless bypass access is established before induction.
- Inhalation induction is preferred to maintain spontaneous ventilation usually with the head of bed elevated or in the preferred position by the patient.
- Airway can be managed with a supraglottic airway device or reinforced endotreacheal tube (ETT) after achieving deep levels of anesthesia.

Maintenance of anesthesia
- The use of airway regional techniques to facilitate intubation or neuroaxial techniques to facilitate surgical anesthesia are advantageous as they decrease the requirement of anesthetics and may reduce adverse events such as laryngospasm.
- Spontaneous ventilation under general anesthesia should be maintained, this is typically achieved with the use of inhaled anesthetics and small doses of opioids or a combination of propofol and ketamine. Dexmedetomidine and ketamine have been used successfully for sedation to obtain percutaneous biopsies.
- Continuous positive airway pressure (CPAP) may help to maintain functional residual capacity and stent open the airway.
- In cases of airway collapse, the patient should be placed in a position which relieved airway obstruction preoperatively (sitting, lateral decubitus, or prone), in an attempt to relieve mass compression.

Extubation and postoperative care
- Extubation depends on the course of the procedure. If surgical edema or hemorrhage is suspected, then keeping the patient intubated should be strongly considered. Tumor therapy should be started and extubation attempted only after demonstration of tumor regression in the following few days when the patient is breathing spontaneously with an adequate airway leak around the tracheal tube.

Further reading

Coté CJ, Lerman J, Anderson BJ. *Coté and Lerman's A Practice of Anesthesia for Infants and Children*, 5th edition. Philadelphia, PA: Elsevier, 2013; 290–2.

Davis PJ, Cladis FP, Motoyama EK. *Smith's Anesthesia for Infants and Children*, 8th edition. Philadelphia: Elsevier Mosby, 2011; 772–8.

Part C Clinical-based areas in pediatric anesthesiology

Thoracic surgery

Video thoracoscopic procedures/ pectus excavatum

Jagroop Mavi and Senthilkumar Sadhasivam

Video-assisted thoracoscopic surgery in pediatric patients

Indications
- Diagnostic inspection.
- Lung biopsy.
- Lobectomy.
- Sequestration resection.
- Cyst excision.
- Lung decortication.
- Thymectomy.
- Patent ductus arteriosus (PDA) ligation.
- Thoracic duct ligation.
- Esophageal atresia repair.
- Aortopexy.
- Mediastinal mass excision.
- Anterior spinal fusion.

Suggested advantages of thoracoscopic vs. open-chest surgery
- Improved surgical visualization.
- Decreased postoperative pain.
- Decreased surgical stress.
- Decreased ileus.
- Shorter hospitalization.
- Quicker return to baseline activity.
- Fewer long-term complications.
- Cosmetically superior.

Preoperative evaluation
- For elective procedures in healthy pediatric patients, no preoperative testing is required.

Handbook of Critical Incidents and Essential Topics in Pediatric Anesthesiology, ed. David A. Young and Olutoyin A. Olutoye. Published by Cambridge University Press. © Cambridge University Press 2015.

- For patients with complicated medical problems or undergoing complex procedures, preoperative testing should focus on known or suspected physiologic derangements (i.e., hematocrit, blood cross-match, CT scan of chest).
- Focus evaluation on the degree of cardiac and pulmonary dysfunction.
- Blood loss during thoracoscopy is usually minimal, but blood or a type and screen should be considered especially for complex procedures.
- It is preferable to have two intravenous lines in case rapid fluid or blood administration is required.
- Arterial blood pressure monitoring is not routinely used unless indicated by the clinical status of the patient or complexity of the procedure.

Intraoperative management

- Various anesthetic techniques can be employed. These include local anesthesia, regional anesthesia, general anesthesia with one-lung ventilation, and general anesthesia with two-lung ventilation and carbon dioxide insufflation.
- Inhalational anesthetic agents are commonly administered with higher fractions of oxygen (as high as 100%) during maintenance of anesthesia.
- Isoflurane may be preferred due to decreased attenuation of hypoxic pulmonary vasoconstriction. Nitrous oxide is avoided.
- There are three common approached utilized to achieve one-lung ventilation: the use of a double-lumen tube, selective endobronchial intubation with a traditional tracheal tube, and the use of a bronchial blocker.
- The etiology of hypoxemia in patients undergoing thoracoscopy can be secondary to malpositioning of the tracheal tube, inadequate ventilation of the dependent lung, pulmonary disease causing V/Q mismatch, pre-existing pulmonary disease, and obstruction of the tracheal tube.

Perioperative complications

- Subcutaneous emphysema.
- Gas embolism.
- Local infection.
- Cardiovascular compromise secondary to high intrathoracic pressures.
- Pulmonary abscess or empyema.

Pectus excavatum repair

- Most common type of chest wall deformity (accounts for over 90% of congenital chest wall deformities). Many patients may be clinically asymptomatic.
- Patients present with a constellation of symptoms including dyspnea upon exertion, a feeling of heaviness in the chest, air hunger, and exercise intolerance. Most patients report they have worsening dyspnea as the defect progressively deepens.

Indications for surgery

- Exercise intolerance.

- Body image issues.
- Pain.
- Exercise-induced asthma.
- Compression of the right atrium or right ventricle.

Surgery
- The Nuss procedure is the surgical technique of choice for correction of this deformity.
- It is a minimally invasive technique in which rigid metal bars are placed transthoracically beneath the sternum and costal cartilages for a period of time until permanent remodeling of the chest wall has occurred.
- These bars are passed through the thorax under direct vision using thoracoscopy to reduce the risk of perforation to nearby structures.

Anesthesia management
- Two large-bore intravenous lines for possible fluid resuscitation.
- Increased vigilance is important during surgical dissection across the mediastinum because of arrhythmias and potential for tissue or vessel perforation.
- Significant postoperative pain is expected and management should include non-opioid analgesics, opioids, regional anesthesia, and anxiolytics if indicated.
- Regional anesthesia techniques include wound catheter infusions, bilateral intercostal nerve blocks, paravertebral catheters, and thoracic epidurals. Aggressive physical therapy significantly improves pain control and may decrease the incidence of chronic postoperative pain and length of stay.
- Due to severe postoperative pain, a thoracic epidural has been shown to be the superior form of postoperative pain control for these patients.

These children return for removal of the pectus bar after several years. Occasionally, the bar becomes adherent to the pericardium or surrounding structures, resulting in severe, sudden rupture or perforation. It is prudent to establish ample intravenous access and have increased vigilance during this critical portion of the procedure.

Further reading

Colombani PM. Preoperative assessment of chest wall deformities. *Semin Thoracic Cardiovasc Surg.* 2009; 21:58–63.

Coté CJ, Lerman J, Anderson BJ. *Coté and Lerman's A Practice of Anesthesia for Infants and Children*, 5th edition. Philadelphia, PA: Elsevier, 2013; 18, 278, 578.

Hammer GB, Fitzmaurice BG, Brodsky JB. Methods for single lung ventilation in pediatric patients. *Anesth Analg.* 1999; 89:1426–9.

Nuss D, Kelly RE, Croitoru DP, Katz ME. A 10 year review of a minimally invasive technique for the correction of pectus excavatum. *J Pediatr Surg.* 1998; 33: 545–52.

Rowe R, Andropoulus D, Heard M, et al. Anesthetic management of pediatric patients undergoing thoracoscopy. *J Cardiothorac Vasc Anesthes.* 1994; 8(5):563–6.

Part C: Clinical-based areas in pediatric anesthesiology

Chapter 165: Transplant surgery
General considerations
Paul A. Stricker

Pediatric organ transplantation has become a treatment option for end-organ dysfunction from primary congenital causes and secondary causes of organ failure. Pediatric solid organ transplants performed include kidney, liver, heart, lung, combined heart-lung, and intestinal transplant.

General anesthetic considerations

- Primary effects of organ failure
  - Must consider direct effects of organ failure, e.g., altered pharmacokinetics with liver and renal failure, coagulopathy from hepatic failure, and sensitivity to myocardial depressants in cardiac failure.

- Secondary effects of organ failure
  - Must also consider secondary effects of organ failure on perioperative management, e.g., pulmonary hypertension or hepatorenal syndrome in hepatic failure, hepatic encephalopathy in hepatic failure, and altered pharmacokinetics in cardiac, renal, and liver failure.

- Organs for cadaveric transplantation become available at unpredictable times; adherence to *nil per os* guidelines may not be possible and rapid-sequence induction and intubation may be indicated. Children may also present with presumed full stomachs related to their underlying disease states (i.e., severe ascites from hepatic failure).

- Considerations relating to the impact of surgical management on anesthetic care include:
  - Intraoperative or postoperative anticoagulation may preclude neuraxial analgesic techniques.
  - Cross-clamping of major veins or arteries may mandate intravenous and arterial access in upper extremities.
  - Advance preparation for sudden and severe blood loss.
  - Plans for postoperative ICU care as well as postoperative mechanical ventilation.

- Immunocompromised states: perioperative considerations
  - Children with organ failure can present with preexisting immunocompromised states.

Handbook of Critical Incidents and Essential Topics in Pediatric Anesthesiology, ed. David A. Young and Olutoyin A. Olutoye. Published by Cambridge University Press. © Cambridge University Press 2015.

- Immunosuppressants given to prevent organ rejection also induce further immunocompromise.
- Strict attention to aseptic technique is imperative at all phases of care.
- Immunosuppressive agents
  - Corticosteroids: inhibit T-cell function at multiple sites.
    - Commonly used for induction phase of immunosuppression.
    - Low-dose steroids are a component of maintenance immunosuppression.
    - Treatment of acute rejection.
    - Side effects include hypertension, hyperglycemia, poor wound healing.
  - Antiproliferative drugs: inhibit DNA and RNA synthesis.
    - Azathioprine.
    - Mycophenolate mofetil is the most commonly used antiproliferative agent with improved side-effect profile compared to azathioprine.
    - Side effects include bone marrow depression, hepatic toxicity.
  - Calcineurin inhibitors: inhibit signal transduction mediating T-cell expansion and differentiation.
    - Cyclosporine and tacrolimus.
    - Side effects include nephrotoxicity and neurotoxicity.

Considerations in the post-transplant patient

In addition to the challenges in managing care during transplantation, children who have previously undergone transplantation present both for elective and emergency operations for conditions related to and conditions unrelated to their transplant. Children who have undergone transplantation have essentially replaced one chronic disease (primary organ failure) with another (post-transplant status) and its associated issues:

- Infection – more likely due to immunosuppression.
- Renal insufficiency – secondary to specific immunosuppressive agents.
- Malignancy – transplantation and immunosuppression lead to significantly higher malignancy rates (> 50% will develop at 20 years post-transplantation). Most common is post-transplant lymphoproliferative disease (PTLD), which typically presents within the first 2 years following transplantation.
- Rejection – both acute and chronic forms; children may present for anesthesia to biopsy transplanted organs for rejection surveillance.
- Cardiovascular – hypertension, dyslipidemia, diabetes mellitus.
- Psychosocial – cognitive/developmental delays, depression, anxiety. Previous long-term hospitalizations, extensive prior interactions with medical personnel (positive and negative), and complex relationship dynamics with parents/caregivers all require a thoughtful approach from anesthesiologists.

Further reading

Davis PJ, Cladis FP, Motoyama EK. *Smith's Anesthesia for Infants and Children*, 8th edition. Philadelphia: Elsevier Mosby, 2011; 891–905.

Gregory GA, Andropoulos DB. *Gregory's Pediatric Anesthesia*, 5th edition. Hoboken: Wiley-Blackwell, 2012; 678–719.

Clinical-based areas in pediatric anesthesiology

Transplant surgery
Hepatic
Yang Liu

Common indications for hepatic transplantation

- Chronic liver disease
    - The most common cause for liver transplantation in children is cholestatic disease from biliary atresia.
    - Alagille syndrome.
    - Sclerosing cholangitis.
    - Progressive familial intrahepatic cholestasis.

- Metabolic liver disease
    - Alpha-1-antitrypsin deficiency.
    - Ornithine transcarbamylase deficiency.
    - Glycogen storage disease, type 1a.
    - Wilson disease.
    - Tyrosinemia.
    - Cystic fibrosis.

- Acute hepatic failure
    - Hepatitis including non-A, non-B, non-C hepatitis.
    - Autoimmune hepatitis.
    - Drug and toxin induced.

- Malignancy
    - Hepatoblastoma.
    - Hemangio-endothelioma.
    - Sarcoma.

- Miscellaneous
    - Re-transplantation.
    - Conditions related to total parenteral nutrition.

Handbook of Critical Incidents and Essential Topics in Pediatric Anesthesiology, ed. David A. Young and Olutoyin A. Olutoye. Published by Cambridge University Press. © Cambridge University Press 2015.

Organ allocation for pediatric candidates
- Liver allografts in the USA are allocated to candidates on a waiting list based on the Pediatric End-Stage Liver Disease scoring system (PELD) which considers the following: bilirubin level, albumin level, age, and INR value.

Pathophysiology of end-stage liver disease
- Cardiovascular
    - Decreased systemic vascular resistance.
    - Hyperdynamic circulation.
    - Arteriovenous shunting.
    - Cardiomyopathy.
- Pulmonary
    - Dyspnea related to ascites-induced abdominal distention or pleural effusions.
    - Pulmonary hypertension.
    - Hepatopulmonary syndrome.
- Central nervous system
    - Acute or chronic hepatic encephalopathy.
    - Cerebral edema.
- Gastrointestinal
    - Hepatic dysfunction.
    - Portal hypertension and gastroesophageal varices.
- Renal
    - Renal insufficiency due to hypovolemia, acute tubular necrosis or hepatorenal syndrome.
- Hematologic
    - Coagulopathy due to diminished synthesis of clotting factors and thrombocytopenia.
    - Anemia.
- Fluids, electrolytes, acid–base status
    - Nutritional failure.
    - Metabolic alkalosis.
    - Metabolic acidosis.
    - Hypokalemia.

Transplantation and surgical techniques
- Whole-liver transplantation.
- Reduced-size liver transplantation.
- Split-liver transplantation.
- Living-donor liver transplantation.

Surgical complications

- Hepatic artery thrombosis is one of the most common complications after liver transplantation.
- Acute organ rejection.
- Infections.
- Biliary complications.
- Portal vein thrombosis.

Anesthetic management

- Potential challenges for children undergoing liver transplantation
    - Smaller blood volume.
    - Challenging vascular access.
    - Size restriction of donor graft.
    - Hepatic artery thrombosis.
- Preoperative evaluation
    - Identify the primary cause of liver failure.
    - Identify liver-related and non-liver-related alterations in physiology through a complete review of systems.
    - Obtain baseline laboratory values to evaluate hematology, renal, metabolic and electrolytes.
    - Consider premedication for anxiety for most patients.
    - Most children are considered to have a full stomach.
- Intraoperative management
    - General consideration.
        - Rapid-sequence intravenous induction is typically recommended.
        - Cuffed endotracheal tubes are recommended as high inspiratory pressures may be required.
        - At least two peripheral upper extremity intravenous catheters should be placed together with a central venous line for fluid management and blood transfusion.
        - Lactated Ringer's solution may cause elevation of serum lactate levels and normal saline may cause metabolic acidosis. Therefore, a pH balanced, isotonic crystalloid solution is recommended.
        - The use of 5% albumin should be considered since the albumin level is typically reduced due to poor synthetic function.
        - Basic monitoring should include an electrocardiogram, pulse oximetry, non-invasive blood pressure, invasive arterial blood pressure, central venous pressure, urine output, and temperature.
        - Advanced monitoring such as transesophageal echocardiogram, continuous cardiac output measurement, and venovenous bypass may be useful.
        - Positioning and padding are critical to prevent soft tissue and peripheral nerve injuries.
    - Preanhepatic stage – dissection and removal of diseased liver.

- The clamping of the inferior vena cava (IVC) results in a 50–60% decrease in venous return.
            - Hypotension is common due to IVC clamping and significant blood loss may occur during dissection.
            - Adequate fluid infusion to maintain central venous pressure (CVP) 10–12 mmHg and optimization of hemodynamic status is recommended prior to cross-clamp of the portal vein and the IVC.
        - Anhepatic stage – The anhepatic stage begins with clamping of the portal venous supply to the native liver and the vena cava, and concludes with unclamping of these vessels and reperfusion of the donor liver. Major concerns during this stage include:
            - Metabolic acidosis.
            - Decreased serum ionized calcium level.
            - Hyperkalemia or hypokalemia.
            - Hypoglycemia or hyperglycemia.
            - Hypothermia.
            - Hypocalcaemia and acidosis should be corrected and cardiovascular status should be optimized prior to reperfusion.
        - Reperfusion stage – this involves serial release of the suprahepatic, infrahepatic, and portal vein clamps.
            - After immediate reperfusion, acute systemic hypotension, bradycardia, elevated pulmonary artery pressure (PAP), and dysrhythmias may be encountered.
        - Completion stage – this is marked by reestablishing hepatic artery blood flow and biliary reconstruction.
            - Typically characterized by stable vital signs and immediate function of the graft.
- Postoperative management
    - Many children require mechanical ventilation in the immediate postoperative period.
    - Prevention of hepatic artery thrombosis
        - Prophylactic anticoagulation therapy with heparin infusion may be of benefit.
        - Dopamine may be used to prevent hypotension.
    - Fluid replacement to maintain adequate urine output.

Further reading

Coté CJ, Lerman J, Anderson BJ. *Coté and Lerman's A Practice of Anesthesia for Infants and Children*, 5th edition. Philadelphia, PA: Elsevier, 2013; 597–607.

Emre S. et al. Current concepts in pediatric liver transplantation. *Mt Sinai J Med.* 2012; 79(2):199–213.

Gregory GA, Andropoulos DB. *Gregory's Pediatric Anesthesia*, 5th edition. Hoboken: Wiley-Blackwell, 2012; 682–93.

Part C: Clinical-based areas in pediatric anesthesiology

Chapter 167

Transplant surgery
Renal
Paul A. Stricker

Background

- Transplantation is preferred treatment for end-stage renal disease (ESRD) in children since many etiologies for ESRD in children are curative with transplantation.
- Incidence of ESRD in children is approximately 14 per 1,000,000.
- Many children have never received preoperative dialysis (unlike adults).
- Diabetes mellitus is an uncommon cause for ESRD in children (unlike adults).
- End-graft survival rates at 3 years are 90% (living donor) and 81% (deceased donor).
- Common causes of ESRD in children:
  - Congenital renal/urologic abnormalities (obstructive nephropathy).
  - Chronic vesicoureteral reflux/pyelonephritis.
  - Glomerulonephritis.

Perioperative considerations associated with ESRD

- Cardiovascular
  - Hypertension due to hypervolemia and renin-angiotensin axis activation.
  - Pericarditis and pericardial effusion development.
  - Myocardial dysfunction due to uremia-induced cardiomyopathy.
  - Fluid overload resulting in pulmonary edema.
  - Hypotension if hypovolemia occurs after dialysis.
  - Intraoperative hemodynamic instability mostly presenting as recurring hypotension.
- Impaired renal drug clearance/pharmacokinetics.
- Electrolyte abnormalities (hyperkalemia, hyperphosphatemia, hypocalcemia, metabolic acidosis).
- Anemia of chronic disease due to decreased erythropoietin production.
- Coagulation disturbances (uremia-induced platelet dysfunction, heparinization for hemodialysis).
- Growth and development delays.

Handbook of Critical Incidents and Essential Topics in Pediatric Anesthesiology, ed. David A. Young and Olutoyin A. Olutoye. Published by Cambridge University Press. © Cambridge University Press 2015.

Preoperative assessment

Preoperative assessment should emphasize:
- History: comorbidities, fluid status, last dialysis, risk factors for full stomach, elective vs. deceased donor (will determine if emergent or elective procedure).
- Physical examination: assessment of intravascular volume status.
- Laboratory evaluation: electrolytes (in particular potassium), hemoglobin and platelet count; may have anemia and platelet dysfunction.
- Medication history including antihypertensives and corticosteroids.

Intraoperative management

- Procedure performed
    - Younger/smaller children will have the kidney placed intra-abdominally; the grafts will be anastomosed to the aorta and vena cava, requiring aorta and vena cava cross-clamps and systemic heparinization.
    - Older children will have the donor kidney placed in the iliac fossa; the grafts will be anastomosed to the iliac vessels, similar to what is done for adults.
- Induction of anesthesia
    - Premedication with midazolam is acceptable.
    - Intravenous induction is most common; rapid sequence induction if full stomach precautions required. Comorbidities, volume status, and altered pharmacokinetics should be considered in selection of induction agents.
    - Inhaled induction is also acceptable in many patients.
    - Neuromuscular blocking agents: Avoid long-acting agents such as pancuronium. Succinylcholine may be contraindicated if high serum potassium levels are present. If succinylcholine use is contraindicated, induction may be performed using a nondepolarizing muscle relaxant such as rocuronium (mostly hepatic metabolism).
- Large-bore peripheral IV catheters placed in the upper extremities for potential large volume shifts and need for lower vascular cross-clamps.
- Urinary catheter placement can occur after induction.
- Arterial catheter in children having aortic cross-clamped or as indicated based on patient's medical comorbidities.
- Central venous catheter: many centers direct perioperative fluid administration using central venous pressure (CVP) with goal of liberal fluid administration (titrate to a CVP of 12–14 mmHg) to avoid episodes of hypotension and impaired graft perfusion
- Intraoperative opioids
    - Fentanyl or hydromorphone are most commonly administered; morphine is avoided because of potential for accumulation of morphine-6-glucuronide (active metabolite).
- Immunosuppressant agents administered according to transplant team plan.
- Graft reperfusion: release of the cross-clamps results in washout of ischemic extremities in addition to the washout of preservative solution (contains potassium), which may result in cardiovascular collapse and hypothermia. Creation of relative hypervolemia prior to cross-clamp release reduces instability and also promotes organ perfusion.

- Promoting function of transplanted kidneys
  - Diuretic administration (furosemide, mannitol).
  - Avoid hypotension.
  - Maintain normovolemia.

Immediate postoperative care

- Extubation: most patients are extubated in the operating room. Younger patients may remain mechanically ventilated postoperatively if the larger transplanted kidney interferes with respiratory mechanics or if there is concern for hypervolemia and postoperative pulmonary edema.
- Immunosuppression: the administration of agents for the induction of immunosuppression continues in the immediate postoperative period; careful communication between anesthesiologists and the postoperative medical team is essential.
- Postoperative analgesia: intravenous opioids remain the mainstay for postoperative analgesia, either by patient-controlled analgesia, intermittent bolus, or by continuous infusion (depending on the patient's age). Concerns regarding hypotension and coagulation derangements may limit the use of neuraxial analgesic techniques.
- Increased vigilance should be maintained in infants since they are at particularly high risk for graft loss due to vascular thrombosis.

Further reading

Davis PJ, Cladis FP, Motoyama EK. *Smith's Anesthesia for Infants and Children*. 8th edition. Philadelphia: Elsevier Mosby, 2011; 931–8.

Gregory GA, Andropoulos DB, ed. *Gregory's Pediatric Anesthesia*, 5th edition. Hoboken: Wiley-Blackwell, 2012; 693–7.

Part C Clinical-based areas in pediatric anesthesiology

Chapter 168

Trauma surgery
General considerations
Carlos Rodriguez

- Traumatic injuries are the most common cause of death for children older than 1 year. Motor vehicle accidents, falls, and nonaccidental trauma are the most common categories of pediatric traumatic injuries.
- The role of the anesthesiologist often varies, with simultaneous responsibilities including management of airway, resuscitation, and performing procedures (both therapeutic and diagnostic). The anesthesiologist may need to quickly prioritize management decisions as well as integrate effectively with other members of the trauma team.
- The American College of Surgeons developed the widely accepted and utilized Advanced Trauma Life Support (ATLS) course; this course is also utilized in pediatric trauma.
- Initial evaluation of a trauma patient is considered the primary survey. Vital signs are obtained, intravenous access is achieved, and basic neurologic status is determined using the Glasgow Coma Scale (GCS). Resuscitation including airway management and volume administration occur during this phase of care. Transition to the secondary survey occurs when the patient has been stabilized. Emergent transfer to the operating room may occur if the patient is refractory to resuscitation.
- The secondary survey includes a head-to-toe examination including removal of all clothing. Diagnostic testing such as laboratory values and radiographs are ordered.
- Appropriate vascular access is crucial but many times difficult to achieve in trauma patients. If peripheral vascular access is difficult to achieve, options include placement of central venous access, use of ultrasound guidance, and insertion of an intraosseous infusion device.
- Trauma patients should be considered to have a full stomach and rapid sequence induction should be performed in the absence of a suspected difficult airway. In-line stabilization should be maintained in most trauma patients since cervical spine injuries have not typically been excluded when airway management is required. After removal of the cervical collar for tracheal intubation, the cervical collar should remain in place until definitive clearance has occurred; clearance typically occurs in the postoperative period. For those patients with airway trauma, the possibility of a difficulty airway should be suspected. Appropriate equipment (e.g., rigid bronchoscope, tracheostomy set) and surgical colleagues (i.e., surgeon capable of performing surgical airway) should be immediately available.
- Patients who experience traumatic brain injury (TBI) may present with a variety of symptoms including vomiting, photophobia, altered mental status, decreased

Handbook of Critical Incidents and Essential Topics in Pediatric Anesthesiology, ed. David A. Young and Olutoyin A. Olutoye. Published by Cambridge University Press. © Cambridge University Press 2015.

consciousness, and seizures. Initial evaluation and determination of the GCS is extremely important for determination of a baseline state. It is crucial to maintain adequate cerebral blood flow; this is accomplished by having sufficient cerebral perfusion pressures. To achieve this, it is recommended to maintain a mean arterial pressure of 60 mmHg for children and 85 mmHg for adolescents. Appropriate medications (e.g., propofol, lidocaine, opioids) should be administered to help reduce increases to intracranial pressure (ICP) during events with increased stimulus such as tracheal intubation. Propofol and etomidate may be beneficial during induction by reducing both ICP and cerebral oxygen consumption. To help reduce brain edema, isotonic intravenous fluid administration should be judiciously administered, particularly in isolated TBI. Strategies to reduce ICP include osmotic diuresis, head-up positioning, drainage of cerebral spinal fluid, and modest hyperventilation (with the goal for an end-tidal CO_2 value of 30–35 mmHg).

- Many blunt abdominal injuries (e.g., liver laceration) may be managed conservatively without surgical intervention. Laparoscopy (diagnostic and therapeutic) may be selected in place of laparotomy in stable patients. Patients that require control of hemorrhage and penetrating injuries will likely have a laparotomy performed.
- Skeletal injury may be the most common type of traumatic injury encountered by pediatric anesthesiologists. Fractures range from isolated extremity fractures to pelvic and facial bone fractures. Patients who suffer complex traumatic injuries may not have simple fractures repaired until the patient is stable and other life-threatening injuries have been addressed. Patients who have pelvic or femur fractures are at risk of major blood loss; the anesthesiologist should be prepared to transfuse blood in these patients.
- These are some possible requirements for the anesthesiologist taking care of the pediatric patient with traumatic injuries:
  - Personnel: Trauma patients can be critically ill and often it is challenging to accomplish multiple tasks without the help of others. Many trauma centers have integrated teams readily available to assist in the perioperative care of a trauma patient.
  - Appropriate set-up: Every operating room should be equipped with age-appropriate equipment (preferably set up in advance), multiple types of intravenous fluids, intra-arterial pressure and central venous pressure transducers, and warming devices (fluid warmers and warming blankets).
  - Blood bank: Blood products including packed red blood cells, fresh frozen plasma, platelets, and cryoprecipitate should be readily available for transfusion. The anesthesiologist should be very cognizant of their institutional massive transfusion protocol.
  - Laboratory: Frequent evaluation of hemoglobin, arterial blood gas parameters, and coagulation status may be indicated and requires effective integration with ancillary departments including the laboratory.

Further reading

Coté CJ, Lerman J, Anderson BJ. *Coté and Lerman's A Practice of Anesthesia for Infants and Children*, 5th edition. Philadelphia, PA: Elsevier, 2013; 789–803.

Davis PJ, Cladis FP, Motoyama EK. *Smith's Anesthesia for Infants and Children*, 8th edition. Philadelphia: Elsevier Mosby, 2011; 971–1000.

Gregory GA, Andropoulos DB. *Gregory's Pediatric Anesthesia*, 5th edition. Hoboken: Wiley-Blackwell, 2012; 908–16.

Part C — Clinical-based areas in pediatric anesthesiology

Chapter 169

Trauma surgery
Burn surgery
Carlos Rodriguez

- According to the Centers for Disease Control (CDC), children of age 4 years and under are at highest risk for burn injuries. There is an estimated 15,000 children hospitalized each year in the United States due to burn injuries.
- Burns are classified by severity:
  - 1st degree – epidermis only is affected.
  - 2nd degree – epidermis + superficial or deep dermis is affected.
  - 3rd degree – epidermis + full thickness dermis involvement occurs.
  - 4th degree – fascia, muscle, and bone are all injured.
- Classification of burns is important in the treatment of burn injuries. The percentage of body surface area involvement provides survival rate information; it also dictates initial fluid resuscitation and long-term nutritional support. Younger patients have more surface area on their head and less surface area in their lower extremities; therefore a similar sized burn in different locations would result in dissimilar percentages burned in a child when compared to an adult. The rule of 9's is not valid for the estimation of pediatric burn injuries due to this disproportionate distribution. Several formulas and charts have been devised to help estimate the amount of surface area involvement.
- Burn injury may result in an inflammatory reaction referred to as the systemic inflammatory response syndrome (SIRS). This generalized response eventually produces varying degrees of shock. Proinflammatory cytokines and other inflammatory mediators contribute to the development of systemic disease. Manifestations of SIRS may include tachycardia, tachypnea, fever, hypotension, and cardiopulmonary failure. SIRS may eventually progress to the development of multiple organ dysfunction syndrome (MODS) which is associated with high morbidity and mortality.
- Physiologic changes after a major burn injury usually occurs in two phases. The first set of changes (acute phase) occurs early after the injury (first couple of days). The later phase (hypermetabolic) usually takes place later in the disease process (5+ days later).
- Acute phase
  - Cardiovascular
    - Depressed myocardial function resulting in decreased cardiac output.
    - Decreased preload from varying degrees of hypovolemia.

Handbook of Critical Incidents and Essential Topics in Pediatric Anesthesiology, ed. David A. Young and Olutoyin A. Olutoye. Published by Cambridge University Press. © Cambridge University Press 2015.

- Pulmonary
    - Decreased pulmonary and chest-wall compliance.
    - Decreased functional residual capacity.
    - Increased atelectasis.
    - Increased potential for hypoxemia.
    - High suspicion for inhalation injuries (early).
    - High suspicion for carbon monoxide toxicity (early).
- Hematologic
    - Increased blood viscosity with subsequent anemia.
    - Thrombocytopenia.
    - Coagulopathies.
- Renal
    - Decreased glomerular filtration rate associated with decreased renal blood flow.
    - Impaired function also associated with myoglobinuria/hemoglobinuria.
- Neurologic
    - Hypoxic/burn encephalopathies: hallucinations, delirium, seizures, and coma.
    - Cerebral edema and possibility for consequential increased intracranial pressure.
- Gastrointestinal
    - Ileus ensues from initial injury with function typically returning after 48–72 hours.
    - Gastric acid prophylaxis should be used to decrease incidence of gastroduodenal ulcerations.
    - Abdominal compartment syndrome may occur after aggressive fluid resuscitation.
- Metabolic/Endocrine
    - Increased oxygen demand and increased carbon dioxide production occurs.

- Hypermetabolic phase
    - Cardiovascular
        - Increased cardiac output.
        - Reduced peripheral vascular resistance.
        - Hypertension.
    - Pulmonary
        - Increased respiratory dysfunction.
        - Increased risk for pulmonary infections.
        - Decreased chest wall expansion.
    - Renal
        - Increased glomerular filtration rate (GFR) due to increased cardiac output.
    - Hepatic (injury due to hypoxemia and hypoperfusion)
        - Increased hepatic flow due to increased cardiac output.
        - Increased synthetic functions such as protein synthesis and gluconeogenesis.
    - Psychiatric

- Post-traumatic stress disorder.
- Delirium.
    - Metabolic/Endocrine
        - Increased stress hormones are present up to 9–12 months.
        - Degree of hypermetabolism is directly proportional to burn size.
- The clinical response from many medications can be unpredictable. Reasons include:
    - Fluid shifts within the intravascular compartment change the volume of distribution.
    - Levels of unbound drug concentrations change due to varying amounts of binding proteins.
    - The absolute number of binding receptors may also be modified.
    - Acute phase: Hypovolemia leads to impaired organ perfusion as well as decreased uptake and drug clearance.
    - Late phase: Hypermetabolism leads to increased drug clearance.
- Airway management should initially focus on the evaluation for the presence of inhalation injuries. Early placement of a definitive airway should be strongly considered in any patient with a suspected inhalational injury.
- Carbon monoxide (CO) poisoning is possible even without appearance of thermal injury. It should be highly suspected in closed-space fires. It is important to note that CO has a much greater affinity for hemoglobin than oxygen. The half-life of carboxyhemoglobin is greatly reduced with administration of 100% oxygen. Pulse oximetry is not reliable in these patients because standard oximeters cannot differentiate between oxyhemoglobin and carboxyhemoglobin.
- Succinylcholine is contraindicated due to the risk of severe hyperkalemia from increased extrajunctional acetylcholine receptors. Succinylcholine may only be utilized early after the original injury (several sources site within the first 12 hours).
- Resistance to nondepolarizing neuromuscular blocking agents should be anticipated, resulting in increased dosing requirements.
- The development of a perioperative pain management plan should incorporate strategies to address increased dosing demands, the possibility of opioid tolerance, need for frequent painful procedures, as well as possible anxiolytic requirements.
- Anesthetic management in the pediatric patient can be very challenging. These patients likely will return multiple times for procedures to have dressing changes, skin grafts, etc. Patients will likely require psychological support. Post-traumatic stress disorder may be present; family members will also be coping with loss, grief, and guilt.
- Measures should be taken to minimize heat loss such as prewarming operating rooms, use of warming blankets, and fluid warmers. Wrapping extremities with sterile plastic bags is an accepted technique to maintain normothermia.
- There should be heightened vigilance and advanced preparation for significant fluid shifts and blood loss. Arterial and central venous access should be strongly considered in many patients. Volume resuscitation requirements are typically substantial when compared with traditional dosing. The Parkland formula is one of the more common strategies for guiding volume resuscitation in burn patients. The fluid requirement is 4 mL/kg for each percentage of estimated burn area. Half of this amount is to be

administered over the first 8 hours; the remaining is to be administered over the next 16 hours. It is critical to utilize several parameters on a regular basis to evaluate and possibly modify volume resuscitation requirements (i.e., urine output, blood pressure, lactate level).

Further reading

Coté CJ, Lerman J, Anderson BJ. *Coté and Lerman's A Practice of Anesthesia for Infants and Children*, 5th edition. Philadelphia, PA: Elsevier, 2013; 712–30.

Davis PJ, Cladis FP, Motoyama EK. *Smith's Anesthesia for Infants and Children*, 8th edition. Philadelphia: Elsevier Mosby, 2011; 1003–22.

Gregory GA, Andropoulos DB. *Gregory's Pediatric Anesthesia*, 5th edition. Hoboken: Wiley-Blackwell, 2012; 896–908.

Part C — Clinical-based areas in pediatric anesthesiology

Chapter 170

Urologic surgery
General considerations
Kha M. Tran

Preoperative considerations
- Majority of patients are healthy.
- Most urology procedures are elective, therefore there is time to optimize the medical management of patients with medical comorbidities:
  o Renal disease with sequelae such as hypertension should be optimized before elective cases.
  o Renal failure
    . Assess degree of renal function by determining the following:
      - Does the patient make urine?
      - Is the patient on dialysis? If yes, what is the dialysis schedule, when was last dialysis?
        . Recently dialyzed patients may be hypovolemic.
  o Review complete blood cell count (rule out severe anemia), check electrolytes especially potassium, and acid–base status.
  o Certain syndromes are associated with urologic anomalies:
    . Trisomy 18: cardiac defects, micrognathia.
    . Branchio-oto-renal syndrome – bronchial cleft cysts, hearing loss and other ear abnormalities, abnormal kidney structure and function.
    . Myelomeningocele with neurogenic bladder predisposes to stones.

Emergency urology procedures
- Testicular torsion.
- Priapism reduction.

Common urology procedures
- Circumcision.
- Chordee repair.
- Hypospadias repair.
- Hernia repair.

Handbook of Critical Incidents and Essential Topics in Pediatric Anesthesiology, ed. David A. Young and Olutoyin A. Olutoye. Published by Cambridge University Press. © Cambridge University Press 2015.

- Orchiopexy for undescended testes.
- Cystoscopy for vesico-ureteral reflux.
- Uteropelvic junction obstruction.
- Kidney bladder stone removal.
- Dialysis catheter placement.
- Posterior urethral valve incisions.

Intraoperative considerations
- Avoid nephrotoxic drugs.
- Avoid (or administer cautiously) drugs excreted or metabolized by the kidney.
- Surgeries can be quite variable in length, position, complexity, invasiveness.
- Communication with surgical team with regards to discussion about procedure and surgical technique is important.
- Some procedures are of short duration and may be performed with a supraglottic airway device while others may require endotracheal intubation.
- Regional anesthetic techniques are commonly utilized in children undergoing urologic surgery – penile block, ilioinguinal/iliohypogastric nerve block, single shot or continuous caudal anesthesia.
- Position for surgery may be supine, lateral, lithotomy or prone.
- Patients should be carefully positioned, with appropriate padding, to avoid brachial plexus and peroneal nerve injuries.

Further reading

Coté CJ, Lerman J, Anderson BJ. *Coté and Lerman's A Practice of Anesthesia for Infants and Children*, 5th edition. Philadelphia, PA: Elsevier, 2013; 572–3.

Gregory GA, Andropoulos DB. *Gregory's Pediatric Anesthesia*, 5th edition. Hoboken: Wiley-Blackwell, 2012; 744–8.

Index

4–2–1 rule 212, 214

abdominal surgery, laparoscopic, *see* laparoscopic procedures
abdominal trauma, blunt 491
abdominal tumors 331
 neuroblastoma 331
 Wilms tumor (nephroblastoma) 331
abdominal wall defects 413
absorption of drugs 181
acetaminophen 193, 451
acid–base balance 323
acidosis
 metabolic 116–17
 respiratory 37–8, 291
acquired heart disease 297–8
 endocarditis 297
 myocarditis 297–8
 pericarditis 298
acute adrenal insufficiency 89–90
acute kidney injury (AKI) 324–5
acute life-threatening events (ALTE), infants 286
acute pain management, *see* pain management
acute respiratory failure 267
acyanotic lesions 371–4
 anesthetic considerations 372
 aortopulmonary window 374
 atrial septal defect 372
 atrioventricular canal (AVC) 373
 left-to-right shunt pathophysiology 295, 371
 patent ductus arteriosus, *see* patent ductus arteriosus (PDA)
 ventricular septal defect 372–3
adenosine, resuscitation 245
adenotonsillectomy 439–41
 perioperative anesthetic management 439
 post-anesthetic management 440–1
 premedication and anesthesia 440
adolescence 169–70
adrenal cortex 339, 340
adrenal disorders 352

adrenal insufficiency 345, 353
 acute 89–90
 diagnostic evaluation 353–4
 pheochromocytoma 353
 preoperative and intraoperative management 354
adrenal medulla 339, 340
α-adrenergic receptors 198
β-adrenergic receptors 198
age-related risk factors 256
agitation, emergence, *see* emergence agitation
air embolism
 craniofacial reconstruction 461
 venous 82–3
airway(s)
 anatomy 173–4
  blood supply 173–4
  developmental, of larynx 173
  epiglottis 174
  innervation 173
  neonates 408
  pediatric *vs.* adult 173
  subglottic region 174
  vocal cords 174
 conditions/critical incidents
  airway fire 5–6
  bronchospasm 9–10
  difficult airway 11–13
  difficult ventilation 14–16
  foreign body 7–8, 444–5
  hemoptysis 17–18
  hypercarbia 19–21
  hypocarbia 22–3
  hypoxemia 24–5
  increased peak airway pressures 26–7
  laryngospasm 28–9
  pulmonary aspiration of gastric contents 30–2
  respiratory acidosis 37–8
  respiratory alkalosis 39–40
  stridor 33–4, 231
  tension pneumothorax 35–6
  upper airway obstruction 41–2
 difficult 11–13, 236
 edema 262
 foreign body 444–5

 management 445
 increased peak airway pressures 26–7
 lesions, fetal surgery 396
 obstruction, *see* upper airway obstruction
 physiology 231
  lower airway 231
  upper airway 231
 postoperative problems 262–3
 preoperative examination 255
 resuscitation 244
airway management 231–3
 burns 494
 craniofacial reconstruction 461
 direct techniques 234–5
  general 234
  specific devices 234–5
 endotracheal tubes 232
 indirect techniques 236–9
  fiberoptic-guided intubation 237
  flexible fiberoptic bronchoscope 236–7
  general background 236
  lighted stylet 238
  optical stylets 237–8
  specific tools/devices/ techniques 236–8
  ultrasound-guided intubation 238
  video/indirect laryngoscopes 237
 laryngoscope blades 232
 mask ventilation 231, 232
 nasopharyngeal airways 232
 oral airways 232
 resuscitation, no-flow/low-flow phase 244
 supraglottic airway devices 232, 237
airway surgery 442–5
 choanal atresia 444
 foreign body 444–5
 laser 442
 subglottic stenosis 443–4
 tracheostomy 442–3
albumin, colloid solution 215
albuterol 208

499

alkalosis
  metabolic 118–19
  respiratory 39–40
allergies, preoperative
  evaluation 255
altered mental status 123–4
amiodarone 202, 245
analgesia, *see* pain management
analgesics
  adjuvant, preemptive
    analgesia 448
  non-opioid, *see* non-opioid
    analgesics
  opioids, *see* opioid(s)
anaphylaxis 43–4
anatomy, pediatric *vs.* adult 171–2
  head, neck, chest 171, 173
  see also individual systems
anesthesia
  machine failure 145–6
  peripheral, *see* peripheral
    anesthesia
  regional, *see* regional anesthesia
  in remote locations, *see* remote
    anesthesia locations
anesthetic agents
  in cardiac surgery 370
  inhaled, *see* inhaled anesthetic
    agents
  local, *see* local anesthetics
  local toxicity, cardiac 59–61
Angelman syndrome 276
ankle block 229
anterior commissure scope 235
anterior mediastinal mass,
    see mediastinal masses
anticholinergic agents 206
anticholinesterase agents 197
antidiuretic hormone (ADH)
    (vasopressin) 200
  excess, syndrome (SIADH)
    346, 349
antiemetics 266
anxiety, preoperative 258–9
see also separation anxiety,
    preoperative
anxiolytics, *see* hypnotics and
    anxiolytics
aortic insufficiency (AI) 302
aortic stenosis 303
aortopulmonary window 374
apnea
  central 286
  neonates 408
  post-operative in infants 286

sleep, *see* obstructive sleep
    apnea (OSA)
appendicitis 330
aqueous humor, production and
    drainage 424
arachnoid cyst 315
Arndt endobronchial blocker
    471–2
Arnold Chiari malformation 316
arrhythmias, *see* rhythm disorders
    (cardiac)
arteriovenous malformations
    (AVMs) 317
arthrogryposis multiplex congenita
    (AMC) 432
asphyxia 267
aspiration of gastric contents 30–2
asthma/reactive airway
    disease 290–1
  medications 291
asystole 45–6
atracurium 195–6
atresia, bowel 329
atrial fibrillation 305
atrial flutter 305
atrial septal defect (ASD) 372
atrioventricular (AV) blocks 304
atrioventricular canal (AVC) 373
atrioventricular nodal reentrant
    tachycardia (AVNRT) 305–6
atrioventricular reentrant
    tachycardia (AVRT) 305
atropine, resuscitation 245
autism 321
awareness, intraoperative 134–5
axillary nerve 179
axillary nerve block 228

barbiturates 186
  methohexital 186
  thiopental 186
benzodiazepines 186–7, 451
  diazepam 187
  flumazenil 187
  midazolam 187
Berry's method, fluid
    replacement 214
beta-adrenergic receptors 198
biliary system, physiology 334
birth, transitional circulation 294
bispectral index (BIS) monitor
    249, 251–2
blindness, postoperative 125–6
blood flow
  ductal-dependent 369–70

pulmonary to systemic,
    ratio 369
  in utero 293
blood groups 217
blood loss
  craniofacial reconstruction 461
  scoliosis surgery 435
blood pressure
  non-invasive monitoring 247
  normal ranges by age 296
  post-resuscitation care 246
blood products 217–20
  applied immunology 217
  cardiac surgery 369
  cryoprecipitate 219
  estimated blood volume
    210–11, 218
  fresh frozen plasma (FFP) 218
  graft versus host disease 220
  packed red blood cells (PRBC)
    217–18
  platelets 219
  transfusion complications
    219–20
  trauma patients 491
  see also transfusion
blood supply, to airway 173–4
blood transfusions, *see* transfusion
blood volume
  estimated 210–11, 218
  preterm infants and term
    infants 357
body water, total 210
brachial plexus
  anatomy 178–9
  surgery 459
bradycardia 47–8
brain
  anatomy 312–13
  traumatic injury 490–1
  vascular anatomy 313
brainstem auditory evoked
    responses (BAER) 251
brain tumors 316, 420–2
  infratentorial 316, 421
  supratentorial 316, 420–2
  midline 421–2
  surgery 420–2
    anesthesia induction/
        maintenance 420–1
    postoperative
        management 421
    preoperative assessment 420
  symptoms 316
bronchial blockers 471

Index

bronchopulmonary dysplasia 287–8
bronchoscope, flexible fiberoptic 236–7
bronchospasm 9–10, 291
burns 492–5
  acute phase 492–3
  classification of burns 492
  hypermetabolic phase 493–4
  response to medications 494
butyrylcholinesterase polymorphisms 275

caffeine–halothane contracture test 241–2
calcium, as an inotrope 199
calcium chloride, resuscitation 245
capnography, monitoring 248
carbon dioxide, pneumoperitoneum 406
carbon monoxide poisoning 494
cardiac arrhythmias, see rhythm disorders (cardiac)
cardiac critical incidents
  anaphylaxis 43–4
  asystole 45–6
  bradycardia 47–8
  heart failure 49–51
  hypertension 52–3
  hypotension 54–6
  inability to obtain vascular access 57–8
  local anesthetic toxicity 59–61
  myocardial ischemia 62–4
  pericardial tamponade 65–6
  prolonged QT interval 67–8
  pulmonary hypertensive crisis 69–71
  pulseless electrical activity 72–3
  sinus tachycardia 74–5
  supraventricular tachycardia 76–7
  tetralogy of Fallot, spell 78–9
  thrombotic pulmonary embolism 80–1
  venous air embolism 82–3
  ventricular fibrillation 84–5
  ventricular tachycardia 86–7
cardiac output, neonates 409
cardiac surgery
  acyanotic lesions, see acyanotic lesions
  anesthetic agent selection 370
  cardiopulmonary bypass, see cardiopulmonary bypass (CPB)
  cyanotic lesions, see cyanotic lesions
  ductal-dependent blood flow 369–70
  general considerations 367–70
  non-cardiac surgery and 379–82
    endocarditis prophylaxis 381
    preoperative planning 380
    risk and outcomes 379
    single ventricle palliation 379, 380–1
  pacemaker/ICD, see pacemaker/implantable cardioverter defibrillator (ICD)
  planned, considerations for 367–9
  preoperative assessment 367
  pulmonary to systemic blood flow ($Q_p:Q_s$) ratio 369
  transplantation, see cardiac transplantation
cardiac tamponade 65–6, 299–300
cardiac transplantation 391–5
  anesthetic management 394
  common diagnoses in recipients 391
  contraindications 391–2
  indications 391
  late anesthetic considerations 395
  listing status 393
  post-transplantation anesthetic considerations 394
  pre-transplant evaluation 393–4
  recipient evaluation 392–3
cardiac tumors 300
cardiogenic shock 269
cardiomyopathies (CM) 298–9
  heart failure due to 309
cardiopulmonary bypass (CPB) 387–90
  basic circuit set-up 387
  complications 390
  management 388–9
  patient preparation 388
  weaning 389
cardiopulmonary resuscitation (CPR) 267–8
cardiovascular agents 198–202
  chronotropes 200
  inotropes, see inotropes
  receptor pharmacology 198
    α-adrenergic receptors 198
    β-adrenergic receptors 198
  rhythm agents 202
  vasoconstrictors, see vasoconstrictors
  vasodilators, see vasodilators
cardiovascular system
  anatomy and physiology 172, 293–6
    fetal circulation 293–4
    innervation 295
    neonatal myocardium 295
    normal physiologic variables 296
    patent ductus arteriosus 295
    persistent fetal circulation 294–5
    transitional circulation 294
  genetic syndromes 282
  medical conditions 297–300
    acquired heart disease, see acquired heart disease
    cardiomyopathies 298–9
    heart failure, see heart failure
    intracardiac masses 300
    pericardial disease 299–300
    pulmonary hypertension, see pulmonary hypertension
    rhythm disorders, see rhythm disorders (cardiac)
    valvular disorders, see valvular disorders
  postoperative instability 263
  preoperative examination 255
catheters
  extracorporeal membrane oxygenation 271
  sizes, cardiac surgery 368
caudal blockade 225, 451
caudal space anatomy 176
central apnea 286
central blockade, see also regional anesthesia
central core disease 241
central nervous system (CNS)
  anatomy 172, 175–7
  congenital anomalies 176–7
  intracranial compartment 175
  monitoring 248–9
  vertebral column, see vertebral column
cerebral autoregulation 313–14
cerebral blood flow (CBF) 313
cerebral palsy 320–1
  orthopedic surgery 431–2
cerebral perfusion pressure (CPP) 313

cervical collar 490
CHARGE association
 syndrome 280
chest anatomy 171
Chiari malformations 177
choanal atresia 444
cholelithiasis 336
cholinesterase, deficiency 194
chronic kidney disease (CKD) 325
chronic lung disease (CLD),
 neonates 408
chronic pain management, *see* pain
 management
chronotropes 200
circulation
 fetal 293–4
 in resuscitation 244
 transitional 294
cisatracurium 196
clearance/metabolism of
 drugs 181–2
cleft lip and palate surgery 463–5
 anesthetic considerations 464
 emergence and extubation 464–5
 postoperative care and
  considerations 465
 surgical repair 463
coagulation 356
coagulopathy 151–2
colloids 212, 215
 crystalloids *vs.* 216
 natural protein 215
 synthetic 215
common peroneal nerve 180
complex regional pain syndrome
 (CRPS) 454
computed tomography (CT) 467
conduction disorders
 (cardiac) 304
congenital diaphragmatic hernia
 (CDH) repair 410–11
congenital heart disease
 acyanotic lesions, *see* acyanotic
  lesions
 cyanotic lesions, *see* cyanotic
  lesions
constrictive pericarditis 299
continuous positive airway
 pressure (CPAP) 440
cosmetic procedures 459
COX isoenzymes 192–3
cranial trauma 318
craniofacial reconstruction 460–2
 air embolism 461
 airway management 461
 anesthetic considerations 460
 bleeding and transfusion 461

metabolic disturbances 461
outcome and prognosis 462
pain management 462
postoperative care 462
preoperative assessment 460
prolonged surgery 462
craniosynostosis 317
craniotomy 414–16
 anesthesia induction 414–15
 anesthesia maintenance 415
 monitoring 415
 patient position 415
 postoperative management
  415–16
 preoperative assessment 414
crisis management, general
 principles 3–4
 management 4
 presentation 3
 prevention 4
 risk factors 3–4
critical care, pediatric 267–9
 acute respiratory failure 267
 cardiopulmonary
  resuscitation 267–8
 ECMO, *see* extracorporeal
  membrane oxygenation
  (ECMO)
 shock 268–9
cryoprecipitate 219
crystalloids 212, 214–15
 colloids *vs.* 216
cyanotic lesions 375–8
 consequences of cyanosis 378
 cyanosis mechanisms 375
 hypoplastic left heart
  syndrome 377–8
 right-to-left shunts 375
 tetralogy of Fallot 375–6
 total anomalous pulmonary
  venous return 377
 transposition of the great
  arteries 376
 truncus arteriosus 377
CYP2D6 variants 275, 450
cystic fibrosis 290–1
cystic hygromas 458

deep peroneal nerve block 229
delayed emergence 127–8
depolarizing muscle relaxants
 194–5
desflurane 184
developmental milestones 167–70
 adolescence 169–70
 early school years 169
 newborn to 5 years 167

dexamethasone 208
dexmedetomidine 187–8
dextrans 215
dextrose, perioperative 214–15
diabetes insipidus (DI) 346, 348–9
 perioperative management
  348–9
 postoperative management 349
diabetes mellitus 346–8
 hyperglycemia, adverse effects
  of 348
 intraoperative management 347
 postoperative management
  347–8
 preoperative management 347
 types I and II 346–7
diazepam 187
difficult airway 11–13, 236
difficult ventilation 14–16
Di-George (velocardiofacial)
 syndrome 282
dilated cardiomyopathy 298, 309
distribution of drugs 181
distributive shock 269
dobutamine 199
dopamine 199
Down syndrome 277–9
 anesthetic considerations 278–9
  airway/pulmonary 278
  cardiovascular 278
  thyroid disease 279
  vascular access 279
 clinical features 277–8
 etiology 277
drug clearance 181–2
drug metabolism 181–2
 hepatic 334–5
Duchenne's muscular
 dystrophy 275
ductal-dependent blood flow
 369–70
ductus arteriosus 293
 patent, *see* patent ductus
  arteriosus (PDA)
ductus venosus 293, 333
duodenal atresia 329

ear, nose and throat (ENT)
 surgery 437–8
 adenotonsillectomy,
  see adenotonsillectomy
 complications 438
 ECMO, *see* extracorporeal
  membrane oxygenation
  (ECMO)
edrophonium 197
Ehlers–Danlos syndrome 275

electrocardiogram (ECG) 247
electroencephalography (EEG) 251
electrolyte balance 323
electromyography (EMG) 250–1
emergence, delayed 127–8
emergence agitation 129–30, 263, 264
  definition 264
  management 264
  prevention 264
  risk factors 264
encephalocele 176
endocarditis 297
  prophylaxis 297, 381
endocrine system 338
  anatomy 338–9
  medical conditions 342
    adrenal disorders, see adrenal disorders
    diabetes insipidus, see diabetes insipidus (DI)
    diabetes mellitus, see diabetes mellitus
    myxedema coma 344–5
    neonatal hypothyroidism 345
    SIADH 140, 346
    thyroid disorders, see thyroid
  physiology 339–40
    adrenal cortex 340
    adrenal medulla 340
    hypothalamus 339
    parathyroid 340
    pituitary 339
    thyroid 339–40
endotracheal tubes (ETT) 232
  double lumen 472
end-stage liver disease 337, 484
end-stage renal disease (ESRD) 487–9
epidermolysis bullosa (EB) 283
epidural anesthesia 226, 452
epidural space, anatomy 176
epiglottis, anatomy 174
epinephrine 198–9, 245
equipment
  anesthesia machine failure 145–6
  line isolation monitor activation 147–8
  power failure 149–50
erythropoiesis 355
esophageal atresia (EA) 329–30
estimated blood volume (EBV) 210–11, 218
etomidate 189
EXIT (ex-utero intrapartum therapy) procedure 400–2
  anesthetic considerations 401

fetus management 402
indications 400–1
management of mother 401–2
resources required 401
extracorporeal membrane oxygenation (ECMO) 270–3
  bladder, tubing and pump 272
  bridge 272
  catheters 271
  complications 273
  contraindications 270
  ECMO circuit 271
  ECMO circuit emergency 273
  indications 270
  medications 273
  membrane oxygenator 272
  veno-arterial (VA) cannulation 271
  veno-venous (VV) cannulation 271
ex-utero intrapartum therapy (EXIT) procedure, see EXIT
eyes
  postoperative blindness 125–6
  see also entries beginning ophthalmologic

face masks, airway management 231, 232
fascia iliaca block 229
fasting deficit, calculation 212
fasting status, preoperative evaluation 255
fat embolism, orthopedic surgery 431
femoral nerve 179–80
femoral nerve block 229, 452
fentanyl 191
fetal circulation 293–4
  persistent 294–5
fetal development
  circulation 293–4
  physiology 285–6
  respiratory system 285
fetal hematopoiesis 355
fetal hemoglobin 294, 356
fetal surgery 396–9
  anesthetic considerations 397
  anesthetic management 398
  conditions requiring surgery 396–7
  EXIT, see EXIT (ex-utero intrapartum therapy) procedure
  fetal physiology 398
  fetal resuscitation 399
  indications 396

mid-gestation procedures 397
open surgery 398–9
fiberoptic-guided intubation (supraglottic airway) 237
fire, airway 5–6
flexible fiberoptic bronchoscope 236–7
fluid balance 323
  general surgery and 403–4
fluid compartments 210
fluid management 210–13
  blood products, see blood products
  in burn patients 494
  colloids, see colloids
  crystalloids, see crystalloids
  estimated blood volume 210–11, 218
  fasting deficit, calculation 212
  fluid replacement 212
  maintenance fluid 212–13
  perioperative requirements 211, 214
  preoperative assessment 211
  total body water and fluid compartments 210
  water and sodium considerations 211
flumazenil 187
Fogarty catheter 471
fontanels 312
foramen ovale 293
  patent 372
foreign body (FB), airway 7–8, 444–5
4-2-1 rule 212, 214
fresh frozen plasma (FFP) 218

gastric contents, pulmonary aspiration 30–2
gastro-esophageal reflux 329
gastrointestinal system
  anatomy and embryology 327–8
  medical conditions 329–32
    abdominal tumor, see abdominal tumor
    appendicitis 330
    atresia 329
    esophageal atresia 329–30
    gastro-esophageal reflux 329
    Hirschsprung's disease 331
    inguinal and umbilical hernia 331
    intussusception 329
    malrotation and volvulus 330
    Meckel's diverticulum 330
    necrotizing enterocolitis 330–1

gastrointestinal system (*cont.*)
  pyloric stenosis 330
  physiology 328
gastroschisis 413
general surgery 403–4
  elective *vs.* emergent 403
  fluid status 403–4
  laparoscopic/abdominal procedures, see laparoscopic procedures
  open *vs.* minimally invasive surgery 403
  perioperative analgesia 404
genes 274
genetic diseases 275–6, 280
  cardiac syndromes 282
  CHARGE association syndrome 280
  cystic fibrosis 291–2
  Di-George (velocardiofacial) syndrome 282
  Down syndrome, see Down syndrome
  epidermolysis bullosa 283
  Goldenhar syndrome 281–2
  micrognathia syndromes 281
  Noonan syndrome 283
  Pierre Robin sequence 281
  Treacher Collins syndrome 281
  VACTERL/VATER syndrome 281
  Williams syndrome 282
genetics
  basic concepts 274–6
  pharmacogenetics, see pharmacogenetics
genomics, anesthesia and 275
glomerular filtration rate (GFR) 322
glucose, control, post-resuscitation care 245
glucose- 6-phosphate dehydrogenase (G6PD) deficiency 359
Goldenhar syndrome 281–2
graft versus host disease 220
granulocytopoiesis 355
greater auricular nerve 178
greater occipital nerve 178

hand surgery 459
head anatomy 171, 178
heart
  innervation 295
  see also entries beginning cardiac

heart disease
  acquired, see acquired heart disease
  congenital, see acyanotic lesions; cyanotic lesions
heart failure 49–51, 308–9
  causes 308–9
  classification 308
  definition 308
heart rate, normal ranges by age 296
hemangiomas 458–9
hematology system
  blood volume 357
  critical incidents
    coagulopathy 151–2
    massive hemorrhage 153–5
    sickle cell crisis 156–7
    transfusion reaction 158–60
  development 355
    erythropoiesis 355
    granulocytopoiesis 355
    hemoglobin 355–6
    thrombopoiesis 355
  hemostasis 356
  medical conditions 358–61
    G6PD deficiency 359
    hemolytic anemia 358
    hemophilia 364–5
    hereditary spherocytosis 358–9
    sickle cell disease 362–3
    thalassemia 360
    thrombocytopenia 361
    Von Willebrand disease 363–4
  neonatal physiology 356–7
  normal values by age 356
hematopoiesis 355
hemifacial microsomia (HM) 457
hemoglobin (Hgb) 355–6
  fetal 294, 356
hemoglobinopathies 360
  see also individual disorders
hemolytic anemia 358
hemophilia 364–5
hemoptysis 17–18
hemorrhage, massive 153–5
hemostasis 356
hepatic system
  anatomy 333
  anesthesia and 334–5
    inhalation anesthetics 334
    local anesthetics 335
    neuromuscular blocking agents 335
    opioids 335
    sedatives 334–5

  drug metabolism 334–5
  end-stage liver disease 337, 484
  medical conditions 336–7
    cholelithiasis 336
    congenital disorders 336
    end-stage liver disease 337, 484
    infectious conditions 337
    metabolic diseases 336
  neonatal 409
  physiology 333–4
hepatic transplantation 483–6
  anesthetic management 485–6
  end-stage liver disease, pathophysiology 484
  indications 483
  organ allocation 484
  surgical complications 485
  types and surgical techniques 484
hereditary spherocytosis (HS) 358–9
Hirschsprung's disease 331
history evaluation, preoperative care 254–5
Hurler syndrome 275
hydrocephalus 315, 417–19
  anesthetic considerations 418–19
  special considerations 418–19
  diagnosis 417–18
  etiology 315, 417
  pathophysiology 417
  surgical treatment 418
  VP (ventriculoperitoneal) shunt 418, 419
hydromorphone 192
hydrops fetalis 396
hydroxyethyl starches (HES) 215
hypercalcemia 91–3
hypercarbia 19–21
hyperglycemia 94–5
  adverse effects 348
hyperkalemia 96–7
hypernatremia 98–9
hypertension 52–3
  postoperative (cardiac surgery) 368
hyperthermia 100–1
  malignant, see malignant hyperthermia
hyperthyroidism (thyrotoxicosis) 120–2, 342–3, 351–2
hypertrophic cardiomyopathy 298
hypnotics and anxiolytics 186–9
  barbiturates, see barbiturates

benzodiazepines,
  see benzodiazepines
  dexmedetomidine 187–8
  etomidate 189
  ketamine 188–9
  propofol 188
hypocalcemia 102–3
hypocarbia 22–3
hypoglycemia 104–5
  neonatal 409
hypokalemia 106–7
hypomagnesemia 108–9
hyponatremia 110–11
hypoplastic left heart
  syndrome 377–8
hypotension 54–6
  regional anesthesia 223
hypothalamus 338, 339
hypothermia 112–13
  neonatal 409
  postoperative 263
  post-resuscitation care 245
hypothyroidism 343–4, 352
  neonatal 345
hypovolemic shock 269
hypoxemia 24–5
hypoxia, neonates 286

idiopathic thrombocytopenic
  purpura (ITP) 361
ilioinguinal/iliohypogastric
  block 228–9
immunocompromised patients,
  transplant surgery 481–2
implantable cardioverter
  defibrillator (ICD) 383–5
  indications 383
  see also pacemaker/
    implantable cardioverter
    defibrillator (ICD)
infants
  head, neck, chest, respiratory
    system anatomy 171
  respiratory system physiology
    285–6
  see also neonate(s)
infectious diseases
  cardiovascular 297–8
  liver 337
informed consent 256
infraclavicular block 228
infraorbital nerve 178
infratentorial tumors 316, 421
inguinal hernia 331
inhaled anesthetic agents 183–5
  desflurane 184

general concepts 183–4
  hepatic metabolism 334
  isoflurane 185
  nitrous oxide 184
  sevoflurane 184
inhaled nitric oxide 201
inotropes 198–9
  calcium 199
  dobutamine 199
  dopamine 199
  epinephrine 198–9
  milrinone 199
intermediate-acting
  nondepolarizing muscle
  relaxants 195–7
interscalene block 228
intracardiac masses 300
intracranial compartment 312
  anatomy 175, 312
intracranial pressure (ICP)
  increased 131–3
  trauma patients 491
intraocular pressure (IOP) 423–4
intraoperative awareness 134–5
intussusception 329
isoflurane 185
isoproterenol 200
isotonic normal saline 214

junctional rhythms 304
junctional tachycardia 305

ketamine 188–9
ketorolac 193
kidney transplant, see renal
  transplantation
King–Denborough syndrome 241

labetalol 207
laboratory testing, preoperative 256
lactated Ringer's solution 214
laparoscopic procedures
  abdominal 405–7
  complications 407
  physiologic
    considerations 406–7
  pneumoperitoneum 405–6
  positioning 406
  types of procedures 405
  open procedures vs. 403
laryngomalacia 442
laryngoscope blades 232
laryngoscopes, video/indirect 237
laryngospasm 28–9, 286, 437
larynx, anatomy 173
laser surgery 440–1

lateral femoral cutaneous nerve 180
left ventricular noncompaction
  cardiomyopathy 309
lidocaine, resuscitation 245
lighted stylet, indirect airway
  management 238
line isolation monitor
  activation 147–8
liver, see hepatic system
liver transplant, see hepatic
  transplantation
local anesthetics 203–5
  binding 204
  elimination 204
  hepatic metabolism 335
  major classification 203
  mechanism of action 203–4
  overview 203
  toxicity 59–61
  ultrasonography and 221
long-acting nondepolarizing
  muscle relaxants 195
lower extremity nerve blocks 228–9
lumbar plexus anatomy 179–80
lung
  collapse in infants 286
  lesions, fetal surgery 397
  single, ventilation
    management 472
lung isolation 471–3
  alternative options 471–2
  main stem 471
  pain management 472–3
  single lung ventilation
    management 472

Macintosh blade 234
magnesium sulfate,
  resuscitation 245
magnetic resonance imaging
  (MRI) 468
maintenance fluid 212–13
malignant hyperthermia
  114–15, 240–2
  associated conditions 241
  clinical presentation 241
  genetics 240
  pathophysiology 240
  testing 241–2
  genetic test 242
  treatment 241–2
malrotation, abdominal
  contents 330
masks, ventilation 231
  face 232
massive hemorrhage 153–5

Meckel diverticulum 330
median nerve 179
mediastinal masses 474–7
  anatomy, etiology and classification 474
  anterior 474, 475–6
    anesthesia maintenance 476
    extubation and postoperative care 476
    perioperative aspects 475
    preinduction and induction 476
    preoperative evaluation 475
    presentation, pathophysiology 475
  middle 474
  posterior 474
medical devices, preoperative examination 255–6
medical genetics, see genetic diseases; genetics
medical history 254–5
membrane oxygenator, in ECMO 272
mental status, altered 123–4
meperidine 191
metabolic acidosis 116–17
metabolic alkalosis 118–19
metabolic critical incidents
  acute adrenal insufficiency 89–90
  hypercalcemia 91–3
  hyperglycemia 94–5
  hyperkalemia 96–7
  hypernatremia 98–9
  hyperthermia 100–1
  hypocalcemia 102–3
  hypoglycemia 104–5
  hypokalemia 106–7
  hypomagnesemia 108–9
  hyponatremia 110–11
  hypothermia 112–13
  malignant hyperthermia 114–15
  metabolic acidosis 116–17
  metabolic alkalosis 118–19
  thyrotoxicosis 120–2
  see also each specific incident
metabolic diseases, of liver 336
methadone 191
methohexital 186
micrognathia syndromes 281
midazolam 187
midface procedures (plastic surgery) 457–8
Miller blade 234
milrinone 199

minimally invasive procedures, see laparoscopic procedures
mitral regurgitation 301
mitral stenosis 302–3
monitoring 247–9
  capnography 248
  central nervous system 248–9
  electrocardiogram 247
  near-infrared spectroscopy (NIRS) 249, 251
  neurophysiologic, see neurophysiologic monitors
  non-invasive blood pressure 247
  pulse oximetry 247
  temperature 248
morphine 190–1
  see also opioid(s)
motor evoked potentials (MEP) 250
  acute loss, differential diagnosis 252
  management of acute loss 252
Moyamoya disease 317
mucopolysaccharidoses 275
multiminicore disease 241
muscle relaxants, see neuromuscular blocking agents
musculocutaneous nerve 179
myelodysplasia 177
myelomeningocele 317, 422
myocardial ischemia 62–4
myocarditis 297–8
myocardium, neonatal 295
myxedema coma 344–5

nalbuphine 192
naloxone 192, 245
nasopharyngeal airways 232
nausea, postoperative,
  see postoperative nausea and vomiting (PONV)
near-infrared spectroscopy (NIRS) 249, 251
neck anatomy 171, 178
necrotizing enterocolitis (NEC) 330–1, 412–13
neonate(s) 408
  airway anatomy 408
  apnea 408
  cardiac output 409
  developmental milestones 167
  head, neck, chest, respiratory system anatomy 171
  hematology system physiology 356–7
  hypothyroidism 345

myocardium 295
respiratory system
  physiology 285–6
surgery
  abdominal wall defects 413
  congenital diaphragmatic hernia repair 410–11
  general considerations 408–9
  necrotizing enterocolitis 412–13
  patent ductus arteriosus ligation 410
neostigmine 197
nephroblastoma (Wilms tumor) 331
nerve injury, peripheral 136–8
nervous system
  anatomy 312–13
  critical incidents, see neurologic critical incidents
  medical conditions 315–18
    arachnoid cyst 315
    Arnold Chiari malformation 316
    autism 321
    brain tumors, see brain tumors
    cerebral palsy 320–1
    cranial trauma 318
    craniosynostosis 317
    hydrocephalus 315
    seizure disorder 319–20
    spinal cord tumors 318
    spinal dysraphism 177, 317
    spine injury 318
    vascular malformations 316–17
  neurophysiology 313–14
  surgery, see neurosurgery
neural tube defects 422
  myelomeningocele 422
  spina bifida 177, 317
neuraxial blockade 224–6, 451–2
neuroblastoma 331
neurologic critical incidents
  altered mental status 123–4
  blindness, postoperative 125–6
  delayed emergence 127–8
  emergence agitation 129–30
  increased intracranial pressure 131–3
  intraoperative awareness 134–5
  loss of somatosensory/motor evoked potentials 252
  peripheral nerve injury 136–8
  seizure 139–40

stroke 141–3
neuromuscular blocking
    agents 194–7
    depolarizing muscle
        relaxants 194–5
        succinylcholine 194–5
    hepatic metabolism 335
    intermediate-acting
        nondepolarizing muscle
        relaxants 195–7
        atracurium 195–6
        cisatracurium 196
        rocuronium 196–7
        vecuronium 196
    long-acting nondepolarizing
        muscle relaxants 195
        pancuronium 195
    reversal agents 197
        anticholinesterase agents 197
neurophysiologic monitors 250–3
    bispectral index (BIS) 249,
        251–2
    brainstem auditory evoked
        responses 251
    electroencephalography
        (EEG) 251
    electromyography (EMG) 250–1
    motor evoked potentials,
        see motor evoked
        potentials (MEP)
    near-infrared spectroscopy
        (NIRS) 251
    somatosensory evoked
        potentials, see somatosensory
        evoked potentials (SSEP)
neurosurgery 414–16
    brain tumors, see brain tumors
    cranial procedure, see cranial
        procedures
    hydrocephalus,
        see hydrocephalus
    neural tube defects, see neural
        tube defects
    spine procedure 416
nicardipine 207
nitric oxide (NO) 201, 206–7
nitroglycerin 201, 207
nitroprusside 201
nitrous oxide 184
no-flow/low-flow phase,
    resuscitation, see resuscitation
nondepolarizing muscle relaxants,
    see neuromuscular blocking
    agents
non-opioid analgesics 190, 192–3
    acetaminophen 193, 451

acute pain management 451
adenotonsillectomy 440
    ketorolac 193
    preemptive analgesia 448
    non-steroidal anti-inflammatory
        drugs (NSAIDs) 192–3
Noonan syndrome 283
norepinephrine 200

obstructive shock 269
obstructive sleep apnea (OSA) 262,
    288, 439
    adenotonsillectomy 439–41
    ENT surgery indication 437
obturator nerve 180
occult spinal dysraphism 177, 317
oculocardiac reflex (OCR) 424, 428
oliguria 161–2
omphalocele 413
ondansetron 208
ophthalmologic medications 424
ophthalmologic physiology 423–4
    aqueous humor production and
        drainage 424
    intraocular pressure 423–4
    medications and 424
    oculocardiac reflex 424, 428
ophthalmologic surgery 423
    anesthesia 425
    postoperative nausea and
        vomiting 425, 428–9
    preoperative assessment 424
    retinopathy of prematurity,
        see retinopathy of
        prematurity (ROP)
    strabismus, see strabismus
        surgery
opioid(s) 190
    acute pain management 450
    regional analgesia 451
    adenotonsillectomy, limitations
        in 440–1
    adjunctive agents with 451
    adverse effects 450
        management 450–1
    agonist-antagonists 192
        nalbuphine 192
    agonists 190–2
        fentanyl 191
        hydromorphone 192
        meperidine 191
        methadone 191
        morphine 190–1
        oxycodone 191
        tramadol 192
    antagonists 192

naloxone 192
chronic pain management 453–4
hepatic metabolism 335
long-term, for chronic
    pain 453–4
preemptive analgesia 447
OPRM1 gene 275
optical stylets, indirect airway
    management 237–8
oral airways 232
orbital hypertelorism 458
orthognathic surgery 458
orthopedic surgery
    arthrogryposis multiplex
        congenita 432
    cerebral palsy 431–2
    fat embolism 431
    general considerations 430
    osteogenesis imperfecta 432
    pain control 431
    scoliosis, see scoliosis surgery
    tourniquet use 430–1
orthopedic trauma 491
osteogenesis imperfecta (OI) 432
otolaryngology, see ear, nose and
    throat (ENT) surgery
oxycodone 191
oxygen desaturation, infants 285

pacemaker/implantable
    cardioverter defibrillator
    (ICD) 383–5
    electromagnetic interference 385
    indications 383
    intraoperative management 384
    magnet use 385
    pacemaker codes 383, 384
    postoperative management 384
    preoperative management 384
packed red blood cells (PRBC)
    217–18
pain 446
    assessment 446, 449–50
    neurophysiology and
        perception 447
    postoperative, evaluation 263
pain management
    acute pain 449–52
        pharmacologic
            interventions 450–1
        preoperative history and
            assessment 449–50
        regional analgesia 451–2
    adenotonsillectomy 440
    burn patients 494
    chronic pain 453–6

pain management (*cont.*)
  complex regional pain
    syndrome 454
  long-term opioid
    analgesics 453–4
  perioperative
    management 455
  phantom limb pain 454–5
  craniofacial reconstruction 462
  general considerations 446–8
  lung isolation and thoracic
    surgery 472–3
  preemptive analgesia and
    multimodal approach 447–8
  see also non-opioid analgesics;
    opioid(s)
pancuronium 195
parathyroid gland 339, 340
Parkland formula 494
patent ductus arteriosus (PDA) 374
  left-to-right shunting 295
  ligation 410
  neonatal surgery 410
patient (proxy) controlled analgesia
  (PCA) 450
peak airway pressures,
  increased 26–7
pectus excavatum repair 479–80
  anesthetic management 480
pediatric advanced life support
  (PALS) 267–8
pericardial disease 299–300
pericardial tamponade 65–6,
  299–300
pericarditis 298
periodic breathing 286
perioperative fluid requirements
  211, 214
perioperative pain
  management 455
peripheral anesthesia 227–30
  acute pain management 452
  lower extremity blocks 228–9
  truncal blocks 228
  upper extremity blocks 228
peripheral nerve injury 136–8
peripheral nervous system
  anatomy 178–80
  brachial plexus 178–9
  head and neck 178
  lumbar plexus 179–80
  sacral plexus 180
persistent fetal circulation 294–5
phantom limb pain (PLP) 454–5
pharmacodynamics 182
pharmacogenetics 274–6

anesthesia and genomics 275
pharmacokinetics 181–2
  absorption 181
  clearance/metabolism 181–2
  distribution of drugs 181
pharmacology 181–2
  pharmacodynamics 182
  pharmacokinetics,
    see pharmacokinetics
  see also specific drugs/drug groups
phentolamine 201
phenylephrine 200
pheochromocytoma 353
physical examination,
  preoperative 255–6
Pierre Robin sequence 281
pituitary gland 338, 339
placenta 398
plastic surgery
  brachial plexus surgery 459
  cleft lip/palate, *see* cleft lip and
    palate surgery
  cosmetic procedures 459
  craniofacial, *see* craniofacial
    reconstruction
  cystic hygromas 458
  general considerations 457–9
  hand surgery 459
  hemangiomas 458–9
  hemifacial microsomia 457
  midface procedures 457–8
  orbital hypertelorism 458
  orthognathic surgery 458
  tissue expanders 459
platelets, transfusion 219
pneumoperitoneum 405–6
pneumothorax, tension 35–6
polyuria 163–4
popliteal fossa block 229
post-anesthesia care unit (PACU)
  chronic pain management 455–6
  discharge from 263
  evaluation and management
    in 262–3
postoperative apnea 286
postoperative care 262–3
  blindness 125–6
  discharge criteria 263
  emergence agitation,
    see emergence agitation
  vital signs and oxygenation 262
postoperative nausea and vomiting
  (PONV) 263, 265–6
  clinical and economic
    implications 265
  ENT surgery 438

incidence 265
ophthalmologic surgery
  425, 428–9
prophylactic and therapeutic
  antiemetics 266
risk factors 265
risk prediction and scoring
  system 265
strategies to reduce risk 265–6
potassium, excretion/balance 323
power failure 149–50
Prader Willi syndrome 276
preoperative care 254–7
  age-related risk factors 256
  fluid status assessment 211
  history evaluation 254–5
  informed consent 256
  laboratory testing 256
  physical examination 255–6
  psychological preparation 256–7
  separation anxiety, *see* separation
    anxiety, preoperative
  see also specific conditions
pressure overload 308
prolonged QT interval 67–8
propofol 188, 434
prostaglandin E_1 201
psychological preparation,
  preoperative 256–7
pulmonary artery pressure
  (PAP) 309
pulmonary edema,
  postoperative 263
pulmonary embolism,
  thrombotic 80–1
pulmonary hypertension 309–11
  acute crisis 69–71, 310–11
  chronic 311
  etiology 309–10
  mechanisms of cardiovascular
    risk in 310–11
  perioperative
    considerations 311
  post-bypass 368–9
  transplantation
    contraindication 391
pulmonary system, *see* airway(s)
pulmonary to systemic blood flow
  (Q_p:Q_s), ratio of 369
pulmonary vascular resistance
  (PVR) 69, 369, 392
pulmonic insufficiency (PI) 302
pulmonic stenosis (PS) 303
pulseless electrical activity 72–3
pulse oximetry 247
pyloric stenosis 330

Index

QT interval, prolonged 67–8

radial nerve 179
radiation therapy 467
rapid sequence induction, in trauma 490
reactive airway disease/asthma 290–1
receptor pharmacology 198
rectus sheath block 228
reentrant supraventricular tachycardia 305
regional anesthesia 221–3
  acute pain management 451–2
  advantages 221
  central blockade 224–6
    caudal block 225
    epidural 226
    hypotension and 223
    peripheral blocks vs. 222
    spinal blockade 224–5
  neuraxial blockade 224–6, 451–2
  pediatric vs. adult 222–3
  peripheral, see peripheral anesthesia
  safety 221
  test dose, use of 222
  ultrasonography 221–2
regurgitant lesions 301
remote anesthesia locations 466–8
  anesthetic management 467–8
  common off-site procedures 467–8
  limitations 466–7
  standards, and setup checklist 466
renal disease, end-stage (ESRD) 487–9
renal system
  anatomy and physiology 322–3
    developmental anatomy 322
    neonatal 409
    physiology 322–3
  anesthetic considerations
    intraoperative 325–6
    postoperative 326
    preoperative 325
  critical incidents
    oliguria 161–2
    polyuria 163–4
  medical conditions 324–6
    acute kidney injury (AKI) 324–5
    chronic kidney disease (CKD) 325
renal transplantation 487–9

intraoperative management 488–9
  perioperative considerations 487
  postoperative care 489
respiratory acidosis 37–8, 291
respiratory alkalosis 39–40
respiratory distress syndrome 408
respiratory failure, acute 267
respiratory system
  anatomy and physiology 171, 285–6
    fetal development 285
    neonates 408
  critical incidents, see airway(s)
  in laparoscopic procedures 406
  medical conditions 287–9
    bronchopulmonary dysplasia 287–8
    cystic fibrosis 290–1
    obstructive sleep apnea, see obstructive sleep apnea (OSA)
    reactive airway disease/asthma 290–1
    respiratory acidosis 37–8
    respiratory alkalosis 39–40
    respiratory failure, acute 267
    sleep-disordered breathing 288
  preoperative examination 255
respiratory tract infections, upper, see upper respiratory tract infection
restrictive cardiomyopathy 298–9, 309
resuscitation 243–6, 490
  cardiopulmonary and advanced life support 267–8
  epidemiology 243
  fetal 399
  no-flow/low-flow phase 244–5
    airway and ventilation 244
    circulation 244
    medications 245
    vascular access 244–5
  post-resuscitation care 245–6
  pre-arrest phase 243
retinopathy of prematurity (ROP) 409, 426–7
  anesthetic management 427
  definition 426
  pathophysiology 426
  risk factors 426
  treatment and classification 426–7
return of spontaneous circulation (ROSC) 267

rhabdomyoma 300
rhythm disorders (cardiac) 304–7
  conduction disorders 304
  medications 202
  supraventricular arrhythmias 304–6
  ventricular arrhythmias 306
rocuronium 196–7

sacral plexus anatomy 180
saphenous nerve block 229
sciatic nerve 180
sciatic nerve block 229, 452
scoliosis surgery 433–6
  anesthetic management 434–5
  intraoperative blood loss 435
  intraoperative complications 435
  positioning 434
  postoperative care 435–6
  preoperative evaluation 433–4
  technique 433
sedatives, hepatic metabolism 334–5
seizure(s) 139–40
seizure disorder 319–20
  anesthetic management 319–20
  surgical management 320
separation anxiety, preoperative 258–9
  behavioral interventions 259
  expected outcomes 258
  incidence/risk factors 258
  pharmacologic interventions 259
serum osmolality 323
sevoflurane 184
shock 268–9
  cardiogenic 269
  distributive 269
  hypovolemic 269
  obstructive 269
  uncompensated 268–9
sickle cell crisis 156–7
sickle cell disease 362–3
sildenafil 208
single nucleotide polymorphism (SNP) 274
single ventricle, palliation 379, 380–1
sinus node dysfunction 304
sinus tachycardia 74–5
sleep apnea, obstructive, see obstructive sleep apnea
sleep-disordered breathing 288
sodium nitroprusside 207
sodium reabsorption/balance 323

somatosensory evoked potentials (SSEP) 250
  acute loss, differential diagnosis 252
  management, loss of 252
spina bifida 177, 317
spinal blockade 224–5
spinal canal 312–13
spinal cord
  anatomy 175–6
  tumors 318
spinal dysraphism 177, 317
spinal muscular atrophy 276
spinal surgery
  loss of somatosensory/motor evoked potentials 252
  procedures 416
spine
  injury 318
  preoperative examination 256
status epilepticus 319
stenotic lesions 302–3
strabismus surgery 427–8
  associated conditions 427–8
  oculocardiac reflex 428
  topical eye medications 428
stridor 33–4, 231
  post-extubation, Down syndrome 278
stroke 141–3
subglottic region
  anatomy 174
  stenosis 443–4
succinylcholine 194–5, 494
superficial peroneal nerve block 229
superior vena cava (SVC) syndrome 475
supraclavicular block 228
supraglottic airway devices 232
  fiberoptic-guided intubation 237
supraorbital nerve 178
supratentorial tumors, *see* brain tumors
supratrochlear nerve 178
supraventricular arrhythmias 304–6
supraventricular tachycardia (SVT) 76–7, 304–5
  reentrant 305
sural nerve block 229
surfactant 231
syndrome of inappropriate antidiuretic hormone secretion (SIADH) 346, 349

systemic inflammatory response system (SIRS) 492

temperature, monitoring 248
tension pneumothorax 35–6
tetralogy of Fallot 375–6
  spells 78–9, 376
thalassemia 360
thermoregulation 172
thiopental 186
thoracic surgery 469–73
  indications 469–70
  intraoperative considerations 470–1
  lung isolation, *see* lung isolation
  mediastinal masses, *see* mediastinal masses
  pathophysiology 470
  pectus excavatum repair 479–80
  preoperative considerations 469
  preoperative preparation 470
  video thoracoscopic procedures, *see* video-assisted thoracoscopic procedures
thrombocytopenia 361
thrombocytopenic purpura, idiopathic (ITP) 361
thrombopoiesis 355
thrombotic pulmonary embolism 80–1
thyroid gland 339–40
  disorders 351–2
    Down syndrome and 279
    hyperthyroidism (thyrotoxicosis) 120–2, 342–3, 351–2
    hypothyroidism 343–4, 345, 352
    perioperative management 352
    thyroid storm 343
thyrotoxicosis (hyperthyroidism) 120–2, 342–3, 351–2
tibial nerve 180
tibial nerve block 229
tissue expanders 459
tonsillitis, recurrent 439
total anomalous pulmonary venous return 377
total body water and fluid compartments 210
total intravenous anesthesia (TIVA), scoliosis surgery 434
tourniquet use, orthopedic surgery 430–1
tracheostomy 442–3

tramadol 192
transfusions 217, 218
  compatibility, red cell antigens and 217
  complications 219–20
  craniofacial reconstruction 461
  rationale 218
  reactions 158–60
  sickle cell disease 363
  see also blood products
transitional circulation 294
transplant surgery 481
  cardiac, *see* cardiac transplantation
  general anesthetic considerations 481–2
  hepatic, *see* hepatic transplantation
  post-transplant patient 482
  renal transplant surgery, *see* renal transplantation
transposition of the great arteries 376
transversus abdominis plane (TAP) block 228, 452
trauma surgery 490–1
  burns, *see* burn surgery
  traumatic brain injury (TBI) 490–1
Treacher Collins syndrome 281
tricuspid regurgitation (TR) 301–2
tricuspid stenosis 303
truncal blocks 228
truncus arteriosus 377
tumors
  abdominal, *see* abdominal tumor
  brain, *see* brain tumors
  cardiac 300
  spinal cord 318
twins, fetal surgery indications 396

ulnar nerve 179
ultrasonography
  guided intubation, airway management 238
  peripheral nerve blocks 227
  regional anesthesia 221–2
umbilical hernia 331
Univent tube 472
upper airway obstruction 41–2
  adenotonsillectomy and 440
  Down syndrome 278
upper extremity blocks 228
upper respiratory tract infections 259–61
  ENT surgery and 437

intraoperative management 260–1
preoperative assessment 260
urologic surgery 496–7
  common procedures 496–7
  emergency procedures 496
  intraoperative
    considerations 497
  preoperative considerations 496

VACTERL/VATER syndrome 281
valvular disorders 301–4
  aortic insufficiency 302
  mitral regurgitation 301
  pulmonary stenosis 303
  pulmonic insufficiency 302
  regurgitant lesions 301, 302
  stenotic lesions 302–3
  tricuspid regurgitation 301–2
vascular access
  Down syndrome 279
  inability to obtain 57–8
  renal transplantation 488
  resuscitation 244–5, 268
  trauma patients 490
vascular malformations 316–17
vasoconstrictors 200
  norepinephrine 200

phenylephrine 200
vasopressin 200
vasodilators 201
  inhaled nitric oxide 201
  nitroglycerin 201
  nitroprusside 201
  phentolamine 201
  prostaglandin E_1 201
  vasopressin 200
vecuronium 196
vein of Galen malformations 317
velocardiofacial (Di-George)
  syndrome 282
veno-arterial (VA) cannulation,
  ECMO 271
venous air embolism 82–3
veno-venous (VV) cannulation,
  ECMO 271
ventilation
  difficult 14–16
  resuscitation 244
  see also airway management
ventricular arrhythmias 306
ventricular fibrillation 84–5, 306
ventricular septal defect
  (VSD) 372–3
ventricular tachycardia 86–7, 306

ventriculoperitoneal (VP) shunt
  418, 419
vertebral column
  anatomy 175
  caudal space anatomy 176
  epidural space anatomy 176
  spinal cord 175–6
video-assisted thoracoscopic
  procedures 478–9
  advantages 478
  complications 479
  pre-/intraoperative
    management 478–9
vocal cords, anatomy 174
volume overload 308
volvulus 330
vomiting, postoperative,
  see postoperative nausea and
    vomiting (PONV)
Von Willebrand disease (vWD)
  363–4

water, see fluid management
Williams syndrome 282
Wilms tumor
  (nephroblastoma) 331
Wis-Hipple blade 235